21 世纪高等医学院校教材

供基础、临床、预防、口腔、影像、护理等专业使用

THE GUIDE OF PATHOLOGY EXPERIMENT AND EXAMINATION

病理学实验与考试指导

（双语版）

主编　陈　莉

科学出版社

北京

内　容　简　介

本书根据医学基础、临床、预防、口腔、影像、护理等专业培养的目标和要求,按照相关专业的教学大纲,在病理学多年来双语教学实践的基础上,采用中英文双语编写。全书共十五章,包括病理实验和考试训练的内容。病理实验部分包括对组织大体标本、显微镜下组织结构和病变特点的描述,有助于学生对病理学基本知识的掌握,培养学生的实践能力和创新能力。病理学考试训练包括每个章节的阶段性训练和学习结束后的综合性训练,结合临床着重于病例讨论和病理分析,采用选择题和问答题的形式编写,适当编入了部分较难试题,以培养学生良好的学习习惯,形成独立思考、分析问题、解决问题的能力,掌握病理学基本知识的同时学习和应用医学专业英语,为今后的工作打好基础。

本书可以配合双语版《病理学》同时使用,亦可单独使用。可作为医学基础、临床、预防、口腔、影像、护理等专业病理教学的实验用书,亦可用于留学生的病理教学,同时也适用于长学制教学和临床病理医生学习的参考用书。

图书在版编目(CIP)数据

病理学实验与考试指导/陈莉主编.—北京:科学出版社,2006

21世纪高等医学院校教材

ISBN 978-7-03-017412-3

Ⅰ.病⋯　Ⅱ.陈⋯　Ⅲ.病理学-实验-医学院校-教学参考资料-汉、英 Ⅳ.R36-33

中国版本图书馆 CIP 数据核字(2006)第 061735 号

责任编辑:胡治国/责任校对:陈丽珠

责任印制:徐晓晨/封面设计:黄　超

科 学 出 版 社 出版

北京东黄城根北街 16 号

邮政编码:100717

http://www.sciencep.com

北京盛通商印快线网络科技有限公司 印刷

科学出版社发行　各地新华书店经销

*

2006 年 7 月第 一 版　　开本:787×1092　1/16

2019 年 7 月第十三次印刷　　印张:18

字数:424 000

定价:59.80元

(如有印装质量问题,我社负责调换)

《病理学实验与考试指导》编委会

主　编　陈　莉
副主编　王桂兰　曹晓蕾　陆　鹏
编　者　(以姓氏笔画为序)
　　　　王东林　王　酉　王桂兰　刘　俊
　　　　李杏玉　陈　莉　陆　鹏　邵伟伟
　　　　严　桥　季俐俐　秦　婧　曹晓蕾
　　　　潘宏佳

前　言

　　病理学作为医学的主干学科，是研究疾病病因、发生、发展规律，及其形态功能变化的一门科学。在病理学习中包括病理理论学习、标本与切片观察、病理讨论与分析。作者根据医学基础、临床、预防、口腔、影像、护理等专业培养的目标和要求，按照相关专业的教学大纲，坚持教材的科学性、启发性、先进性和适用性的原则，在病理学双语教学多年教学实践的基础上，编写了这本双语版《病理学实验与考试指导》。本书作为二十一世纪教材，重点体现病理基础理论、基本知识和基本技能的训练。

　　病理实验课是病理教学的重要组成部分，医学生在实验课中通过对组织大体标本、显微镜下组织结构和病变特点的观察，联系其机能代谢变化及临床特征，有助于对病理学基本知识的理解和掌握，有助于实践能力和创新能力的培养。

　　病理学考试不仅是医学生必须经过的学习训练过程，而且是毕业后执业医师考试、研究生入学医学综合考试、临床基础知识与技能考试的主要内容。作者将病理实验与考试训练合并编写，在每章后均配有思考题和病理讨论，在全书最后有综合性测验，特别编写了密切结合临床的病例讨论、病理分析和一部分较难试题，其目的就是让学生在实践中应用理论知识，指导实践，以培养学生独立思考、分析问题、解决问题的能力，使学生能够把病变组织的形态变化和机能、代谢以及临床表现有机地结合起来，并进行归纳总结，达到掌握病理学知识的目的。学生在病理学习中通过动眼、动手、动脑的训练，培养他们形成良好的学习习惯，提高学习病理的兴趣。

　　本书共十五章全部采用中英文双语编写，这将有利于学生在学习、掌握病理学基本知识的同时学习和应用医学专业英语，为今后的工作打好基础。

　　本书可以配合双语版《病理学》同时使用，亦可单独使用。可作为医学基础、临床、预防、口腔、影像、护理专业病理教学的实验用书，亦可作为留学生的病理教学用书，同时也适用于长学制教学和临床病理医生学习的参考书。

　　由于编写双语版病理学实验教材还没有经验，又限于编者的水平，肯定不无缺憾，恳请读者批评指正。本教材是在各位编者密切合作的基础上共同完成，同时得到了南通大学领导的支持与帮助，在此致以衷心的谢意。

陈　莉

2006 年 4 月 8 日

目 录
Contents

病理学实验规章

一、实验课的目的和意义

病理学实验课在病理学教学中的作用至关重要。实习课中,学生通过对病变器官、组织形态学的观察,联系其机能、代谢的变化以及临床症状、体征,一方面有利于系统掌握病理学基本知识,同时也有助于培养学生独立思考、分析问题和解决问题的能力,为以后临床课的学习奠定一个良好的基础。

二、实验课的内容和方法

病理学实验内容包括大体标本观察、组织切片观察,观看幻灯片、投影片和电视录像,进行尸体解剖、临床病理讨论及动物实验等,其中最主要的是对大体标本和组织切片的观察。

（一）大体标本观察

1. 首先识别标本属何种器官及其大体结构。

2. 观察该器官或组织的大小、形状、色泽是否正常(与相应的正常脏器和组织比较)。

3. 表面和切面状况

（1）光滑度:平滑或粗糙。

（2）透明度:器官的包膜是菲薄、透明,还是增厚、混浊。

（3）颜色:暗红或苍白、灰白或灰黑、深黄或棕黄等。

（4）质地:软、硬、韧、松脆等。

4. 病灶的情况

（1）分布与位置:观察病灶在器官的哪一部位及其分布情况。

（2）数量:单个或多个,局限或弥散。

（3）大小:体积以长×宽×厚表示,面积以长×宽表示,均以厘米为计量单位。也可以用常见的实物大小来形容,如米粒大、黄豆大、鸡蛋大、成人手拳大等。

（4）颜色:正常器官应保持其固有的色泽,如有不同着色,则往往是由于内源性或外源性色素的影响比如暗红色表示含血量多、黄绿色表示含胆汁、黄色表示含有脂肪或类脂等。

（5）形状:圆形、不整形、乳头状、菜花状、结节状等。

（6）病变与周围组织的关系:境界清楚或模糊,有无压迫或破坏,有无包膜、包膜是否完整,脏器间有无粘连等。

对空腔性器官检查要注意器官壁增厚或变薄、内壁粗糙或平滑,有无突起等,腔内物质颜色、性质、容量,器官外壁有无粘连等情况。

（说明:实验室中的大体标本,一般经过 10% 甲醛溶液固定,其大小、颜色、硬度与新鲜标本有所不同）

（二）组织切片观察

1. 先用肉眼观察组织切片的形状、颜色，并进一步确定病变的部位。

2. 显微镜下观察　注意切勿将切片放反，以免压碎玻片。

（1）低倍镜是镜检的主要手段，可以洞察全局，了解组织结构的改变。确定病变部位与性质，了解病变与周围组织的关系。观察时上下左右扫视全片，确认是何种组织、病变的部位和性质，并明确病变与周围组织的关系。切忌一开始即用高倍镜观察。

（2）高倍镜主要观察组织和细胞的微细结构和形态变化。

三、描述、诊断原则及绘图

对病理标本的描述一定要真实，不可主观臆造，亦不可照抄书本。语言要精炼，层次要清楚，从局部到整体，由里到外，由上到下，逐次描述。

对病理标本作诊断时，要细致观察，结合病史，联系理论知识，综合分析。诊断原则是，器官或组织名称+病理变化，如脾梗死、支气管鳞状上皮化生等。

病理绘图十分重要，学生通过绘图可加强对病变的观察、理解和记忆，也是能力训练的一个重要环节。绘图的方法是：首先仔细观察病变的镜下表现，找出比较典型的区域，然后用铅笔淡淡勾出轮廓（注意各种成分的位置、比例、关系等）。对草图满意后，再用红蓝彩笔分别涂出细胞质、间质和细胞核等，落笔由轻到重，色彩由浅入深，画图要有边框（圆形或方框）和注解（写于一侧或底部）。教材上的图谱可供参考，但决不可不看显微镜就临摹教科书的图片。

四、实习注意事项

1. 爱护显微镜、教学标本和病理切片以及实验室其他用具不得损坏。

2. 实习前仔细阅读实习指导，复习有关理论，了解实习目的与要求。

3. 保持实验室安静，在实验室内应专心实验，不许做其他工作。

4. 实行卫生值日制，保持实验室整洁。

5. 遵守实验室各项规章制度。

Notices For the Experiment Class

The objectives for the class

The pathological experiment class plays a key roll in the process of pathological teaching. During the class, students can observe the diseased organs macroscopically and histologically in combination with body metabolism and clinical symptoms and signs, which can help the student to master the pathological basic knowledge as well as training the students's ability of independently thinking, analyzing and solving of problems. Moreover by the means of the classe the students are able to gain the strong foundation for further study in medicine.

Learning methods and contents

The pathological experiment class consists of the observing gross appearance of the diseased organs, histological slides, watching videos, doing autopsies, holding clinical pathology symposiums and undertaking animal experiments. The major task of the class is to observe gross appearance of the diseased organs and histological slides.

Gross appearance observing

1. Firstly identifying the organ or architecture.

2. Observing the shape, size and color of the organ, and finding out if it is normal (in com-parison with the corresponding normal organ or tissue)

3. The surface and cut surface

(1) Smoothness: Smooth or rough.

(2) Transparency: The capsule is thin or thick, clear or turbid.

(3) Color: Dark red or pale, gray or black, deep yellow or buffy.

(4) Texture: Soft, hard, tenacious or fragile, etc.

4. Focuses of the disease

(1) Distribution and location: Identifying the location of the focuses, and how the focuses are distributed in the organ.

(2) Quantity: Single or multiple, focal or diffuse.

(3) Size: The volume is represented as length×width×thickness. The area is represented as length×width. The measuring unit is centimetre (cm). You could also describe it as a real object, for example, as big as a grain of rice, a soy bean, an egg or an adult's fist, etc.

(4) Color: Normal organ should keep the natural color of itself. Otherwise, it may be influenced by the endogenous or exogenous pigment. For instance, the dark red represents the increasing blood flow, the flavo-green represents the existence of bile, and yellow represents the deposit of fat or lipoid.

(5) Shape: Round, irregular, papillary, cauliflower like or nodular.

(6) The relationship between the focus and the adjacent tissue: Well bordered or ill bor-

dered, compressed or destroyed, encapsuled or not, and whether the encapsulation is integrity. Is there adhesion to other organs.

As for the hollow organ, you should pay attention to the organ wall because it can become thicker or thinner. You should also identify whether the inner wall is smooth or rough, is there a pustute, and the color, character, capacity of the intracavitary matters. Finally, is there any adhesion on the parietal wall.

(Notice: The organs for the experiment has been fixed in formalin, and the color, size, hardness are different from the fresh ones.)

Histological slides observing

1. Firstly, observing the shape and the color of the slides macroscopical, and further defining the pathological area.

2. Observing with microscope: Do not make the sections up side down. Otherwise it can be broken.

(1) Low power lens is mainly used to inspect the overall situation of the tissue, and to observe the changes of histological structure, identifying the location and the nature of the focus, and the correlation to the adjacent tissues. The observing directions should be like this: From upward to downward, and from the left to the right. You shall not use the high power lens at the beginning.

(2) High power lens is mainly used to observe the fine structures and the morphologic changes of the tissues and cells.

Description, diagnosis principle and picture drawing

The description of the specimen should be ingenuous. Never make it with subjective views ot feelings, and do not transcript it from the book. The description should be purificate and understandable. From part to whole, from inside to outside, from upward to downward.

When diagnosing a specimen, you should observe it carefully, associate the case history and the theory, and do the aggregate analysis.

The diagnosis principle is: the name of the organ or the tissue + pathological change. For example: Spleen infarction, Squamous metaplasia of respiratory epithelium and so on.

Drawing pathological pictures are very important. The students could strengthen the observation, comprehension and memorization of the pathology by doing this. It is also a training of the students' ability. The procedure should be like this: firstly observing the pathological change with microscope, finding out the typical area. Then sketching it lightly, take notice of the position, proportion and correlation. If you are satisfied with the rough sketch, paint the cytoplasm and the mesenchyma with pink pencil, the nucleus with violet pencil. Picture should be situated in the frame (square or round), and illustration (seated in one side or the bottom of the frame). You could use the pictures in the teaching book as references. But do not imitate them without microscopic observation.

Practice announcement

1. Taking care of the microscopy, specimen, pathological slides and other experimental instrument. Especially the slides. For they are very valuable, and the relevant patient is not available

currently. Once destroyed it maybe never obtained again.

2. Reading the practice instruction before you take the class. Reviewing the relevant theory and understanding the requirement and objective of the class.

3. Keeping the classroom quiet, paying attention to the experiment, and avoiding distractions.

4. Keeping the classroom clean. And 3 or 4 students being on duty for the day.

5. Obeying the laboratory rules and regulations.

第一章 细胞、组织的适应和损伤

大体观察

1. 子宫萎缩
2. 肾脏萎缩
3. 心肌肥大
4. 前列腺结节性增生
5. 宫颈糜烂伴鳞状上皮化生
6. 肾脏混浊肿胀
7. 脂肪肝
8. 脾包膜的玻璃样变性
9. 肺炭末沉着症
10. 眼黑色素瘤
11. 脾凝固性坏死
12. 肾脏干酪样坏死
13. 脑液化性坏死
14. 足干性坏疽

镜下观察

1. 睾丸萎缩
2. 前列腺结节性增生
3. 子宫内膜增生(单纯性增生)
4. 子宫颈糜烂伴鳞状上皮化生
5. 支气管鳞化
6. 食管上皮柱状上皮化生
7. 胃上皮的肠化
8. 肾脏细胞水肿(混浊肿胀)
9. 肝细胞脂肪变性(脂肪肝)
10. 血管壁透明变性
11. 结缔组织透明变性
12. 肺炭末沉着症
13. 眼恶性黑色素瘤
14. 肝脏疟色素沉积(疟原虫色素)
15. 病理性钙化
16. 心肌梗死(凝固性坏死)
17. 肺结核干酪样坏死
18. 脓肿(液化性坏死)
19. 细胞凋亡

一、大 体 观 察

1. 子宫萎缩

(1) 简要说明:病因:老年性、炎症晚期、激素失调以及理化因素。

(2) 大体所见:由于子宫肌壁纤维化导致子宫体积缩小,子宫质地变硬。

2. 肾脏萎缩　肾脏体积缩小、质地变硬,多由于高血压引起。

3. 心肌肥大

(1) 简要说明:病因:高血压及某些心脏疾病。

(2) 大体所见:心脏体积比正常增大、重量增加、心室扩大、心室壁增厚。

4. 前列腺结节性增生

(1) 简要说明

1) 前列腺间质及上皮细胞增生(多位于尿道周围区域)多见于50岁以上的男性。

2）尿道部分或完全梗阻。

（2）大体所见：境界清楚、大小不一的结节。切面观：间质增生形成的海绵状小结节、灰白色、质地硬；腺体增生形成黄色小结节、质地软。新鲜标本中可见乳白色液体流出。

5. 宫颈糜烂伴鳞状上皮化生

（1）简要说明

1）鳞化被定义为分泌黏蛋白的柱状上皮被覆层鳞状上皮取代。

2）病因：局部环境因素（阴道）、外伤、慢性炎症刺激、子宫颈感染。

（2）大体所见：子宫颈内膜呈红色、绒毛样外观，与邻近的粉红色、半透明的鳞状上皮形成鲜明的对比。

6. 肾脏混浊肿胀

（1）简要说明

1）水变性或空泡变性。

2）当细胞无法维持离子和液体内环境稳定时发生。

3）几乎是各种形式的细胞损伤最早期的表现。

4）是可逆性损伤。

（2）大体所见：颜色苍白、包膜紧张、体积增大。

7. 脂肪肝

（1）简要说明

1）病因：酗酒、肥胖、非酒精性肝炎。

2）肝细胞内中性三酰甘油的异常蓄积，病变严重时可损伤细胞功能。

（2）大体所见：轻度脂肪变性时没有大体改变。进展期改变为肝脏体积增大，颜色变黄。重度改变为体积增大、颜色苍白或淡黄色、质地软、有油腻感，重量可达 3~6kg。

8. 脾包膜的玻璃样变性　脾脏包膜的纤维性渗出未完全吸收，随后发生机化。脾脏包膜增厚，呈现均质的、玻璃样的外观。

9. 肺炭末沉着症

（1）简要说明

1）肺脏和淋巴结内炭粉尘的沉积。

2）单纯性炭末沉着症源于吸烟及城市环境的污染。

（2）大体所见：肺野内散在分布局灶性的炭末色素沉着，绝大多数位于肺上下叶的上部区域。

10. 眼黑色素瘤

（1）简要说明

1）白种人眼内黑色素瘤较常见。

2）该肿瘤发生于眼的色素膜（包括虹膜；睫状体；脉络膜），眼睑皮肤，眼结膜及眼眶内。

（2）大体所见：显著的黑色素沉着。

11. 脾凝固性坏死　坏死灶呈苍白色锥形，灰白干燥，质地硬。锥形坏死的尖断指向器官的门部。

12. 肾脏干酪样坏死　坏死灶呈微黄白色,与周围正常组织分界清楚。坏死组织质地疏松,颗粒状,易碎,形似干酪。

13. 脑液化性坏死　坏死区质地软,坏死中心液化形成一个由厚囊壁包裹的囊腔。

14. 足干性坏疽　大片的坏死区(整个足)呈深黑色,干燥。

二、镜下观察

1. 睾丸萎缩

(1) 生精小管内可见睾丸支持细胞,但无精子发生。精原细胞变性消失。

(2) 曲细精管变细并且被纤维分隔。

(3) 基底膜增厚,明显的间质细胞增生和纤维化。

2. 前列腺结节性增生

(1) 腺体增生,或扩张的巨大腺泡可向内折叠形成乳头状皱褶。

(2) 一些腺泡上皮由双层细胞构成,内层淡染的柱状或立方形腺上皮细胞,及外层深染的小肌上皮细胞。

(3) 腺体及间质增生。

3. 子宫内膜增生(单纯性增生)

(1) 腺体增生,互相拥挤,大小及形状各异。

(2) 腺体上皮为单层扁平或立方或柱状上皮构成,细胞核位于基底部。

(3) 混合性的上皮和间质增生。

4. 子宫颈糜烂伴鳞状上皮化生

(1) 鳞状上皮代替子宫颈内黏膜柱状上皮,随后柱状上皮变性脱落,由扁平的鳞状上皮取代分泌黏液的柱状上皮。

(2) 子宫颈内腺体的囊性扩张,被称为宫颈腺体囊肿。

5. 支气管鳞化　慢性支气管炎时,支气管的柱状上皮转化为鳞状上皮。

6. 食管上皮柱状上皮化生　慢性胃反流性炎症时,食管下段鳞状上皮由胃或肠柱状上皮替代。

7. 胃上皮的肠化　慢性胃炎,胃壁细胞及主细胞消失,由薄层的组织结构取代,该组织由柱状细胞及杯状细胞组成的小腺体构成。该组织类似萎缩的小肠黏膜。

8. 肾脏细胞水肿(混浊肿胀)

(1) 细胞肿胀,胞浆含有粗颗粒。近曲小管内皮细胞肿大,胞浆内充满嗜伊红染颗粒。

(2) 光镜下细胞核无改变。

(3) 红细胞管型(红色)及透明管型(粉色至紫色)。

其他描述:

(1) 细胞水肿为细胞损伤的最初表现,病变可逆。

(2) 细胞内水分增加是因为细胞膜离子转运功能的改变。

(3) 病因:感染,理化损伤(中毒),局部缺血。

9. 肝细胞脂肪变性(脂肪肝)

(1) 许多小球状胞浆空泡,因细胞内脂肪聚集而将核挤至一侧。

（2）邻近的细胞破裂形成脂囊。

其他描述：

核周胞浆内脂肪空泡可以通过制作冷冻切片苏丹Ⅲ或苏丹黑染色证明。

10. 血管壁透明变性　小动脉壁呈现为均质粉红色玻璃样外观。血管壁增厚，管腔狭窄。

11. 结缔组织透明变性　胶原纤维融合并且发生透明变性，仅有少量或无血管。

12. 肺炭末沉着症　含有大量碳粉尘的巨噬细胞位于邻近细支气管，肺动脉，胸膜下间质以及肺门淋巴结内。

13. 眼恶性黑色素瘤　如果不去除黑色素很难鉴别细胞形状或类型。

其他描述：

（1）眼部恶性黑色素瘤起源于葡萄膜黑色素细胞，包括虹膜、睫状体、脉络膜。

（2）视网膜色素上皮细胞，大多数来自脉络膜后方。

14. 肝脏疟色素沉积（疟原虫色素）

（1）肝血窦充血，肝细胞索紊乱。

（2）肝内枯否细胞增生，这些细胞胞质内含有被疟原虫吞噬了的红细胞和未被吞噬的红细胞、残留的寄生虫、疟原虫色素颗粒，偶尔可见含铁血黄素。

15. 病理性钙化　血管壁内可有异常的钙盐沉积（蓝色）。

16. 心肌梗死（凝固性坏死）

（1）凝固性坏死灶表现为嗜伊红染的颗粒状外观，坏死区仍可保留细胞外形及组织结构轮廓。

（2）坏死区周围可见炎症细胞浸润及出血反应带。

17. 肺结核干酪样坏死

（1）坏死灶呈嗜伊红染的颗粒无定形的碎屑或无结构坏死。

（2）可见上皮样细胞的朗汉斯巨细胞。

（3）坏死区周围可见有淋巴细胞及纤维细胞。

18. 脓肿（液化性坏死）　组织变性伴有大量中性粒细胞浸润。

19. 细胞凋亡　圆形或椭圆形境界清楚的细胞团块，胞浆呈强嗜伊红染色，核染色质浓缩并向细胞边缘聚集，可以形成凋亡小体。

三、思 考 题

（一）选择题

选一个字母代表的最合适答案。

1. 活检送病理检查应该以何种方式固定最常用？
　　A. 在10%甲醛溶液中固定　　B. 在90%乙醇溶液中固定　　C. 在0.9%盐溶液中保存
　　D. 冰冻　　　　　　　　　　E. 在普通的固定剂中

2. 送活检时应该同时有以下信息，除了
　　A. 病人的年龄和性别　　B. 活检部位　　　　　C. 相关实验室检验结果
　　D. X线检查　　　　　　E. 家族史

（二）问答题

1. 萎缩和退化的区别是什么？

2. 什么是肾积水？

3. 什么是瘘管？

4. 什么是溃疡？

5. 肥大和增生的区别是什么？

6. 如何证实淀粉样物质？

7. 什么是淀粉样变性？什么情况下发生？

8. 最常发生脂肪变性的细胞有哪些？

9. 哪些细胞核的形态学变化显示细胞已经死亡？

10. 什么是坏疽？有哪些类型？

11. 什么是病理性钙化？

12. 什么是化生？请举例。

13. 凋亡和坏死的区别。

14. 细胞老化的形态学变化是什么？

Chapter 1 Cell and Tissue Adaptation and Injury

Gross Findings
1. Atrophy of uterus
2. Atrophy of kidney
3. Hypertrophy of myocardium
4. Nodular hyperplasia, Prostate
5. Cervical erosion with squamous metaplasia
6. Cloudy swelling, Kidney
7. Fatty liver, Liver
8. Hyaline degeneration of spleen capsule
9. Lung Anthracosis
10. Eye Melanin (Malignant melanoma)
11. Coagulation necrosis of spleen
12. Caseous necrosis of kidney
13. Liquefaction necrosis of brain
14. Dry gangrene of foot

Micro Findings
1. Atrophy of testis
2. Prostate nodular hyperplasia
3. Endometrial hyperplasia (simple)
4. Cervical erosion with squamous metaplasia
5. Bronchial epithelium squamous metaplasia
6. Columnar epithelium metaplasia, esophagus
7. Intestinal metaplasia of gastric epithelium
8. Cell edema, Kidney (Cloudy swelling)
9. Fatty degeneration, Liver (Fatty liver)
10. Vessel wall hyaline degeneration
11. Hyaline degeneration of connective tissue
12. Anthracosis, Lung
13. Melanin, Eye (Malignant melanoma)
14. Malaria pigment, Liver (Hemozoin)
15. Pathological calcification
16. Coagulation necrosis myocardium infarction
17. Caseous necrosis, Lung tuberculous
18. Liquefaction necrosis, abscesses
19. Apoptosis

Gross Findings

1. Atrophy of uterus

(1) Brief Descriptions: Cause: senility, end stage of inflammatory or chitis, hormones imbalance, and physico-chemical effects.

(2) Gross Findings: Small in uterus size and firm in consistency is caused by uterus fibrosis.

2. Atrophy of kidney   Small in kidney size and firm in consistency result from hypertention.

3. Hypertrophy of myocardium

(1) Brief Descriptions: Cause: hypertension and several heart diseases.

(2) Gross Findings: The heart size is larger than normal. The weight increased and ventricle is enlargement, and the wall of ventricle become thicken.

4. Nodular hyperplasia, Prostate

(1) Brief Descriptions

1) Hyperplasia of prostate stromal and epithelial cells(always in the periurethral region).

Common in male over 50 years old.

2）Partial or complete obstruction of urethra.

（2）Gross Findings：Well-defined, variously sized nodules. Cut surface: small nodules, spongy, gray and tough (stromal proliferation) to yellow and soft with milky white fluid oozing out (glandular hyperplasia).

5. Cervical erosion with squamous metaplasia

（1）Brief Descriptions

1）Squamous metaplasia is defined by replacement of mucin-secreting columnar epithelium by stratified squamous epithelium.

2）Cause: local (vaginal) environmental factors, trauma, chronic irritation, cervical infection.

（2）Gross Findings：When viewed with naked eye, the endocervical mucosa appears as a red, velvety zone, sharply contrasting with the neighboring pink, translucent squamous epithelium.

6. Cloudy swelling, Kidney

（1）Brief Descriptions

1）Hydropic change or vacuolar degeneration.

2）Appears whenever cells are incapable of maintaining ionic and fluid homeostasis.

3）The first manifestation of almost all forms of cell injury.

4）Reversible injury.

（2）Gross Findings：Pallor, increased turgor, and increased in weight.

7. Fatty liver, Liver

（1）Brief Descriptions

1）Cause: alcoholic,obesity,non-alcoholic hepatitis.

2）Abnormal accumulation of neutral triglyceride (fat) in hepatocytes, when severe may impair cellular function.

（2）Gross Findings：Mild fatty change: no gross change. Progressive change: enlarges and getting yellow.Severe: enlarge,pale or bright yellow,soft,greasy and may even weigh 3~6kg.

8. Hyaline degeneration of spleen capsule   The capsular fibrin exudates of spleen is not completely obstruted following organiration. The capsule thickening with homogenous, glassy appearance.

9. Lung Anthracosis

（1）Brief Descriptions

1）Deposition of coal (carbon) dust in the lung and lymph nodes.

2）Simple anthracosis resulting from smoking and urban living.

（2）Gross Findings：Focal black pigmentation scattered through the lung fields,most numerous in the upper zones of the upper and lower lobes.

10. Eye Melanin (Malignant melanoma)

（1）Brief Descriptions

1）Intraocular melanoma is common in Caucasians.

2）It occurs on the uveal tract (the iris; ciliary body; and choroids), on the skin of lid, on the conjunctiva and with in the orbit.

（2）Gross Findings：Striking black in pigmentation.

11. Coagulation necrosis of spleen   The necrotic foci are pale,tapper,hoary dry and hard.The

tip of taper pattern point to portal of organ.

12. Caseous necrosis of kidney   Foci are yellowish white and well circumscribed from the surrounding normal tissues.The necrotic tissue is soft, granular and friable, reminiscent of dry cheese.

13. Liquefaction necrosis of brain   The necrotic area is soft and the center is liquefied, a cystic space is formation with thicken cystic wall.

14. Dry gangrene of foot   Huge necrotic area (all foot) is dark black color with dry.

Micro Findings

1. Atrophy of testis

(1) The tubules show Sertoli cells but no spermatogenesis. Degeneration and disappearance of spermatogonial cells

(2) Small and far apart of seminiferous tubules.

(3) Thickening of basement membrane. Prominent of interstitial cells (Leydig's cells) and fibrosis.

2. Prostate nodular hyperplasia

(1) Glandular proliferation or dilation, large acini with papillary infoldings (star shape).

(2) Some acini lined with pale columnar to cuboidal cells and small dark cells in outer row (two-cell type).

(3) Gland and stroma proliferation.

3. Endometrial hyperplasia (simple)

(1) Crowded glands varying in size and shape.

(2) Glands lined by a single layered flattened (cystic change) to cuboidal or columnar epithelium with uniformed basal seated nuclei.

(3) Mixed epithelial and stromal proliferation.

4. Cervical erosion with squamous metaplasia

(1) Squamous epithelial cells growth under the columnar endocervical mucosa, then the columnar cells degenerate and sloughed.The replacement of mucin-secreting columnar epithelium by stratified squamous epithelium.

(2) Cystic dilation of endocervical glands known as Nabothian cysts.

5. Bronchial epithelium squamous metaplasia   In chronic bronchitis, the brochial mucous membranes epithelium undergo metaplastic transformation to the replacement of squamous cells.

6. Columnar epithelium metaplasia,esophagus   In chronic gastric reflux, the normal stratified squamous epithelium of the lower esophagus may undergo metaplastic transformation to the replacement of gastric epithelium with columnar and goblet cells of intestinal variety.

7. Intestinal metaplasia of gastric epithelium   In chronic gastritis parietal and chief (oxyntic) cells of stomach have disappeared and instead there is a much thinner structure composed of short glands lined by columnar cells and goblet cells. The tissue resembles atrophic small intestinal mucosa.

8. Cell edema, Kidney(Cloudy swelling)

(1) Cell swelling, cytoplasm contains coarse granules. The individual tubular lining cells are enlarged and filled with eosinophilic granules in cytoplasm.

(2) Nucleus not affected in light microscopy.

(3) Pigmented (RBC) cast (red color) and hyaline cast (pink to purple color).

Others:

(1) The first manifestation of cell injury and is reversible.

(2) Increasing hydration of the cell due to alteration in ion transport at cell membrane.

(3) Cause: infection, physico-chemical injury (toxic), ischemia.

9. Fatty degeneration, Liver (Fatty liver)

(1) Many small globular intracytoplasmic clear space, may accumulate and displace the nucleus to the periphery.

(2) Contiguous cells may rupture to produce fatty cyst.

Others:

(1) Fat vacuoles in the cytoplasm around the nucleus.

(2) Prepare by frozen section and stained by Sudan Ⅲ or Sudan black.

10. Vessel wall hyaline degeneration   A homogenous glassy pink appearance in the arteriolar wall That result in thicken and stenosis of the blood vesels.

11. Hyaline degeneration of connective tissue   Collagenous fibrous fused and hyalinized with few or no blood vessls.

12. Anthracosis, Lung   Coal dust-filled macrophages located interstitially adjacent to bronchioles, pulmonary arteries, subpleurally and within hilar lymph nodes.

13. Melanin, Eye (Malignant melanoma)   It is hard to identify the cell shape or type without remove the melanin.

Others:

(1) Origin of melanoma of the eye Melanocytes of the uvea (iris、ciliary body、choroid).

(2) Pigmented epithelium of the retina. Mostly from posterior choroid.

14. Malaria pigment, Liver (Hemozoin)

(1) Congested sinusoids, and some disarrangement of hepatic cords.

(2) Hypertrophy Kupffer cells containing parasitized or unparasitized RBC, remnants of parasites, hemozoin granules, and occasional hemosiderin.

15. Pathological calcification   There are abnormal deposition of calcium salts (blue) in blood vessels wall

16. Coagulation necrosis myocardium infarction

(1) Foci of coagulation necrosis expressed eosinophilic granular with recogniting the cell outline and tissue architecture.

(2) Inflammatory cells and hemorrhage reponse zone around necrotic areas.

17. Cascous necrosis, Lung tuberculous

(1) Foci of necrosis show eosinophilic granular as amorphous debris or unstructured necrosis.

(2) Epitheliod and Langhais giant cell may be seen.

(3) lymphocyte and fibrocyte around necrotic areas.

18. Liquefaction necrosis, abscesses   Tissue degeneration with numerous leukocytes.

19. Apoptosis   Round or oval well-delimited masses with intensely eosinophilic ctroplasm, nuclear chromatin condensed and aggregates peripherally, may be formed apoptotic bodies.

Study Questions

Choose Tests

Directions: Each of the numbered items or incomplete statements in this section is followed by answers or by completions of the statement. Select the one lettered answer or completion that is best in each case.

1. A biopsy should be sent to pathology in which of the following modes?
   A. Fixed in 10% formalin   B. Fixed in 90% alcohol   C. Fresh in 0.9% saline
   D. Frozen   E. Fixed in a generic fixative
2. All of the following information should accompany a biopsy EXCEPT
   A. patient age and sex   B. biopsy site   C. pertinent laboratory values
   D. x-ray findings   E. family history

Questions

1. What is the difference between atrophy and involution?
2. What is hydronephrosis?
3. What is a fistula?
4. What is an ulcer?
5. What is the difference between hypertrophy and hyperplasia?
6. How is the confirm of amyloid substance made?
7. What is amyloidosis and in what conditions does it occur?
8. Which are the commonest cells in which fatty change is seen?
9. What morphological changes in the nucleus indicate that a cell is dead?
10. What is gangrene and in what types does if occur?
11. What is pathologic calcification?
12. What is metaplasia? Give examples.
13. What is the difference between necrosis and apoptosis?
14. What morphological changes occur in the cell aging?

第二章　损伤的修复

大体观察	镜下观察
1. 皮肤角质层的肥厚性瘢痕	1. 肉芽组织
2. 粘连和机化	2. 瘢痕组织
3. 骨折愈合	

一、大 体 观 察

1. 皮肤角质层的肥厚性瘢痕

大体所见:胶原纤维组织过度增生导致瘢痕的过度形成。皮肤角质层苍白,质硬,生长超过了上皮水平。

2. 粘连和机化　结核性胸膜炎表现为胸膜腔内过量的液体渗出,当炎症愈合时渗出液吸收不完全则可以形成肉芽组织及纤维组织的增生,导致组织机化,胸膜粘连引起的胸腔部分或完全性闭塞。

3. 骨折愈合　分为以下四个阶段

(1) 血肿的形成和机化。

(2) 纤维性骨痂形成(暂时骨痂)。

(3) 骨性骨痂形成(永久骨痂)。

(4) 骨痂改建或再塑。

二、镜 下 观 察

1. 肉芽组织

(1) 成纤维细胞增生和大量薄壁毛细血管的形成。

(2) 组织水肿,炎症细胞浸润。

2. 瘢痕组织

(1) 胶原网的蓄积依赖梭形纤维细胞。

(2) 有少量的或无血管。

三、思 考 题

(一) 选择题

选一个字母代表的最合适答案。

一旦组织或器官被破坏后自身重建,下列细胞能够重建组织除外

A. 肝细胞　　　　　　　B. 结肠黏膜细胞　　　　　　　C. 血管内皮细胞

D. 心肌细胞　　　　　　　E. 骨髓原始细胞

（二）问答题

1. 伤口愈合的过程中是如何进行收缩的?
2. 骨折愈合的主要事件有哪些?
3. 纤维细胞和纤维母细胞的区别是什么?
4. 肉芽组织的结构和作用是什么?

Chapter 2　Repair for injury

Gross Findings
1. Hypertrophic scar, Skin keratoid
2. Adhesion and organization
3. Fracture healing

Micro Findings
1. Granulation tissue
2. Scar tissue

Gross Findings

1. Hypertrophic scar, Skin keratoid(stratum corneum)
Gross Findings:Collaginous fibrous tissue are overproliferation with overscar formation
Skin keratinize are pale,hard, growth over epithelial level.

2. Adhesion and organization　Tubercule pleurisies express effusive fluid exudates in the pleural space when healing with no complete absorb forming the proliferations of granulation and fibrisos tissue, resulting in tissue organization and adhesion of pleura with partial or complete obliteration of the pleural cavity.

3. Fracture healing　There are four steps
(1) Hematoma formation and organization.
(2) fibrocartilagineus callus.(provisional callus)
(3) Osseous callus.(definitive callus)
(4) Remodeling.

Micro Findings

1. Granulation tissue
(1) Fibroblasts proliferation and numerous thin walled,delicate capillaries
(2) Tissue edema and some inflammatory cells.
2. Scar tissue
(1) Net collagen accumulation depends with spindle shaped fibrocytes.
(2) A few or no blood vessels.

Study Questions

Choose Tests
Directions: Each of the numbered items or incomplete statements in this section is followed by answers or by completions of the statement. Select the one lettered answer or completion that is best in each case.

Once damaged, a tissue or organ usually attempts to regenerate itself. All of the following cell types are capable of regenerating tissue EXCEPT

A. hepatocytes   B. colonic mucosal cells   C. vascular endothelial cells
D. myocardial cells   E. bone marrow myelobtasts

Questions

1. How does a wound contract with healing?
2. What are the main events in the healing of a fracture?
3. What is the difference between a fibrocyte and a fibroblast?
4. What is granulation tissue and what effects does it occur?

第三章　局部循环和血流动力学障碍

大体观察	镜下观察
1. 肺充血水肿(褐色硬化)	1. 肺淤血心衰细胞
2. 肝脏心源性淤血	2. 肝脏心源性淤血
3. 槟榔肝(中心性坏死)	3. 肝淤血及凝固性坏死
4. 脑出血	4. 心源性肝硬化
5. 动脉血栓	5. 静脉血栓(混合血栓)
6. 静脉血栓	6. 血栓的机化与再通
7. 附壁血栓	7. 肺水肿
8. 肺动脉栓塞	8. 瘤栓,肝癌转移到肺
9. (肝细胞癌)门静脉栓塞	9. 脾梗死
10. 脾或肾贫血性梗死	10. 回肠出血性梗死
11. 肠出血性梗死	

一、大体观察

1. 肺充血水肿(褐色硬化)

大体所见:长期持续性的肺间质充血水肿导致肺泡壁纤维化,随即含铁血黄素沉积,肺组织变硬呈褐色(褐色硬化)。

2. 肝脏心源性淤血

(1) 简要说明

1) 肝脏慢性被动性淤血,称为槟榔肝。

2) 病因:右心衰竭,肝脏慢性被动性淤血。

(2) 大体所见:肝小叶中央静脉周围的区域因淤血和出血颜色深,而小叶周边门管区因肝细胞发生脂肪变性而呈淡黄色。

3. 槟榔肝(中心性坏死)

(1) 简要说明:右心衰竭→肝脏被动性淤血→肝小叶中心肝血窦允血→肝小叶中心肝细胞萎缩。

左心衰竭→肝血流灌注不足→肝小叶中心坏死,肝小叶中心出血性坏死;槟榔肝。

(2) 大体所见:肝小叶中心区域呈明显的红褐色并有轻微的凹陷,与周边未发生淤血的脂肪变性的肝细胞形成红黄相间像槟榔一样。

4. 脑出血　侧脑室有大量的出血。

5. 动脉血栓　动脉管腔内可见有一血栓。

6. 静脉血栓

（1）血栓与受损的血管壁黏附。

（2）血栓外观上为明暗交替的层状结构。

7. 附壁血栓 血栓牢固地附着在血管壁上。

8. 肺动脉栓塞 在肺淋巴管内可见有大量的癌性栓子。

9.（肝细胞癌）门静脉栓塞 肝门静脉内可见巨大的癌性栓子伴栓塞。

10. 脾或肾贫血性梗死

简要说明：几乎99%的梗死是来源于血栓性栓塞，而且绝大多数为动脉的阻塞。贫血性梗死或白色梗死发生于实体性组织合并动脉阻塞的情况下。梗死区颜色呈灰白色，与周围组织分界清楚（炎症反应充血带）。梗死呈楔形，顶端指向血管阻塞处。当梗死底部累及浆膜时，引起纤维素渗出。梗死侧面边缘不规则，反映了邻近血管的侧支血供。

11. 肠出血性梗死

（1）简要说明：出血性梗死或红色梗死一般发生于以下情况：①静脉闭塞；②组织疏松；③组织有双套血液供应；④组织原有淤血。

肠道的三支主要供应血管（腹主动脉,肠系膜上动脉及肠系膜下动脉）中的一支发生急性闭塞将导致肠出血性梗死。

（2）大体所见：梗死的肠道呈现明显的淤血，颜色暗红色或紫红色，管壁水肿增厚，橡胶样，有出血。

二、镜 下 观 察

1. 肺淤血心衰细胞

（1）淤血心衰细胞在肺泡腔内，是吞噬了含铁血黄素的巨噬细胞。

（2）淤血和出血：肺泡腔内充满水肿液伴褐色的心衰细胞；肺泡间隔增厚。

2. 肝脏心源性淤血

（1）淤血性改变,在肝小叶中央区域加重,而肝小叶周边区域为苍白色缺氧改变。

（2）在严重的病例中,小叶中央区域坏死常伴有肝血窦持续性淤血,随后发生硬化 →心源性硬化。

肝脏正常结构破坏,尤其是中央静脉周围区域。

肝血窦淤血,中央静脉附近的肝细胞坏死。

3. 肝淤血及凝固性坏死

（1）肝小叶中心区出现坏死并有轻微的炎症反应（细胞轮廓保存,核溶解消失）。肝小叶中心区的缺血将导致肝索的凝固性坏死。门静脉区周围的肝细胞尚保存。

（2）坏死区与正常组织间有明显的界限。

4. 心源性肝硬化

（1）邻近腺泡的小叶中央区纤维化将相互联合或向门管区延伸。纤维组织将肝实质分隔成不规则结节,从中心区域发生的纤维化间隔相互延伸连接。

（2）纤维分隔间有少量的炎症细胞浸润。胆小管增生不显著。

5. 静脉血栓(混合血栓)

(1) 血栓附着在受损的静脉管壁上。

(2) 血栓表现为层状结构,由混有纤维蛋白的血小板梁(灰白色)与较多红细胞、变性白细胞(暗红色)组成。

6. 血栓的机化与再通

(1) 血栓机化:血栓内有肉芽组织的形成并替代血栓。使其与血管壁牢固地黏附。

(2) 血栓再通:血栓内出现裂隙,内皮细胞长入覆盖裂隙表面形成新的血管腔,使血流再通。

7. 肺水肿 因为肺淤血,肺泡腔内充满浆液性水肿液(粉红色)。

8. 瘤栓,肝癌转移到肺 在肺淋巴管内可见有大量的癌细胞栓子。

9. 脾梗死

(1) 坏死区呈现均质的粉红色外观。

(2) 切片中可见有含铁血黄素结晶。吞噬了含铁血黄素的巨噬细胞更多见于纤维化区域(梗死与正常组织结合处)。

(3) 炎症细胞位于梗死区的边缘。

10. 回肠出血性梗死

(1) 肠壁水肿:增厚,橡胶样,肠黏膜出血性坏死。

(2) 间质出血:黏膜层及黏膜下层炎症反应。

三、思 考 题

(一) 选择题

选一个字母代表的最合适答案。

1. 下肢末梢血栓性静脉炎引起的最严重的并发症是

    A. 脑梗死　　　　　　　　B. 肾梗死　　　　　　　　C. 心肌梗死

    D. 肺梗死　　　　　　　　E. 消化道梗死

2. 血栓闭塞性脉管炎通常发生于以下病人

    A. 先天性心房缺陷　　　　B. 动脉粥样硬化性心脏病　　C. 高脂饮食

    D. 严重吸烟患者　　　　　E. 低运动量病人

(二) 问答题

1. 什么是水肿?

2. 什么是血栓?

3. 血栓形成的原因是什么?

4. 肺循环中的栓子有哪些类型?

5. 栓子有哪些种类,其主要的栓塞途径有哪些?

6. 什么是弥散性血管内凝血(DIC)?

7. 什么是减压病?

8. 贫血性梗死与出血性梗死的鉴别。

9. 什么是血栓(性)静脉炎?

10. 闭塞性动脉内膜炎的病理学变化是什么? 在哪种情况下会发生?

Chapter 3   Local Fluid and Hemodynamic Derangement

Gross Findings	Micro Findings
1. Pulmonary congestion and edema (brown induration)	1. Heart failure cell, Lung
2. Cardiac congestion, Liver	2. Cardiac congestion, Liver
3. Nutmeg liver (Central necrosis), Liver	3. Congestion and coagulative necrosis Liver
4. Hemorrhage of brain	4. Cardiac cirrhosis, Liver
5. Thrombus of artery	5. Venous thrombosis (mixed thrombus)
6. Thrombus of vein	6. Organization and recanalization of thrombus
7. Mural thrombus	7. Pulmonary edema
8. Embolism of pulmonary artery	8. Tumor embolus liver cancer matastasis to lung
9. Embolism(hepatocellular carcinoma) of portal vein	9. Splenic infarction
10. Splenic or kidney anemic infarction	10. Hemorrhagic infarction, Ileum
11. Hemorrhagic infarction of intestine	

Gross Findings

1. Pulmonary congestion and edema (brown induration)

Gross Findings: Long persistence septal congestion and edema often induces fibrosis within the alveolar wall. With hemosiderin deposition.The lung become harder and brown (brown induration).

2. Cardiac congestion, Liver

(1) Brief Descriptions: Chronic passive congestion of the liver ; so-called nutmeg liver.

Cause: Right-side heart failure, chronic passive congestion of the liver.

(2) Gross Findings: Dark congested and hemorrhagic perivenular areas with pale zone (yellowish tinge due to fatty change) of periportal areas.

3. Nutmeg liver (Central necrosis), Liver

(1) Brief Descriptions: Right-sided cardiac failure→ passive congestion of the liver→congestion of centrilobular sinusoid→ centrilobular hepatocytes become atrophic.

Left-sided cardiac failure → hepatic hypoperfusion → centrilobular necrosis. Centrilobular hemorrhagic necrosis; nutmeg liver.

(2) Gross Findings: In liver the central regions of the hepatic lobules are grossly red brown and slightly depressed,and are accentuated against the surrounding zones of uncongested tan with fatty liver.Red brown and yellow do in turn likely nutmeg.

4. Hemorrhage of brain   There are a amount of bleeding in side ventricle.

5. Thrombus of artery   Thrombus is seen in the artery.

6. Thrombus of vein.

（1）Thrombi adherent to the injured venous wall.

（2）Thrombi apparent laminations with pale layer and darker layer.

7. Mural thrombus   Thrombus is firmly adherent to the vessel wall.

8. Embolism of pulmonary artery   Numerous carcinoma embolus in lymph tubes of lung.

9. Embolism(hepatocellular carcinoma) of portal vein   Huge carcinoma embolus in portal vein of liver with embolism.

10. Splenic or kidney anemic infarction

Brief Descriptions:Nearly 99% of infarcts are caused by thromboembolic events, and almost all are the result of arterial occlusions.

White infarcts are encountered with arterial occlusion and in solid tissues. Infarcts area show pale yellow-gray, and the margins of infarct tend to defined will time by a narrow rim of inflammtion and hyperemia.The infart area tends to be wedge shaped, with the occluded vessel at the apex. When infarct base influence over serosal surface, there are often an fibrinous exudates. The lateral margins may be irregular, reflecting the pattern of vascular supply from adjacent vessels.

11. Hemorrhagic infarction of intestine

（1）Brief Descriptions:Red or hemorrhagic infarcts are encountered usually

①with venous occlusions,②in loose tissues,③in tissues with a double circulation, and④in tissues previously congested.

Acute occlusion of one of the three major supply trunks of the intestines (celiac, superior and inferior mesenteric arteries) may lead to infarction of intestine.

（2）Gross Findings:The infarcted bowel appears intensely congested and dusky to purple-red and the wall becomes edematous, thickened, rubbery, and hemorrhagic.

Micro Findings

1. Heart failure cell, Lung

（1）Congestion. Heart failure cells as hemosiderin laden macrophages in the alveolar spaces.

（2）Congestion and hemorrhage. The alveolar spaces are filled with edematous fluids and brownish heart failure cells; note thickened alveolar septi.

2. Cardiac congestion, Liver

（1）Congestive changes and accentuation of the centrilobular areas surrounded by paler hypoxic regions.

（2）In severe form: central lobular necrosis appear along with sinusoidal congestion with persistence, it become sclerotic → cardiac cirrhosis.

Destruction of regular liver structure especially in the central areas (perivenular areas).

Sinusoidal congestion and necrosis of hepatocytes in the perivenular areas.

3. Congestion and coagulative necrosis Liver

（1）Central area show necrosis (preservation of cellular contour with disappearance of nucleus)with slight inflammation. Ischemia of centrilobular area resulting in coagulative necrosis of hepatic cords. Preserved periportal area.

（2）Sharp demarcation between necrotic and viable area.

4. Cardiac cirrhosis, Liver

（1）Centrilobular zone: Fibrosis in adjacent acini may link up or extend to connect with portal tracts.

Liver parenchyma is segregated into irregular areas by fibrous tissue. The fibrosis initiated from centrilobular area spreads out to connect with each.

(2) Few inflammatory cells in fibrous septi. Inconspicuous proliferation of bile ductules.

5. Venous thrombosis (mixed thrombus)

(1) Thrombi adherent to the injured venous wall.

(2) Thrombi apparent laminations with pale layer of platelets admixed with some fibrin, and darker layer containing more red cells and degenerating leukocytes.

6. Organization and recanalization of thrombus

(1) Organization of thrombus: Granulation grow in the thrombus and replace thrombus. Let it firmly adherent to the vessel wall.

(2) Recanalization of thrombus: There are some split cover endothelium form space,which running blood flow again.

7. Pulmonary edema　The alveolar spaces are filled with serous edematous fluids (pinkish appearance) with congestion.

8. Tumor embolus, liver cancer metastasis to lung　Numerous carcinoma embolus in lymph tubcs of lung.

9. Splenic infarction

(1) Necrotic area with homogenous pinkish appearance.

(2) Hematoidin crystals can be found in this section. Hemosiderin laden macrophages in the more fibrous areas (junction of infarction).

(3) Inflammatory cells seated on the margin of infarct area.

10. Hemorrhagic infarction, Ileum

(1) The bowel wall becomes edematous, thickened, rubbery, and hemorrhagic necrosis of the mucosa.

(2) Interstitial hemorrhage. Inflammatory response into mucosa and submucosa.

Study Questions

Choose Tests

Directions: Each of the numbered items or incomplete statements in this section is followed by answers or by completions of the statement. Select the one lettered answer or completion that is best in each case.

1. The most common serious complication of lower extremity thrombophlebitis is

　A. cerebral infarction　　　　B. kidney infarction　　　　C. myocardial infarction

　D. pulmonary infarction　　　E. intestinal infarction

2. Thromboangiitit, obliterans occurs predominantly in people with

　A. congenital cardiac atrial defects　　　　B. atherosclerotic heart disease

　C. diets high in saturated fats　　　　D. heavy cigarette-smoking habits

　E. low exercise tolerance

Questions

1. What is oedema?

2. What is a thrombus?

3. What causes thrombosis?

4. What types of emboli lodge in the pulmonary circulation?

5. Are there what kinds of embolus and what pathways of embolism?

6. What is disseminated intravascular congulation (DIC) ?

7. What is decomression sickness?

8. To make a comparism between the anemic and hemorrhagic infarct.

9. What is thrombophlebitis?

10. What is the pathology of endarteritis obliterans and in what conditions does it occur?

第四章 炎 症

大体观察

1. 纤维素性渗出性心包炎
2. 白喉
3. 肠道的假膜性炎
4. 胆囊积脓
5. 输卵管积脓
6. 急性化脓性阑尾炎(蜂窝织炎)
7. 阿米巴肝脓肿
8. 化脓性脑脊髓膜炎
9. 肠出血性炎
10. 结肠息肉
11. 宫颈息肉
12. 慢性胃溃疡

镜下观察

1. 炎症细胞包括中性粒细胞,嗜酸粒细胞,单核细胞(巨噬细胞),淋巴细胞,浆细胞
2. 肠纤维素性炎(假膜性炎)
3. 胆囊表面积脓
4. 输卵管积脓
5. 急性化脓性阑尾炎(阑尾蜂窝织炎)
6. 乳腺脓肿
7. 异物肉芽肿性炎
8. 感染性肉芽肿性炎(结核性干酪性肉芽肿)
9. 子宫颈息肉

一、大体观察

1. **纤维素性渗出性心包炎** 心包浆膜面形成富含纤维蛋白的渗出。心脏表面毛巾头样,又被称为绒毛心。

2. **白喉** 在咽,喉,气管,支气管黏膜表面形成一层假膜,属于纤维素性炎。

3. **肠道的假膜性炎** 渗出液富含纤维蛋白。在肠道的黏膜面形成一层假膜。假膜主要由坏死的上皮细胞,中性粒细胞,细菌,以及纤维素网眼内网罗的红细胞构成。

4. **胆囊积脓** 肉眼观察,胆囊腔内有积脓。胆囊壁增厚,胶状脓液积聚。

5. **输卵管积脓** 输卵管管腔扩张,管腔内充满脓液。

6. **急性化脓性阑尾炎(蜂窝织炎)**

(1)简要说明

1)病因:与阑尾阻塞性疾病相关(粪石,胆石,肿瘤或肠蛔虫团块)。

2)肠壁脓肿形成,肠黏膜化脓性坏死。

(2)大体所见

1)淤血肿胀

2)阑尾腔扩张,内含脓液,粪石,或二者兼有。

3)浆膜面有纤维蛋白或脓性纤维素性渗出或脓液渗出。

7. **阿米巴肝脓肿** 阿米巴肝脓肿病灶位于肝右叶,脓肿有一个厚包膜,直径可以超过

10cm,囊腔内充满了巧克力色,无臭的囊液。

8. 化脓性脑脊髓膜炎　脓性渗出液位于脑组织的表面,并可见脑血管的扩张淤血。

9. 肠出血性炎　肠壁呈黑色,肠腔内有大容量的出血。

10. 结肠息肉　结肠内可见一肿块凸出在肠黏膜面,并且有一蒂与黏膜相连。

病因:炎性增生或肿瘤。

11. 宫颈息肉　可见一肿块凸出在宫颈黏膜面,并有一蒂与子宫颈相连。

12. 慢性胃溃疡

(1) 由于胃黏膜的炎性坏死导致胃黏膜表面有一缺损。

(2) 溃疡将胃肌层破坏,溃疡底部由坏死碎屑及致密的纤维组织所构成。溃疡周边部区域可以形成纤维化、瘢痕化及慢性炎症反应。

二、镜 下 观 察

1. 炎症细胞包括中性粒细胞,嗜酸粒细胞,单核细胞(巨噬细胞),淋巴细胞,浆细胞。这些细胞有着不同的形态和功能。

2. 肠纤维素性炎(假膜性炎)　肠黏膜面形成渗出性炎,渗出物中形成的纤维素网包括坏死的上皮组织,中性粒细胞和细菌。

3. 胆囊表面积脓

(1) 在胆囊黏膜面形成溃疡中伴急性或慢性炎症细胞浸润。

(2) 胆囊结石伴脓液形成,以及异物型多核巨细胞的浸润。

4. 输卵管积脓

(1) 输卵管皱襞肿胀水肿。

(2) 输卵管管腔内脓液积聚。输卵管腔及输卵管褶处可见有坏死碎屑及中性粒细胞的积聚。

(3) 输卵管管壁增厚伴有急性或慢性炎症细胞的浸润。

5. 急性化脓性阑尾炎(阑尾蜂窝织炎)

(1) 黏膜溃疡形成:中性粒细胞,嗜酸粒细胞,浆细胞,淋巴细胞浸润至阑尾各层;并常浸润至浆膜层。

(2) 炎症进展期:由于炎症使肠壁增厚,肠壁组织可以部分发生坏死或梗死(此处为肠穿孔的好发部位)。

6. 乳腺脓肿

(1) 乳腺实质炎症使其中央形成脓,腔内充满脓液。

(2) 多个腺叶及周围残留导管间质的炎性细胞浸润。

(3) 局部扩张的导管中可见有泡沫型组织细胞。

7. 异物肉芽肿性炎　由异物,异物型巨细胞,上皮样组织细胞,淋巴细胞,浆细胞,中性粒细胞共同构成肉芽肿。

8. 感染性肉芽肿性炎(结核性干酪性肉芽肿)　肉芽肿结节由中心区的干酪样坏死物,浸润的上皮样组织细胞,朗汉斯巨细胞。在结节周边部可有淋巴细胞浸润。

9. 子宫颈息肉　息肉有一个结缔组织构成的完整的蒂,表面覆盖增生的宫颈鳞状上皮。

三、思 考 题

(一)选择题

选一个字母代表的最合适答案。

1. 急性炎症时聚集的液体中含有的蛋白成分超过 3g/dl 而且比重超过 1.015 时,称为:

    A. 水肿   B. 渗出   C. 漏出液   D. 血清   E. 渗出液

2. 哪种类型的细胞能分化为产生免疫球蛋白的细胞,此种细胞形态具有特征性?

    A. 中性粒细胞   B. 嗜碱性细胞   C. B 细胞   D. T 细胞   E. 浆细胞

3. 在进入血管外间隙之前,中性粒细胞和单核细胞与血管内皮黏附,这被称为

    A. 边集   B. 血球渗出   C. 附壁   D. 白细胞游出   E. 凝结

4. 损伤后发生的旺盛的增生和胶原化反应称为

    A. 胼胝   B. 瘢痕   C. 挛缩   D. 瘢痕疙瘩   E. 粘连

5. 具有噬菌作用的细胞包括

    A. 中性粒细胞、巨噬细胞、嗜酸粒细胞   B. 淋巴细胞、肥大细胞

    C. T 细胞、裸细胞   D. 嗜碱性细胞、干细胞

    E. 内皮细胞、浆细胞

6. 白细胞朝靶部位单向移动称为

    A. 血球渗出   B. 趋化现象   C. 调理作用   D. 内吞作用   E. 边集

7. 在炎症组织的活检中发现嗜酸粒细胞和肥大细胞,最可能发生以下哪种免疫反应?

    A. Ⅰ型   B. Ⅱ型   C. Ⅲ型   D. Ⅳ型   E. Ⅴ型

8. 在试验动物中网状内皮组织系统清除血液中黑碳粒子,可见于以下的器官除外

    A. 淋巴结窦   B. 肾小球   C. 肠上皮   D. 肝窦   E. 脾索

9. 下列有关白细胞从炎症区域血管移动的描述中是正确的除外

    A. 白细胞穿过血管内皮细胞之间的间隙   B. 中性粒细胞是首先移出

    C. 白细胞伸出伪足以协助移动   D. 白细胞移动伴有少量液体丢失

    E. 伴有红细胞被动性丢失

10. 炎症反应有以下有利因素除外

    A. 感染组织的分离   B. 致炎因素的失活   C. 中和毒素

    D. 清除失活组织碎片   E. 瘘管形成

给每一题选出最接近的答案。每个选项可选一次,多次或不选。

问题 11~15. 给下列炎症细胞的描述匹配最合适的细胞类型:

    A. 巨噬细胞   B. 肥大细胞   C. 中性粒细胞   D. 嗜酸粒细胞   E. 嗜碱粒细胞

11. 这些细胞首先到达损伤的部位

12. 这些细胞能抑制超敏反应

13. 这些细胞有异染颗粒而且主要见于组织内

14. 这些细胞参与Ⅰ型和Ⅱ型超敏反应

15. 这些细胞对于细胞内或有包囊的微生物特别有效

（二）问答题

1. 什么是炎症？

2. 急性和慢性炎症的病理学区别是什么？

3. 单核细胞、组织细胞和巨噬细胞的关系是什么？

4. 什么是趋化现象？

5. 炎症反应中最重要的化学介质是什么？

6. 哪里可以见到肥大细胞？可通过什么来识别肥大细胞？肥大细胞的功能是什么？

7. 葡萄球菌可以引起哪些皮肤病损？它们有何特点？

8. 什么是卡他性炎？

9. 脓肿与蜂窝织炎如何区别？

10. 什么是假膜性炎？

11. 什么是积脓？引起积脓的原因有哪些？

12. 胸腔积液的病因是什么？

13. 什么是淋巴结反应性增生？

Chapter 4　Inflammation

Gross Findings	Micro Findings
1. Fibrinous pericarditis	1. Inflammatory cells include neutrophils, eosinophils, mo-
2. Diphtheria	noncytes (macrophages), lymphocytes, plasma cells
3. Pseudomembranous inflammation of bowel	2. Fibrinous inflammation (pseudomembranous inflamma-
4. Empyema, Gallbladder	tion) bowel
5. Pyosalpinx, Fallopian tube	3. Empyema, Gallbladder
6. Acute suppurative appendicitis,(Phlegmonous)	4. Pyosalpinx, Fallopian tube
7. Amebiic liver abscess	5. Acute suppurative appendicitis (phlegmonous inflam-
ma-	
8. Suppurative cerebrospinal meningitis	tion of Appendix)
9. Hemorrhagic inflammation of intestine	6. Breast abscess
10. Polyps in the colon	7. Foreign body granulomatous inflammation
11. Cervical polyp	8. Infective granulomatous inflammation (tubercle, caseous
12. Chronic ulcer of stomach	granuloma)
	9. Cervical lopyp

Gross Findings

1. Fibrinous pericarditis　The exudates with rich in fibrin happen in serous membrance(pericarditis).The surfaces of heart appear toweliod, named toweloid heart.

2. Diphtheria　There are false membrane in the surfaces of the pharynx, laryns, trachea, bronchi, that belongs to fibrinous inflammation.

3. Pseudomembranous inflammation of bowel　The exudates are rich in fibrin. In bowel mucous surfaces form the false membrane consisted of necrotic epithelium, neutrophils,bacteria and RBC in the fibrinous meshs.

4. Empyema, Gallbladder　Present of macroscopically identifiable pus in the lumen of the gallbladder.

Wall is thickened and has a rubbery pus accumulates.

5. Pyosalpinx, Fallopian tube　Distention of the tube which is filled with pus.

6. Acute suppurative appendicitis(Phlegmonous)

(1) Brief Descriptions

1) Cause: It is associated with obstruction (fecalith, gallstone, tumor or ball of worms).

2) Abscess formation within the wall and focal suppurative necrosis in the mucosa.

(2) Gross Findings

1) Congested and swollen.

2) Dilated appendix lumen contain pus, or a fecalith, or both.

3) Serosa coated with fibrin, fibrinopurulent exudate, or pus.

7. Amebiic liver abscess   Amebiic liver abscess focal localized in right lobar of liver with thick capsule, it may be exceeding 10cm in diameter and full of chocolate-colored, odorless, pus.

8. Suppurative cerebrospinal meningitis   Suppurative exudates in surface of brain with blood vessels dilatation and congestion.

9. Hemorrhagic inflammation of intestine   The intestinal wall appear dark black color with a large volume of bleeding in the lumen of the intestine.

10. Polyps in the colon   A mass that projects above the mucosal surface with stem occur in colon.

Cause: It is inflammation proliferation or is neoplastic.

11. Cervical polyp   A mass that projects above the mucosal surface with stem occur in cervical.

12. Chronic ulcer of stomach

(1) A defect on the surface of stomach owing to inflammatory necrosis of the mucosa.

(2) The ulcer has destroyed the muscle coats of the stomach. The floor of the ulcer consists of necrotic debris and dense fibrous tissue. The area surrounding the ulcer develops fibrosis, scarring and chronic inflammatory reaction.

Micro Findings

1. Inflammatory cells include neutrophils, eosinophils, mononcytes (macrophages), lymphocytes, plasma cells, which are vary appearance and different functions.

2. Fibrinous inflammation (pseudomembranous inflammation) bowel   Exudative inflammation in mucous surfaces, where contain coagulates, enclosing necrotic epithelium, neutrophils bacteria, form fibrinous meshs.

3. Empyema, Gallbladder

(1) Mucosal ulceration with acute and chronic inflammatory infiltration.

(2) Entrapped bile stones with abscess formation and foreign body type multinucleated giant cells.

4. Pyosalpinx, Fallopian tube

(1) Swelling and edema in the plicae of the tube.

(2) Pus in the lumen. Accumulation of necrotic debris and leukocytes in the lumen and the plicae.

(3) Thickened tubal wall with infiltration of acute and chronic inflammatory cells.

5. Acute suppurative appendicitis (phlegmonous inflammation of Appendix)

(1) Mucosal ulceration and infiltration by PMNs, eosinophils, plasma cells, and lymphocytes throughout all layers and frequently into serosa.

(2) More advanced stage, the inflammatory process involved the full thickness of wall, with partial necrosis or infarction of wall (perforated areas).

6. Breast abscess

(1) A central cavity fill with pus surround with inflamed breast parenchyma.

(2) Inflammatory infiltration with involvement of gland buds and surrounding stroma with residual ducts.

(3) Foamy histiocytes in regional dilated ducts.

7. Foreign body granulomatous inflammation   Foreign bodies, foreign body-type giant cells,

epithelioid histiocytes, lymphocytes, plasma cells,neurophils form granuloma.

8. Infective granulomatous inflammation (tubercle, caseous granuloma)   The nodule is composed of caseous necrotic debris in the center, infiltrated by epithelioid histiocytes and Langhans' giant cells surrounded by lymphocytes at peripheral.

9. Cervical lopyp   It has a pedicle of delicate connective tissue covered with cervical squamous epithelial cells with proliferation.

Study Questions

Choose Tests

Directions: Each of the numbered items or incomplete statements in this section is followed by answers or by completions of the statement. Select the one lettered answer or completion that is best in each case.

1. Fluid that collects during acute inflammation and that has a protein content exceeding 3g/dl and a specific gravity exceeding 1.015 is referred to as
   A. edema   B. an effusion   C. a transudate   D. serum   E. an exudate

2. Which cell type differentiates into morphologically distinct cells capable of immunoglobulin production?
   A. Neutrophils   B. Basophils   C. B cells   D. T cells   E. Plasma cells

3. The adherence of neutrophils and monocytes to the vascular endothelium prior to movement into the extravascular space is called
   A. margination   B. diapedesis   C. pavementing   D. emigration   E. clotting

4. An exuberant, hypertrophic, collagenous reaction that can occur following an injury is referred to as
   A. a callus   B. a cicatrix   C. a contracture   D. a keloid   E. an adhesion

5. Cells that are capable of phagocytosis of particulate matter include
   A. neutrophils, macrophages, eosinophils   B. lymphocytes, mast cells
   C. T cells, null cells   D. basophils, stem cells
   E. endolhelial cells, plasma cells

6. The unidirectional migration of leukocytes toward a target is referred to as
   A. diapedesis   B. chemotaxis   C. opsonization   D. endocytosis   E. margination

7. If eosinophils and mast cells are identified in a tissue biopsy from an inflammatory process, which type of immune reaction is most likely occurring?
   A. Type I   B. Type II   C. Type III   D. Type IV   E. Type V

8. Black carbon particles, cleared from the blood by the reticuloendothelial system of a laboratory animal, can be seen in cells in all of the following organ components EXCEPT
   A. lymph node sinuses   B. glomeruli   C. intestinal epithelium
   D. liver sinuses   E. splenic cords

9. All of the following statements describing leukocyte emigration from vessels in areas of inflammation are true EXCEPT
   A. leukocytes pass through gaps between the vascular endothelial cells
   B. neutrophils are the first cells to emigrate
   C. leukocytes develop pseudopods to aid in emigration

D. a small loss of fluid accompanies leukocyte emigration

E. accompanying loss of red cells is passive

10. The inflammatory response serves all of the following EXCEPT

    A. isolation of infected tissues   B. inactivation of causative agents

    C. neutralization of toxins   D. removal of devitalized tissue debris

    E. fistula formation

Directions: The group of items in this section consists of lettered options followed by a set of numbered items. For each item, select the one lettered option that is most closely associated with it. Each lettered option may be selected once, more than once, or not at all.

Questions 11~15

Match each description of an inflammatory cell to the most appropriate cell type.

    A. Macrophage   B. Mast cell   C. Neutrophil   D. Eosinophil   E. Basophil

11. These cells are the first to arrive at a site of injury

12. These cells can aborthypersensitivity reactions

13. These cells have metachromatic granules and are found mainly in the tissues

14. These cells are involved in both type Ⅰ and type Ⅱ hypersensitivity reactions

15. These cells are particularly effective against intracellular or encapsulated microbes

Questions

1. What is inflammation?

2. What are the pathological differences between acute and chronic inflammation?

3. What is the relationship between monocytes, histiocytes and macrophages?

4. What is chemotaxis?

5. What are the more important chemical mediators of the inflammatory response?

6. Where are mast cells found? What features make them recognizable and what function do they serve?

7. What skin lesions can be caused by staphylococci? Differentiate them.

8. What is catarrh?

9. How to distinguish between abscess and cellulites?

10. What is pseudomembrauous inflammtion?

11. What is an empyema and what can cause it?

12. What are the causes of pleural effusions?

13. What is meant by reactive hyperplasia of a lymph node?

第五章 肿 瘤

大体观察

1. 结肠管状绒毛腺瘤
2. 皮肤乳头状瘤
3. 甲状腺腺瘤
4. 卵巢囊腺瘤
5. 软组织脂肪瘤
6. 软组织神经鞘瘤(施万细胞瘤)
7. 子宫多发性平滑肌瘤
8. 乳腺纤维腺瘤
9. 皮肤海绵状血管瘤
10. 软骨瘤
11. 皮肤鳞状细胞癌
12. 食管鳞状细胞癌
13. 胃印戒细胞癌
14. 卵巢畸胎瘤(卵巢皮样囊肿)
15. 肝脏转移性黑色素瘤
16. 软组织脂肪肉瘤
17. 软组织平滑肌肉瘤
18. 软组织横纹肌肉瘤
19. 皮肤恶性黑色素瘤
20. 皮内痣
21. 淋巴瘤

镜下观察

1. 结肠管状绒毛状腺瘤
2. 皮肤海绵状血管瘤
3. 软组织神经鞘瘤
4. 唾液腺多形性腺瘤(混合瘤)
5. 腱鞘巨细胞瘤
6. 卵巢畸胎瘤(卵巢皮样囊肿)
7. 胃腺癌伴淋巴结转移
8. 肝转移性恶性黑色素瘤
9. 皮肤上皮内瘤变(Bowen病)
10. 皮肤鳞状细胞癌
11. 乳腺纤维腺瘤
12. 结肠脂肪瘤
13. 软组织脂肪肉瘤
14. 子宫体平滑肌瘤
15. 软组织平滑肌肉瘤
16. 软组织横纹肌肉瘤
17. 皮内痣
18. 皮肤恶性黑色素瘤

一、大 体 观 察

1. 结肠管状绒毛腺瘤

(1) 简要说明:结肠腺瘤在40岁前的发病率大约为20%~30%,而在60岁之后增至40%到50%。

(2) 大体所见:病理变化从有蒂的小瘤体到无蒂的大肿瘤。

2. 皮肤乳头状瘤 境界清楚的乳头状生长的瘤体,不浸润到其周围组织。

3. 甲状腺腺瘤

(1) 女性好发。

(2) 完全由纤维囊包裹的局限的瘤结节。

4. 卵巢囊腺瘤　肿瘤呈多囊状,囊内含有大量的浆液。

5. 软组织脂肪瘤

(1) 软组织脂肪瘤:外观上为淡黄色,圆形,有包膜,在深层结构中也可能有浸润。

(2) 与其他成分结合:例如,血管脂肪瘤,纤维脂肪瘤,血管肌脂肪瘤,黏液脂肪瘤。

6. 软组织神经鞘瘤(施万细胞瘤)

(1) 简要说明

1) 起源于神经嵴来源的雪旺细胞,并与Ⅱ型神经纤维瘤病相关。

2) 临床症状与相关神经的局部压迫有关。

(2) 大体所见:有包膜的肿块,周围神经中的起源于神经的纤维状细胞沿包膜生长,不发生浸润。

7. 子宫多发性平滑肌瘤

(1) 简要说明

1) 女性最常见的肿瘤。

2) 肿瘤为雌激素敏感性;在去势或绝经后可使肿瘤萎缩甚至钙化,而在妊娠期肿瘤体积可迅速增大。

3) 病因:不明

(2) 大体所见:孤立性或多发性,境界清楚,质硬,灰白色,切面可呈漩涡状。

8. 乳腺纤维腺瘤

(1) 简要说明

1) 女性乳腺最常见的良性肿瘤。

2) 多发,双侧,多见于乳腺的外上象限。

3) 肿瘤由纤维组织和腺体组织所构成。

(2) 大体所见

1) 肿瘤结节生长呈球形,境界清楚,可活动。

2) 肿瘤直径大小可从小于1cm到大到10~15cm。

9. 皮肤海绵状血管瘤

(1) 简要说明

1) 正常或异常血管数量增多。

2) 以婴幼儿好发,可自发消退。

(2) 大体所见:红色-蓝色,质地软,海绵状肿块。

10. 软骨瘤　肿瘤向骨表面凸出,有包膜,或囊性变(内含有淡蓝色黏蛋白),或玻璃样透明外观,形似正常的软骨组织。

11. 皮肤鳞状细胞癌

(1) 简要说明

1) 好发于暴露在阳光的皮肤。

2) 危险因素:阳光,工业致癌物(油烟),慢性溃疡,骨髓炎引流,陈旧性瘢痕,砷的吸入,电离辐射,(口腔)烟草,咀嚼槟榔。

(2) 大体所见:浅的溃疡周围有范围较广的,质地硬的边缘,偶尔呈现为真菌样疣状隆起而无溃疡形成。

12. 食管鳞状细胞癌　癌症早期,肿瘤表现为隆起,质地坚硬,串珠状改变,或者表现为黏膜增厚,不规则粗糙不平,乳头状。随着病变的扩大,肿瘤将形成向食管腔内突出的肿块,中心可发生坏死,边缘隆起外翻,质地坚硬。

13. 胃印戒细胞癌

(1) 简要说明:世界卫生组织分类标准将胃癌分为五个亚型:乳头状癌,管状癌,黏液癌,印戒细胞腺癌以及未分化癌。

(2) 大体所见:胃壁增厚变硬,伴或不伴有黏膜溃疡的形成。

14. 卵巢畸胎瘤(卵巢皮样囊肿)

(1) 简要说明

1) 良性囊性畸胎瘤(皮样囊肿)是最常见的卵巢肿瘤,占所有卵巢肿瘤的 25% 以上。

2) 肿瘤由各种成熟组织构成,这些组织起源于一种或一种以上的胚胎生殖细胞层,包括:外胚层,中胚层和内胚层。

3) 分类:成熟畸胎瘤(良性),不成熟畸胎瘤(恶性),单胚层畸胎瘤或高分化畸胎瘤。

(2) 大体所见

1) 囊性肿块内含有稠厚的皮脂样物质和毛发。

2) 囊壁内面光滑,但在一侧常有一个融合的瘤样结节性突起(头嵴)。

3) 突起区域可见软骨、骨,以及成形的牙齿组织。

15. 肝脏转移性黑色素瘤

(1) 肝脏表面可见不对称分布,不规则的色素瘤,瘤体边界不清。

(2) 癌性结节位于肝脏表面,可伴有坏死性缺损(癌脐)。

16. 软组织脂肪肉瘤

(1) 简要说明

1) 成人最常见的软组织肉瘤。

2) 发病高峰见于 40 至 60 岁人群,好发部位位于四肢远端(大腿)及后腹膜腔。

(2) 大体所见:常有完整的包膜,分叶状,并有卫星结节。

17. 软组织平滑肌肉瘤

(1) 简要说明:好发人群为成人,女性多见(发病率 64%),发病部位为下肢,皮下。

(2) 大体所见:境界清楚的肿块(显微镜下有浸润),肿瘤体积大,因伴有出血坏死质地软,有囊性变。

18. 软组织横纹肌肉瘤

(1) 简要说明

1) 最常见的儿童软组织肉瘤。

2) 该病以婴儿及儿童多见,而在 40 岁以上的成人少见。

3) 以头颈部,生殖泌尿道,后腹膜腔及四肢多见。

(2) 大体所见:多结节或息肉状,肿瘤表面凝胶样,颜色灰白。

19. 皮肤恶性黑色素瘤

(1) 简要说明:起源于色素神经上皮层,或葡萄膜色素上皮细胞。

1）病因：日光照射，轻微的色素沉着，原发痣。

2）肿瘤增大，有瘙痒感或疼痛，皮肤新的病灶，边界不规则，颜色呈花斑样。

3）呈放射性和垂直生长。

（2）大体所见：皮肤瘙痒，斑驳，不规则，呈斑丘疹样病灶。

20．皮内痣

（1）简要说明：先天性或获得性。

（2）大体所见：黑褐色，或者比周围正常皮肤颜色稍深，色素均一，为小的扁平的实质性损伤，或隆起于皮肤表面，有或无汗毛。

21．淋巴瘤　淋巴结肿块，切面呈均质，质硬。

二、镜下观察

1．结肠管状绒毛状腺瘤　腺瘤样息肉依据其上皮结构可以分为三种亚型：①管状腺瘤：超过 75% 的上皮呈管型结构；②绒毛状腺瘤：超过 50% 的上皮呈绒毛状结构；③管状绒毛状腺瘤：上皮 25% 至 50% 呈绒毛样结构。

（1）肿瘤（腺瘤）上皮：核增大，核染色深，细胞增大，有核分裂象；细胞不同程度的不典型增生。

（2）管状腺瘤：腺瘤上皮增生形成多个小管（管与管之间被正常固有膜分隔），规则的小管排列成分支状或簇状。

（3）绒毛状腺瘤：呈指状或绒毛状生长，从黏膜肌层向腺瘤顶端垂直生长。

其他描述：

（1）所有的腺瘤样病变都是上皮异常增生的结果，病变程度有轻有重（比如原位癌）。

（2）有证据表明腺瘤是侵袭性结、直肠腺癌的癌前病变。

2．皮肤海绵状血管瘤　病变呈暗红色，楔形。主要由扩张的静脉腔伴有增厚的纤维血管壁构成。有可能是发育中错构瘤性的。

3．软组织神经鞘瘤

（1）束状型区域：细胞呈梭形，胞浆界限不清，细胞排列成相互交叉的条索状结构。

（2）Verocay 小体：细胞核围绕着一片酸性染色的区域排列成栅栏状，而这些酸性染色区域为纤维性胞质向外伸出的位点（类似触觉小体）。

（3）网状型区域：大量水肿样基质伴微囊形成，细胞排列疏松。

（4）肿瘤细胞排列成漩涡状。

其他描述：为良性肿瘤，好发于四肢屈侧，纵隔，颈部，腹膜后腔，脊神经根后角及小脑桥脑角。

4．唾液腺多形性腺瘤（混合瘤）　是最常见的肿瘤，占腮腺肿瘤的 60% ~ 70%，而在其他唾液腺肿瘤中占 40% ~ 70%。

（1）由于肿瘤起源为上皮和间质的混合成分，因此肿瘤呈双向性。

（2）上皮成分

1）腺体（导管）表现鳞状上皮化生。

2）导管内的内层细胞呈扁平或柱状。

3) 导管的外层肌上皮细胞形态可为立方形,扁平形,透明梭形或呈玻璃样外观。有时细胞可增生形成较厚的,境界不清的导管周围鞘,或细胞肿胀水肿形成软骨样的细胞(软骨样改变)。

4) 腺腔内含有透明或伊红染的液体。

(3) 间质:呈非特异性纤维黏液样外观,有大量黏液性变性,并伴有软骨,黏液软骨和钙化。

其他描述:

(1) 是唾液腺尤其是腮腺最常见的肿瘤,生长缓慢。

(2) 增殖的肌上皮细胞呈多形性。

(3) 一些瘤组织类似上皮成分而另外一些类似间质成分(如软骨)。

5. 腱鞘巨细胞瘤　肿瘤由不同比例的单核细胞,类似破骨细胞的多核巨细胞以及大量的间质构成。

6. 卵巢畸胎瘤(卵巢皮样囊肿)　囊性肿块含有不同来源的组织成分。

(1) 皮肤成分(皮肤附属器,例如毛囊,皮脂腺)。

(2) 内胚层来源的组织成分(呼吸道上皮和胃肠道上皮)。

(3) 中胚层来源的组织成分(肌肉,脂肪,软骨)。

(4) 神经胶质成分。

(5) 卵巢皮样囊肿内的成分:可见有皮脂腺,脂肪组织,上皮成分,软骨组织。并可见纤毛上皮。

其他描述:占卵巢肿瘤的 15% ,10% 为双侧性。

7. 胃腺癌伴淋巴结转移　淋巴结内肿瘤细胞的增生导致淋巴结肿大,瘤细胞栓子首先进入淋巴结被膜下窦,随后进入淋巴结周窦,最后浸润整个淋巴结。

8. 肝转移性恶性黑色素瘤　大而不典型的黑色素细胞呈不对称地增殖,肿瘤境界不清。

9. 皮肤上皮内瘤变(Bowen 病)

(1) 表皮层增厚。

(2) 表皮和真皮之间的分界明显。

(3) 整个表皮层,细胞排列紊乱,大量细胞表现为异形性,核大深染。

(4) 在表皮层,有一些分散的细胞表现为不典型的细胞角化(角化不良症)。

(5) 皮肤角质层通常增厚,由大量的角化不全细胞构成,这些细胞具有异形性,核深染。

10. 皮肤鳞状细胞癌

(1) 上皮细胞增生并向真皮层内浸润形成不规则肿块。

(2) 肿瘤结节由不同比例的异形性鳞状细胞构成。

(3) 肿瘤的异形性:细胞大小及形态不一,细胞异常增生,核深染,细胞间桥消失,出现病理性核分裂,细胞角化不良。

(4) 角化不良细胞:个别细胞角化,伴大而圆,胞浆深伊红染色,核深染。

(5) 分化较好的肿瘤细胞有细胞间桥,有角化珠的形成,并有大量部分角化的细胞。

(6) 角化珠:形成一个由鳞状上皮构成的圆形癌巢,其中肿瘤细胞围绕无细胞的角蛋白呈同心圆状排列。

11. 乳腺纤维腺瘤

（1）由纤维包膜包裹的境界清楚的肿瘤结节。

（2）乳腺导管及导管周围的结缔组织增生。其生长方式：

1）管周型：圆形或椭圆形导管。

2）管内型：裂隙状导管。

（3）结缔组织：纤维黏液瘤样基质。

12. 结肠脂肪瘤　瘤组织由成熟的脂肪细胞构成，瘤细胞无异型性。

13. 软组织脂肪肉瘤

（1）五个基本的组织学分类：黏液样脂肪肉瘤，圆形细胞脂肪肉瘤，高分化脂肪肉瘤（包括不典型脂肪瘤），去分化性脂肪肉瘤，多型性脂肪肉瘤。

（2）肿瘤细胞重度异型性，有不同分化程度的脂母细胞及异型的多核瘤巨细胞。核分裂多见。

（3）脂母细胞：核深染，核呈圆齿状，有明显的核仁，胞浆内有含量不等的脂质。

14. 子宫体平滑肌瘤

（1）平滑肌细胞梭形，均匀增生，细胞核呈雪茄烟形状，两端钝圆。

（2）有时可见细胞异型性，尤其是在发生透明变性的区域。

（3）肿瘤可出现红色变性（渐进性坏死），囊变性，透明变性和钙化。

15. 软组织平滑肌肉瘤

（1）恶性的梭形瘤细胞：细胞胞体拉长，核两端钝圆，胞浆嗜酸纤维样。这些钝圆核的梭形瘤细胞有着较高的核分裂活性（>20/50HPF）。

（2）瘤细胞增殖相互交织成束状，核排列成栅栏状。核表现出异型性，核大，核染色质致密。一些圆形的瘤细胞在核周有透明空晕。

16. 软组织横纹肌肉瘤

（1）有四种组织学分型：胚胎性横纹肌肉瘤；葡萄状横纹肌肉瘤（为胚胎性横纹肌肉瘤的变异体）；腺泡型横纹肌肉瘤；多型性横纹肌肉瘤。

（2）肿瘤由大量的圆形或梭形的恶性瘤细胞构成，细胞分布在肿瘤组织黏液样间质中。

（3）横纹肌母细胞体积大，圆形，有大量的深嗜酸性染色胞浆。

17. 皮内痣

（1）真皮层内的痣细胞排列成巢状或束状，其上方的表皮层较薄。

（2）痣细胞。

立方形细胞，细胞核呈规则球形，核染色质密度适中。

1）大细胞型（A型）：可见一些多核的巨黑色素细胞。

2）中间型：小细胞（B型）：似淋巴细胞。

3）梭形细胞（C型）：细胞位于神经束内（推测由施万细胞衍变而来）。

（3）无细胞异型性，交界处无活跃的现象。

（4）交界处活跃：黑色素细胞局限在表皮基底部增殖或垂直于基底部。

其他描述：

（1）黑色素细胞：是神经外胚层来源的细胞，位于皮肤的基底层，皮肤附属器及黏膜内。

（2）能够产生黑色素并通过细胞突起转运至邻近的上皮细胞。

（3）染色：银染，DOPA 染色，S-100 免疫组化染色，弹性蛋白染色。

（4）可以通过高锰酸钾将黑色素去除。

18. 皮肤恶性黑色素瘤

1）黑色素瘤细胞是一些形态奇异的细胞,细胞境界不清,细胞大小和形态不一,有梭形细胞,长形细胞,及黏合细胞,(从界限清楚到界限不清)。胞浆丰富,高染色质性核不规则,有明显的嗜酸染色的核仁。可见多核瘤巨细胞。核分裂多见。

2）瘤细胞成疏松的巢状生长,缺少典型的分化成熟特征。

三、思 考 题

（一）选择题

选一个字母代表的最合适答案。

1. 一名妇女胸膜腔渗出液的细胞学检查有不明来源恶性细胞,其细胞最可能表现为源于以下哪种恶性肿瘤?

    A. 淋巴瘤   B. 间皮瘤   C. 乳癌   D. 肺癌   E. 平滑肌肉瘤

2. 恶性细胞的细胞学异常表现的最佳描述为

    A. 染色体异常   B. 黏液过多   C. 细胞表面改变

    D. 细胞糖原减少   E. 有丝分裂活跃

3. 组织学上的良性肿瘤危及生命时,最可能的原因

    A. 由于广泛出血   B. 多灶性病变   C. 没有引发免疫应答

    D. 妨碍了器官的功能   E. 转变为癌

4. 流行病学揭示了癌和以下因素的关系,除了

    A. 老龄   B. 非遗传性染色体异常   C. 空气污染

    D. 细菌感染   E. 饮食

5. 下列情况可使组织肿块增大,除了

    A. 肥大   B. 炎症   C. 肿瘤   D. 增生   E. 间变

6. 以下肿瘤及其成因匹配都正确,除了

    A. 肝血管肉瘤——砷元素   B. 子宫内膜癌——外源性雌激素

    C. 阴道癌——己烯雌酚   D. 间皮瘤——铍元素

7. 下列关于唾液腺的良性混合性肿瘤的说法都是正确的,除了

    A. 常发生在腮腺   B. 它是快速生长的无症状的肿块

    C. 不浸润皮肤或神经   D. 是常见的唾液腺肿瘤

8. 什么是原发性的恶性黑色素瘤的预后因素

    A. 侵袭的深度   B. 恶性细胞的大小   C. 多核巨细胞的数量

    D. 周围炎症的程度   E. 产生黑色素的多少

9. 皮肤和皮下的软组织病变可包括以下各种,除了

    A. 在躯干的脂肪肉瘤   B. 在手背的上皮性肉瘤

    C. 年长病人头部的血管肉瘤   D. 在颈部的非典型纤维黄色瘤

E. 一个红紫的结节与艾滋病相关的病变

10. 一个 50 岁的老年人在大腿上长了个 10cm 的肿块,下面各项可以解释这个肿块,除了
    A. 肿块可能是恶性纤维组织细胞瘤(MFH)   B. 肿瘤可能已经生长了三个月
    C. 肿瘤可能是良性的   D. 肿瘤可能是反应性的病变
    E. 肿瘤可能钙化

给每一题选出最接近的答案。每个选项可选一次,多次或不选。

11~14. 把以下诊断癌的技术和相应的选项匹配起来
    A. 电子显微镜   B. 免疫组化   C. 两者都是   D. 两者都不是

11. 鉴别前列腺癌和胃癌

12. 鉴别淋巴瘤和癌

13. 鉴别腺癌和间皮瘤

14. 给鳞癌的原发部位定位

问题 15~18 把下列各项和相关类型的癌匹配起来
    A. 恶性淋巴瘤   B. 白血病   C. 宫颈癌   D. 血肿

15. Down 综合征

16. 硬化

17. 人乳头状瘤病毒感染

18. 原发免疫缺陷

问题 19~23 某些癌基因对人类肿瘤有诊断意义,将下列癌基因与其最有关联的肿瘤匹配起来。
    A. 神经母细胞瘤   B. 肺腺癌   C. 乳癌
    D. 伯基特淋巴瘤   E. 视网膜母细胞瘤

19. Ras

20. N-myc

21. RB

22. C-myc

23. C-erb-B$_2$

(二) 问答题

1. 增生和瘤形成的主要区别是什么?

2. 什么是不典型增生? 什么是上皮内瘤变,两者的关系如何?

3. 什么是错构瘤?

4. 肿瘤的含义是什么?

5. 常见致瘤因素有哪些? 会产生哪些肿瘤?

6. 什么是原位癌?

7. 什么是脱落细胞学(细胞病理学)? 其临床应用有哪些?

8. 恶性肿瘤是怎样扩散的?

9. "胚胎性肿瘤"是什么? 好发于什么部位?

10. 生殖细胞会产生哪种肿瘤？

11. 畸胎瘤的特征是什么？

12. 什么是副肿瘤综合征？

13. 什么是 Krukenberg 瘤？

14. 哪种睾丸肿瘤与肿瘤标记物相关？

15. 第一个被描述的职业因素引起的恶性肿瘤是什么？

16. 什么是黏膜白斑病？

17. 良恶性肿瘤的鉴别。

18. 癌和肉瘤的鉴别。

19. 什么是癌前病变？常见的癌前病变有哪些？

Chapter 5   Tumor

Gross Findings	Micro Findings
1. Tubulovillous adenoma, Colon	1. Tubulovillous adenoma
2. Papilloma of skin	2. Hemangioma cavernous
3. Thyroid adenoma	3. Neurilemmoma
4. Cystadenoma of ovary	4. Pleomorphic adenoma (mixed tumor)
5. Lipoma, Soft tissue	5. Giant cell tumor of tendon sheath
6. Neurilemmoma (Schwannoma), Soft tissue	6. Teratoma (Dermoid cyst)
7. Multi leiomyoma, Uterine corpus	7. Gastric adenocarcinoma with metastasis of lymphnode
8. Fibroadenoma, Breas	8. Metastatic melanoma
9. Hemangioma cavernous, Skin	9. Intraepithelum neoplasm Skin(Bowen's disease)
10. Chondroma	10. Squamous cell carcinoma
11. Squamous cell carcinoma, Skin	11. Fibroadenoma
12. Esophageal squamous cell carcinoma	12. Lipoma
13. Signet ring cell carcinoma, Stomach	13. Liposarcoma
14. Teratoma (Dermoid cyst), Ovary	14. Leiomyoma
15. Metastatic melanoma, Liver	15. Leiomyosarcoma
16. Liposarcoma, Soft tissue	16. Rhabdomyosarcoma
17. Leiomyosarcoma, Soft tissue	17. Intradermal nevus
18. Rhabdomyosarcoma, Soft tissue	18. Malignant melanoma
19. Malignant melanoma	
20. Intradermal nevus	
21. lymphoma	

Gross Findings

1. Tubulovillous adenoma, Colon

(1) Brief Descriptions: The prevalence of colonic adenomas is about 20% to 30% before age of 40, arising to 40% to 50% after age of 60.

(2) Gross Findings: Range from small, pedunculated lesions to large neoplasm that are usually sessil.

2. Papilloma of skin   Well-circumscribed masses with papillary growth pattern and without infiltrating the surround tissue.

3. Thyroid adenoma

(1) Predilection for females.

(2) Well-circumscribed nodular mass completely enclosed in a fibrous capsule.

4. Cystadenoma of ovary   Tumor appear multifoci cysts with a large volume of serous in the cysts.

5. Lipoma, Soft tissue

（1）Lipoma of soft tissue: appear bright yellow, round, encapsulated, but maybe a infiltrated pattern in deeper structure.

（2）Combined with other components. Example: angiolipoma, fibrolipoma, angiomyolipoma, myxolipoma.

6. Neurilemmoma（Schwannoma）, Soft tissue

（1）Brief Descriptions

1）Arise from the neural crest-derived Schwann cell and are associated with neurofibromatosis type 2.

2）Symptoms are referable to local compression of the involved nerve.

（2）Gross Findings：Encapsulated mass, with flattened original nerve grow in the periphery nerve along the capsule, not penetrating.

7. Multi leiomyoma, Uterine corpus

（1）Brief Descriptions

1）The most common tumors in women.

2）Estrogen responsive：they regress or even calcify after castration or menopause and may undergo rapid increase in size during pregnancy.

3）Cause: unknown.

（2）Gross Findings：Solitary or multiple circumscribed, firm, grayish-white, whirled appearance in cut surface.

8. Fibroadenoma, Breas

（1）Brief Descriptions

1）Most common benign tumor of the female breast.

2）Frequently multiple and bilateral and occur in the upper outer quadrant.

3）A new growth compose of both fibrous and glandular tissue.

（2）Gross Findings

1）Grow as a spherical nodule which is usually well-circumscribed and freely movable.

2）Vary in size from less than 1cm to giant forms 10~15cm in diameter.

9. Hemangioma cavernous, Skin

（1）Brief Descriptions

1）Increased number of normal or abnormal vessels.

2）Infancy and childhood, regress spontaneously.

（2）Gross Findings：Red-blue, soft, spongy mass.

10. Chondroma　Tumor project from bone surfaces with encapsulated, or cyst change with bright blue muscin, or hyaline appearance, there is alike normal cartilage.

11. Squamous cell carcinoma, Skin

（1）Brief Descriptions

1）Most often occurs on sun-exposed skin.

2）Risk factors: sunlight, industrial carcinogen（tars and oils）,chronic ulcers and draining osteomyelitis,old burn scars, ingestion of arsenicals, ionizing radiation, and（in the oral cavity）tobacco and betel nut chewing.

（2）Gross Findings：A shallow ulcer surrounded by a wide, elevated indurated border, occasionally raised, fungoid, verrucous lesions without ulceration.

12. Esophageal squamous cell carcinoma In the early stage, cancer may appear as raised, firm, pearly plaques or as irregular roughened or verrucous areas of mucosal thickening.

As the lesion enlarge, they may create a protruding masses or undergo central necrosis, rimmed by elevated, firm, and so on.

13. Signet ring cell carcinoma, Stomach

(1) Brief Descriptions: The World Health Organization classification subdivides gastric carcinoma into five subtype : papillary,tubular, mucinous, and signet-ring cell adenocarcinomas and undifferentiated carcinoma.

(2) Gross Findings: Thickened and rigid of gastric walls, with or without mucosal ulceration.

14. Teratoma (Dermoid cyst), Ovary

(1) Brief Descriptions

1) Benign cystic teratoma (dermoid cyst) is the most common ovarian neoplasm, comprising up to 25% or more of all ovarian tumors.

2) Contain various mature tissues derived from one or more of the embryonic germ layers : the ectoderm, mesoderm, and endoderm.

3) Categories:mature(benign), immature(malignant), monodermal or highly specialized.

(2) Gross Findings

1) Cystic mass containing thick sebaceous material and hairs.

2) The internal lining is smooth but frequently has a knob-like nodular protrusion in one.

3) Area (the "umbo"), in which cartilage, bone, and well-formed teeth may be present.

15. Metastatic melanoma, Liver

(1) Asymmetric irregularly pigmented lesions with ill-defined margins in the liver.

(2) Carcinoma nodular located surfaces of liver appearing necrosis remained defect.

16. Liposarcoma, Soft tissue

(1) Brief Descriptions

1) One of the most common soft tissue sarcoma of adulthood.

2) A peak incidence between 40~60 years, with two major sites in the extremities (thigh) and the retroperitoneum.

(2) Gross Findings: Tend to be well circumscribed or encapsulated with a lobulated pattern and satellite nodules.

17. Leiomyosarcoma, Soft tissue

(1) Brief Descriptions: Adult, female (64%), lower extremity, subcutaneous.

(2) Gross Findings: Well-circumscribed (infiltrate microscopically), larger, softer with necrosis, hemorrhage, and cystic degeneration.

18. Rhabdomyosarcoma, Soft tissue

(1) Brief Descriptions

1) The most common soft tissue sarcoma of children.

2) Predominantly in infants and children, and rare in patient older than 40 years.

3) Predominant in the head and neck, genitourinary tract and retroperitoneum, and the extremities.

(2) Gross Findings: Multi-nodular, or polypoid with a glistening, gelatinous, gray-white surface.

19. Malignant melanoma, Skin

(1) Brief Descriptions: Arising from pigmented neuroepithelia or uveal melanocytes.

1) Sunlight, lightly pigmented, preexisting nevus.

2) Enlargement, itching or pain, a new lesion, irregular border, variegation of color.

3) Radial and vertical growth.

(2) Gross Findings: Pruritic, variegated, irregular, maculopapular lesions.

20. Intradermal nevus

(1) Brief Descriptions: Congenital or acquired.

(2) Gross Findings: Tan to brown, or little darker than surrounding skin, uniformly pigmented, small solid lesion of flat to elevated skin, with or without hairs.

21. lymphoma   Lymphadenopathy, the cut surfaces appear uniformly bland with firm.

Micro Findings

1. Tubulovillous adenoma   Adeomatous polyps are segregated into 3 subtypes on the basis of epithelial architecture. ① Tubular adenoma: exhibit greater than 75% tubular architecture. ②Villous adenoma: contain greater than 50% villous architecture. ③Tubulovillous adenoma: contain 25% ~ 50% villous architecture.

(1) Neoplastic (adenomatous) epithelium: enlarged nuclei, hyperchromatic and elongated in shape; stratification of nuclei; varies degree of dysplasia.

(2) Tubular adenoma: proliferation of adenomatous epithelium, that forms tubules (separated from each other by normal lamina propria), regular tubules with little branching or tufting.

(3) Villous adenoma: growth of fine fingerlets or villi that project perpendicularly from the muscularis mucosa to the outer tip of the adenoma.

Others:

(1) All adenomatous lesions arise as the result of epithelial proliferative dysplasia, which may range from mild to severe (as carcinoma in situ).

(2) There is strong evidence that adenoma are precursor lesion for invasive colorectal adenocarcinoma.

2. Hemangioma cavernous   This is a dark red wedge shaped lesion. It consists of large venous channels with thick fibous walls and is probably hamartomatous in nature.

3. Neurilemmoma

(1) Antoni A areas: cellular spindle cells with indistinct cytoplasm which are arranged in intersecting bundles.

(2) Verocay's body: nuclei arranged in palisades around eosinophilic areas towards which the fibrillar cytoplasmic processes are oriented (like tactile corpuscles).

(3) Antoni B areas: abundant edematous stroma with microcystic formation and loosely distributed cells.

(4) Tumor cells in wavy pattern.

Others: Benign, common in flexor surface of extremity, mediastinum, neck, retroperitoneum, posterior spinal roots, and cerebello-pontine angle.

4. Pleomorphic adenoma (mixed tumor)   The most common tumor, according for 60% ~ 70% of all parotid tumors and for 40% ~ 70% of tumors in other glands.

(1) Biphasic appearance resulting from the admixture or epithelial and stroma.

(2) Epithelial component

1) Glandular (ductal) with foci of squamous metaplasia.

2) Inner ductal lining cells from flatten to columnar.

3) Outer myoepithelial cells from cuboidal, flattened, clear spindle shaped or hyaline, sometimes proliferated to form thick, ill-defined sheaths around ducts, or become swollen and hydropic to cartilage-like cells (chondroid change).

4) Lumen may contain clear to eosinophilic fluid.

(3) Stroma: Nonspecific fibromyxoid appearance with abundant myxoid change areas, with clear-cut cartilaginous, myxochondroid, or calcification.

Others:

1) Most common neoplasm of the salivary glands especially parotid gland, with slow growth.

2) Proliferation of myoepithelial cells with pleomorphic appearance.

3) Some mimic epithelial component while others mimic stroma component (cartilage).

5. Giant cell tumor of tendon sheath　Variable proportion of mononuclear cells, multinucleated giant cells resembling osteoclasts and the amount of stroma.

6. Teratoma (Dermoid cyst)　Cystic mass containing heterogeneous component

(1) Skin element (dermal appendages, e.g. Hair follicles, sebaceous glands).

(2) Endodermal element (respiratory and gastrointestinal epithelia).

(3) Mesodermal element (muscle, fat, cartilage).

(4) Glial element.

(5) Dermoid component seen sebaceous gland, adipose tissue, epithelial component, and cartilage are seen in this view Ciliated epithelium.

Others: Account for 15% of ovarian neoplasm, 10% bilateral.

7. Gastric adenocarcinoma with metastasis of lymphnode　Lymph nodes enlarged results from the growth of tumor cells in nodes, tumor emboli lodge in the subcapsular space or peripheral sinus, eventually infiltrate overwhelm the node.

8. Metastatic melanoma　Poorly circumscribed asymmetric proliferation of large atypical melanocytes.

9. Intraepithelum neoplasm Skin(Bowen's disease)

(1) The epidermis is thickened.

(2) The border between the epidermis and dermis appears sharp.

(3) Throughout the epidermis, cells lie in complete disorder, and many of them appear atypical, showing large, hyperchromatic nuclei.

(4) In the epidermis there are scattered cells showing atypical individual cells' keratinization (dyskeratosis).

(5) The horny layer usually is thickened and consists largely of parakeratotic cells with atypical, hyperchromatic nuclei.

10. Squamous cell carcinoma

(1) Irregular masses of epithelial cells proliferate downward into the dermis.

(2) Individual tumor masses composed in varying proportion of atypical squamous cells.

(3) Atypia: varying size and shape, hyperplasia, hyperchromatism, absence of intercellular bridge, presence of atypical mitosis and dyskeratotic cells.

(4) Dyskeratotic cells: individual cell keratinization with large, round and deep eosinophilic

cytoplasm and hyperchromatic nuclei.

(5) Well differentiated cells with intercellular bridge and keratin pearl formation and sheets of partially keratinized cells.

(6) Keratin pearl: a rounded nest of squamous epithelium in which the cells are arranged in concentric circles surrounding a central focus of acellular keratin.

11. Fibroadenoma

(1) A well circumscribed nodule with fibrous capsule.

(2) Proliferation of both duct and periductal connective tissue. Growth pattern: ①Pericanalicular pattern: round or oval duct. ②Intracanalicular pattern: slit-like duct.

(3) Connective tissue: fibromyxomatous stroma.

12. Lipoma   Mature adipose tissue (univacuolar mature adipocytes) with no cellular atypia.

13. Liposarcoma

(1) Five basic histological categories: Myxoid liposarcoma; Round cell liposarcoma; Well-differentiated liposarcoma (including atypical lipoma); Dedifferentiated liposarcoma; Pleomorphic liposarcoma.

(2) An extreme degree of cellular pleomorphism with different differentiated stages of lipoblasts and some bizarre multinucleated tumor giant cells. Mitosis is easily seen.

(3) Lipoblast: hyperchromatic, scalloped nuclei with prominent nucleoli and different content of intracellular lipid material.

14. Leiomyoma

(1) Uniform proliferation of spindle-shaped smooth muscle cells with bilateral blunt and (cigar-shaped) nuclei Tumor is composed of spindle-shaped cells in whorl pattern.

(2) Cytological atypia is sometimes present, particularly in areas of hyalinization.

(3) Degenerative change red degeneration (necrobiosis), Cystic degeneration, Hyalinization,Calcification.

15. Leiomyosarcoma

(1) Malignant spindle cells: elongated, blunt-ended nuclei and acidophilic, fibrillary cytoplasm. Spindle cells with elongated blunt-end nucle with high mitotic activity(>20/50 HPF).

(2) Growth in interlacing cords, with palisading of nuclei. Nuclear atypia, large bizarre nuclei or pyknotosis.Some round cells with clear space surrounding nucleus.

16. Rhabdomyosarcoma

(1) Four histological categories:Embryonal rhabdomyosarcoma; Botryoid rhabdomyosarcoma (variant of embryonal type);Alveolar rhabdomyosarcoma; Pleomorphic rhabdomyosarcoma.

(2) Consist of sheets of both malignant round and spindle cells in a variably myxoid stroma.

(3) The rhabdomyoblasts are large and round and have abundant eosinophilic cytoplasm.

17. Intradermal nevus

(1) Small nests or bundles of nevus cells in dermis with thinned overlying epidermis.

(2) Nevus cells.

Cuboidal cells with regular, spheroid, moderately hyperchromatic nuclei.

1) larger cells (type A) with some multinucleated giant melanocytes.

2) Middle: smaller cells (type B) like lymphocytes.

3) Spindle shaped (type C) in neuroid bundles (presumed schwannian derivation).

(3) No cellular atypia nor junctional activity.

（4）Junctional activity: melanocytes proliferation or dropping off restricted to basal portion.

Others：

（1）Melanocytes: Neuroectodermal derived cells, located in the basal layer of skin, skin adnexae, and mucosal membranes.

（2）Produce melanin and transfer through cytocrinia to adjacent epithelial cells.

（3）Stains: silver, DOPA, S-100, vimentin.

（4）Remove melanin pigments by potassium permanganate.

18. Malignant melanoma

（1）Melanoma cells are very bizarre cells with poorly visualized cell border and variation in size and shape,such as spindle cell, elongated, cohesive cells, (from well-demarcated to poorly cohesive), abundant cytoplasm, hyperchromatic irregular nucleus with prominent eosinophilic nucleoli. Multinucleated tumor giant cells. Frequent mitosis.

（2）They grow as loose nests lacking the typical features of maturation

Study Questions

Choose Tests

Directions：Each of the numbered items or incomplete statements in this section is followed by answers or by completions of the statement. Select the one lettered answer or completion that is best in each case.

1. Cytologic examination of pleural effusions in a woman without a known primary cancer is most likely to reveal cells derived from which of the following malignant tumors?
   A. Lymphoma   B. Mesothelioma   C. Carcinoma of the breast
   D. Carcinoma of the lung   E. Leiomyosarcoma

2. The cytologic abnormalities of malignant cells can be explained best by
   A. chromosomal abnormal B. excessive mucin content C. cell surface alterations
   D. a decrease in cellular glycogen content   E. mitotic activity

3. When histologically benign neoplasms prove fatal, they most likely do so because they
   A. cause extensive bleeding   B. are multifocal
   C. fail to invoke an immune response   D. interfere with organ function
   E. transform into carcinoma

4. Epidemiologic studies reveal a relationship between cancer incidence and all of the following factors EXCEPT
   A. advanced age   B. nonhereditary chromosomal abnormalities
   C. air pollution   D. bacterial infection   E. diet

5. All of the following conditions can increase tissue mass EXCEPT
   A. hypertrophy   B. inflammation   C. neoplasia
   D. hyperplasia   E. anaplasia

6. The tumor and causative agent are correctly matched in all of the pairs EXCEPT
   A. hepatic angiosarcoma—arsenicals
   B. endometrial carcinoma—exogenous estrogens
   C. vaginal carcinoma—diethylstilbestrol (DES)
   D. mesothelioma-beryllium

7. All of the following statements regarding benign mixed tumor (BMT) of the salivary glands are true EXCEPT
    A. it most commonly occurs in the parotid
    B. it is a rapidly growing asymptomatic mass
    C. it does not invade skin or nerves
    D. it is the most common salivary gland neoplasm
8. Which prognostic factor is the most useful for primary malignant melanoma?
    A. Depth of invasion   B. Size of malignant cells
    C. Number of multinucleate giant cells   D. Degree of surrounding inflammation
    E. Amount of melanin produced
9. A soft tissue lesion based in the skin or subcutaneous region can be any of the following EXCEPT
    A. a liposarcoma if on the trunk
    B. an epithelial sarcoma if on the hand
    C. an angiosarcoma if on the head of an elderly patient
    D. an atypical fibroxanthoma if on the neck
    E. an AIDS-associated lesion if a red-purple nodule
10. A 10-cm lump is noted on the thigh of a 50-year-old man. All of the following statements are likely explanations for this lump EXCEPT
    A. the tumor could be a malignant fibrous histiocytoma (MFH)
    B. the tumor could have been there for over 3 months
    C. the tumor could be benign (E.g., a myxoma)
    D. the tumor could be a reactive lesion
    E. the tumor could be calcified

Directions: The group of items in this section consists of lettered options followed by a set of numbered items. For each item, select the one lettered option that is most closely associated with it. Each lettered option may be selected once, more than once, or not at all.

Questions 11 ~ 14

Match each use for cancer diagnostic techniques with the appropriate response.
    A. Electron microscopy (EM)   B. Immunohistochemistry (IHC)
    C. Both   D. Neither
11. Differentiation between prostate cancer and gastric cancer
12. Differentiation between lymphoma and carcinoma
13. Differentiation between adenocarcinoma and mesothelioma
14. Localization of the primary site of a squamous cell carcinoma (SCC)

Questions 15 ~ 18

Match each condition below with the related type of cancer.
    A. Malignant lymphoma   B. Leukemia
    C. Uterine cervical cancer   D. Hematoma
15. Down syndrome
16. Cirrhosis
17. Human papillomavirus (HPV) infection
18. Primary immunodeficiency

Questions 19~23

Certain oncogenes have prognostic implications in human tumors. Match the oncogene with the human tumor that is most commonly associated with it.

A. Neuroblastoma   B. Lung adenocarcinoma   C. Breast carcinoma

D. Burkitt's lymphoma   E. Retinoblastoma

19. ras

20. n-myc

21. Rb

22. c-myc

23. C-erb-B$_2$

Questions

1. What is the main difference between hyperplasia and neoplasia?

2. What is meant by dysplasia or by intraepithelial neoplasia? What is the relationship between dysplasia and intraepithelial neoplasia?

3. What is a hamartoma?

4. What is meant by a tumour?

5. What agents are known to be carcinogenic and what type of tumour is produced?

6. What is carcinoma in situ?

7. What is exfoliative cytology (cytopathology) and what are its clinical applications?

8. How do malignant tumours spread?

9. What is meant by the term "embryonic tumour"? Where do they occur?

10. What tumours are derived from germ cells?

11. What are the features of teratomata?

12. What are paraneoplastic syndromes?

13. What is a Krukenberg's tumour?

14. What type of testicular tumour is associated with the appearance of 'tumour markers'?

15. What was the first occupational cancer described?

16. What is meant by the term 'leukoplakia'?

17. What is the difference between benign and malignant tumors?

18. What is the difference between carcinoma and sarcoma?

19. What is the percancinoma lesion? which are common percancinoma lesions?

第六章　心血管疾病

<table>
<tr><td>大体观察</td><td>镜下观察</td></tr>
<tr><td>1. 动脉粥样硬化</td><td>1. 动脉粥样硬化</td></tr>
<tr><td>2. 心肌梗死</td><td>2. 急性心肌梗死</td></tr>
<tr><td>3. 高血压的心脏</td><td>3. 心肌梗死</td></tr>
<tr><td>4. 高血压的肾脏(原发性固缩肾)</td><td>4. 心内膜弹力纤维增生症</td></tr>
<tr><td>5. 高血压脑出血</td><td>5. 高血压之肾(原发性固缩肾)</td></tr>
<tr><td>6. 夹层动脉瘤</td><td>6. 肾硬化症,肾终末期变化</td></tr>
<tr><td>7. 风湿性心内膜炎</td><td>7. 动静脉畸形(大脑)</td></tr>
<tr><td>8. 慢性风湿性心瓣膜病的心脏</td><td>8. 夹层动脉瘤</td></tr>
<tr><td>9. 亚急性细菌性心内膜炎(SBE)</td><td>9. 风湿性心脏病(风湿性肉芽肿)</td></tr>
<tr><td></td><td>10. 亚急性细菌性心内膜炎(SBE)</td></tr>
<tr><td></td><td>11. 心肌炎</td></tr>
</table>

一、大体观察

1. 动脉粥样硬化

(1) 简要说明

1) 动脉粥样硬化表示动脉变硬。

2) 动脉粥样硬化主要影响大中型肌型动脉和大弹力型动脉,在腹主动脉或冠状动脉中显著地出现灶性的内膜纤维脂质斑块。

3) 主要的危险因子:高血压,糖尿病,吸烟,高胆固醇血症。

(2) 大体所见

1) 脂纹:脂质渗入某些内皮细胞,大量的黄色、扁平的斑点融合成长的条纹——脂纹(动脉粥样硬化的先兆)。

2) 纤维脂质斑块:脂质的进一步累积导致组织变性和纤维化——内膜上灶性纤维脂质斑块。

3) 粥瘤的并发症:粥瘤破裂释放脂质栓子,斑块内出血,钙化,溃疡形成,血栓形成。

2. 心肌梗死

(1) 简要说明

1) 心肌梗死是缺血性心脏病的最重要的形式。

2) 发病机制:冠状动脉阻塞。

3) 危险因素:动脉粥样硬化,衰老,糖尿病,高血压,吸烟,遗传,高胆固醇血症等

（2）大体所见

1）所有的梗死灶往往是形成楔形,闭塞的血管位于其顶端,器官的边缘形成其底部。

2）梗死区灰白。

3）梗死的边缘较清楚。

3. 高血压的心脏　随着心肌细胞的肥大,心室壁变厚,导致心脏重量的增加(超过500g)。早期心脏体积增大,心室不扩张,称为向心性肥大。随着心脏体积的逐渐增大,心室扩张,称为离心性肥大。

4. 高血压的肾脏(原发性固缩肾)　肾体积缩小,质硬,表面颗粒状,切面肾小动脉管壁明显增厚。

5. 高血压脑出血　脑切面上可见出血灶。

6. 夹层动脉瘤

（1）简要说明

1）动脉瘤是血管局部的异常扩张。

2）沿着动脉中层,血管壁内被分离,形成一个充满血液的管道。

3）囊性的动脉中层变性,动脉壁薄弱,血液动力的因子使内膜撕裂,夹层动脉瘤,重新进入血管腔的末梢,形成一个二级管道或穿过血管壁破裂。

（2）大体所见:沿着动脉中层的层面,血管被分解,形成一个充满血液的管道。

7. 风湿性心内膜炎　二尖瓣和主动脉瓣结缔组织变性,增生活跃,瓣膜的闭锁缘形成疣状赘生物,直径1mm,多个,小而附着牢固,表面光滑。

8. 慢性风湿性心瓣膜病的心脏　瓣膜增厚,粘连,回缩,瓣叶缩短,导致瓣膜口狭窄。二尖瓣瓣膜、主动脉瓣、三尖瓣和肺动脉瓣的闭锁不全和狭窄常同时发生。

9. 亚急性细菌性心内膜炎(SBE)

（1）简要说明:感染性心内膜炎(IE):心瓣膜或心内膜壁被微生物侵袭,结果形成含有微生物的质脆的赘生物。

（2）大体所见:一般在心瓣膜上可见质脆,大的含有细菌的赘生物,在SBE时通常不被破坏。

二、镜下观察

1. 动脉粥样硬化

（1）脂纹:内膜聚集着吞噬了脂质的巨噬细胞和平滑肌细胞。

（2）动脉粥样斑块(粥瘤):纤维帽和坏死性中心。

1）表面的纤维帽:平滑肌细胞、吞噬脂质的巨噬细胞(泡沫细胞)、巨噬细胞、淋巴细胞、胶原、弹性蛋白、蛋白多糖。

2）中心性坏死:死亡的细胞、脂质、胆固醇结晶、充满脂质的泡沫细胞、钙化。

3）斑块周围:可见新血管形成。

2. 急性心肌梗死

（1）简要说明:心肌梗死的连续变化(表6-1)。

表 6-1 心肌梗死的连续变化

时间	大体特征	光镜
1~4 小时	无改变	无改变
4~12 小时	无改变	开始出现凝固性坏死,中性粒细胞浸润,水肿,出血。
18~24 小时	苍白	持续的凝固性坏死,边缘收缩,出现坏死带
24~72 小时	苍白,有时充血	心肌细胞的核和条纹消失,中性粒细胞弥漫浸润。
3~7 天	边缘充血,中心呈黄褐色	坏死的心肌纤维崩解,巨噬细胞出现,边缘的组织反应开始出现。
10 天	红褐色,扁平的黄色,柔软的血管化的边缘。	坏死的变化在发展,边缘出现显著的纤维血管反应
第七周	疤痕	纤维化

(2)镜下所见:肌束坏死、变性,伴大量的炎细胞浸润。

3. 心肌梗死

(1)慢性心肌梗死时不规则的纤维束取代心肌。心肌被纤维组织分离、中断。

(2)具有丰富血管网和早期胶原的肉芽组织沉积。伴有毛细血管和轻微的炎症反应,纤维束平行排列,分离和中断心肌。

(3)间质中毛细血管增生。

4. 心内膜弹力纤维增生症

(1)胶原和弹性纤维的显著增加引起心内膜的增厚。

(2)纤维弹力组织层延伸入邻近的心肌的下方。

(3)增厚的心内膜纤维弹力组织的碎片延伸入心肌。

5. 高血压之肾(原发性固缩肾)

(1)动脉和细动脉发生硬化显示玻璃样变性,动脉壁细胞数量减少,嗜酸性内膜增厚。

(2)肾小球显示毛细血管基底膜增厚,玻璃样变性,萎缩。肾小球囊变厚,玻璃样变性。

6. 肾硬化症,肾终末期变化

(1)入球小动脉血管壁增厚,管腔狭窄,伴肾小球退化。

(2)肾小球:血管丛皱缩,缺血,肾球囊增厚,一些肾小球完全玻璃样变和纤维化。

(3)肾小管:萎缩伴基底膜增厚,含透明管型。

(4)血管:玻璃样物质沉积在小动脉的内膜和中层,大血管内皮下纤维化和脂质沉积,硬化的小叶间血管中层变薄,管腔扩张。

(5)间质:纤维化,慢性炎细胞浸润。

其他描述:

(1)高血压肾硬化症(小动脉硬化)/恶性阶段(恶性高血压):当舒张压超过 125mmHg 时,视网膜变化出现。小动脉纤维素样坏死,尤其是在入球小动脉的进入肾小球的分枝点。纤维素样坏死时,基底膜也出现皱纹和增厚。增生性(洋葱皮样)动脉炎和小动脉坏死。

(2)细胞增生,肾小球囊壁形成新月体,炎症通常不明显。

(3)肾小管显著萎缩伴出血(血尿)。

7. 动静脉畸形(大脑)

(1)各种直径的异常血管处于混乱状态,被神经胶质组织分隔,缺乏介于其间的毛细血管床,常有先前出血的证据。在动静脉间有异常的交通支。

（2）一些血管有薄的胶原的血管壁,然而其他血管的肌层和动脉的弹力层结构紊乱。动脉直接连接静脉。静脉动脉化,出现异常的厚壁静脉。

（3）弹性纤维染色识别动脉和灶性的弹性蛋白的缺失或重叠。

（4）血管壁上的新月形的钙化可显示一些血管的轮廓。

（5）不同的神经胶质增生或含铁血黄素的沉积介于脑实质之间。

（6）血管的淤血和血栓形成。

（7）血管周围炎。

8. 夹层动脉瘤

（1）在血管中膜的中间和管壁外 1/3 层分离,形成两个管腔(中间被出血分离;通常与弹性蛋白的断裂和纤维化有关)。真性管腔:内皮衬壁,光滑。假的管腔:红细胞覆盖形成不规则的壁。

（2）动脉粥样硬化性改变的情况:壁上有吞噬了胆固醇的巨噬细胞(泡沫细胞)。

9. 风湿性心脏病(风湿性肉芽肿)

（1）在心肌小血管旁,黏液样变性,纤维素样坏死,围绕着增生的组织细胞(Aschoff 细胞),淋巴细胞,浆细胞或中性粒细胞。

（2）Aschoff 细胞体积大,形状不规则,有多个泡状核,颗粒状嗜碱性胞浆。

10. 亚急性细菌性心内膜炎(SBE)

（1）瓣叶的尖端覆盖有粉染的赘生物,其中含有小的染成蓝紫色的细菌菌落。

（2）赘生物:由纤维蛋白、炎细胞和病原生物组成。瓣膜没有明显的细菌破坏,在瓣叶上有大量的炎细胞浸润。赘生物中呈蓝紫色的是细菌菌落。

11. 心肌炎   炎症累及心肌特征性的白细胞浸润,导致心肌细胞的变性和坏死;或形成明显的脓肿、肉芽肿。

三、思考题

（一）选择题

选一个字母代表的最合适答案。

1. 哪个冠状动脉最常对室间隔后部供血?

    A. 左主冠状动脉　　　　B. 左前降支冠状动脉　　　　C. 左旋冠状动脉

    D. 近侧边缘冠状动脉　　E. 右冠状动脉

2. 心肌梗死时血栓形成最常阻塞哪条冠状动脉?

    A. 左主冠状动脉　　　　B. 左前降支冠状动脉　　　　C. 左旋冠状动脉

    D. 近侧边缘冠状动脉　　E. 右冠状动脉

3. 哪项关于心衰的陈述是正确的?

    A. 前心衰指心室扩大时心脏对胸壁运动的压力

    B. 呼吸困难是由于末端血管血液淤滞

    C. 右心衰可导致肝肿大

    D. 肺心病常由于严重的肺动脉狭窄

E. 临床显示心衰多为右心衰

4. 下列关于继发于急性心肌梗死后的心室壁瘤描述中哪项是正确的?

    A. 摄片见心脏轮廓变小   B. 可能发生肾梗死

    C. 血栓很少形成   D. 出血性肺炎是常见的并发症

    E. 心室瘤壁由少量含胶原的淀粉样蛋白

5. 下列哪一型的炎症是急性风湿热的特征?

    A. 心内膜炎   B. 心肌炎   C. 心包炎   D. 全心炎   E. 脉管炎

6. 急性风湿热的典型组织病变是

    A. Mallory 小体   B. Aschoff 小体   C. 砂粒体   D. Negri 小体   E. Anitschkow 细胞

7. 下列关于感染性心内膜炎的陈述是正确的除了

    A. 最常见由革兰阴性杆菌感染   B. 常包括以前损伤的瓣膜

    C. 可能发生瓣膜穿孔   D. 如不治疗则有生命危险

    E. 在大多数人中左侧瓣膜的损伤较常见

8. 以下是出现于慢性缺血性心脏病的组织学改变,除了

    A. 弥漫性心脏纤维化   B. 瓣膜纤维钙化改变

    C. 小灶心肌疤痕斑   D. 心内膜纤维组织与弹力组织增生

    E. 冠状动脉粥样硬化

9. 心包炎引起的心脏病,形态学检查包括以下几项,除了

    A. 纤维蛋白的渗出   B. 钙化   C. 纤维化

    D. 恶性细胞   E. 血红蛋白沉积

10. 以下都是肾脏调节血压的系统除了

    A. 肾素-血管紧张素系统   B. 醛固酮   C. 前列腺素

    D. 血管紧张素-缓激肽系统   E. 淋巴因子

给每一题选出最接近的答案。每个选项可选一次,多次或不选。

11~15 把以下感染性心脏病的特征同相应的疾病匹配起来

    A. 急性风湿热   B. 慢性风湿性心脏病   C. 急性心内膜炎

    D. 亚急性心内膜炎   E. Libman Sacks 心内膜炎

11. 瓣膜融合

12. A 组 β 溶血性链球菌感染

13. α-草绿色溶血性链球菌感染

14. 葡萄球菌感染

15. 二尖瓣表面疣状赘生物

(二) 问答题

1. Fallot 四联征的病理学和血流动力学的特点是什么?

2. 什么是动脉粥样硬化?

3. 哪些因子促进动脉粥样硬化的发展?

4. 动脉粥样硬化如何导致临床症状的出现?

5. 动脉粥样硬化好发于哪里?

6. 描述动脉粥样硬化的病变过程。

7. 什么是小舞蹈症？

8. 什么是 Monckeberg 硬化症？

9. 主动脉瓣关闭不全的原因是什么？

10. 主动脉瓣狭窄的原因是什么？

11. 动脉瘤的病因有哪些？

12. 什么是瓣膜赘生物？

13. 心脏瓣膜病的病因有哪些？

14. 风湿热的病因是什么？

15. 急性风湿热侵袭心脏的哪个部位？

16. 急性风湿热侵袭的器官和组织有哪些？

17. 慢性风湿性心脏病的特征和并发症？

18. 什么是 Aschoff 小体？

19. Aschoff 小体的组织学表现是什么？

20. 比较急性与亚急性细菌性心内膜炎。

21. 什么是感染性心内膜炎？

22. 冠状动脉闭塞的后果是什么？

23. 什么是心绞痛？

24. 心肌梗死的后遗症是什么？

25. 心肌梗死后多久能在肉眼或镜下看到心肌的变化？

26. 什么样的炎症性疾病可能影响心脏？

27. 什么是心肌病？

28. 心力衰竭的主要病因以及它在临床与病理学上的主要特征？

29. 哪些条件下可以引起心力衰竭？

30. 高血压的病因有哪些？

31. 高血压累及血管和器官的病理变化有哪些？

32. 恶性高血压中肾脏病变的镜下表现是什么？

33. 哪根脑动脉特别易于形成血栓？其后果是什么？

34. 什么是心脏压塞？

Chapter 6 Diseases of the Heart and Blood Vessles

Gross Findings	Micro Findings
1. Atherosclerosis	1. Atherosclerosis
2. Myocardial infarction	2. Acute myocardial infarction
3. Heart of hypertension	3. Myocardial infarction
4. Kindney of hypertension (primary contracted kidney)	4. Endocardial fibroelastosis
ney)	5. Kidney of hypertension (primarily contracted kidney)
5. Brain bleeding in hypertension	6. Nephrosclerosis with ending stage change, Kidney
6. Dissecting aneurysm	7. Arterio-venous malformation(Cerebrum)
7. Rheumatic endocarditis	8. Dissecting aneurysm
8. Chronic rheumatic valvular vitium of heart	9. Rheumatic heart disease (rheumatic granuloma)
9. Subacute bacterial endocarditis (SBE)	10. Subacute bacterial endocarditis (SBE)
	11. Myocarditis

Gross Findings

1. Atherosclerosis

(1) Brief Descriptions

1) Atherosclerosis means hardening of the arteries.

2) Atherosclerosis primarily affects large to medium-sized muscular arteries and large elastic arteries, marked by elevated focal intimal fibrofatty plaques principally in the abdominal aorta or coronary arteries.

3) Major risk factors: hypertension, diabetes mellitus, smoking, hypercholesterolemia.

(2) Gross Findings

1) Fatty streak: Infiltration of lipids into certain intimal cells, multiple yellow、flat spots coalescece into elongated streaks → fatty streak(precursors of atherosclerosis).

2) fibrolipid plaque: Progressive accumulation of lipids causing tissue degeneration and fibrosis → focal intimal fibrolipid plaque.

3) Complicated atheroma: Atheroma break and release lipidoid embolus, internal hemorrhage, calcification, ulceration and thrombus formation.

2. Myocardial infarction

(1) Brief Descriptions

1) Myocardial infarction is the most important form of ischemic heart disease.

2) Pathogenesis: coronary arterial occlusion.

3) Risk factors: atherosclerosis, old age, diabetes mellitus, hypertension, cigarette smoking, genetic hypercholesterolemia, etc.

（2）Gross Findings

1）All infarction tend to forming wedge shaped occluded vessel at apex and the periphery of the organ forming the base.

2）White infarct area.

3）The margin of infarcts become better define.

3. Heart of hypertension   Ventricle wall become thickening with myocytes hypertrophy, result in increasing heart weight（over 500 gm）.In early stage the size of heart is enlarge without Ventricle dilation, which named concentric hypertrophy. And in progressive stage the size of heart increased with Ventricle dilatation, which named eccentric hypertrophy.

4. Kindney of hypertension（primary contracted kidney）   Kidney become atrophy, harder, grunalar in surface, and arteries and aterioles wall thicking in cut surface.

5. Brain bleeding in hypertension   There are hemorrhagic lesions in brain cut surface.

6. Dissecting aneurysm

（1）Brief Descriptions

1）An aneurysm is a localized abnormal dilation of a blood vessel.

2）Dissection of blood vessel along the laminar planes of arterial media with the formation of a blood-filled channel.

3）Cystic medial degeneration weakened arterial wall hemodynamic factors make intimal tear dissecting aneurysm reenter the lumen distally to create a second channel, or rupture through the vessel wall.

（2）Gross Findings：Dissection of blood vessel along the laminar planes of arterial media with the formation of a blood-filled channel.

7. Rheumatic endocarditis   The mitral and aortic valves with degeneration of connective tissue and proliferative activity, verrucous vegetations form at the line of contact of the leaflets,1mm in the free margin,with multiple, firm and small, smooth.

8. Chronic rheumatic valvular vitium of heart   The valves are seen as thickening adhesions retraction, and shortening of the leaflets. There result in narrowing of the valve opening through it. Valvalar insufficiency and stenosis same times happen in mitral, aortic, tricuspid and pulmonary

9. Subacute bacterial endocarditis（SBE）

（1）Brief Descriptions

Infective endocarditis（IE）: colonization of heart valves or mural endocardium by microorganisms leading to the formation of friable vegetations laden with organisms.

（2）Gross Findings：Friable, bulky bacteria-laden vegetations most commonly on the heart valves which is usually not destructed in SBE.

Micro Findings

1. Atherosclerosis

（1）Fatty streak : intimal collections of lipid-laden macrophages and smooth muscle cells.

（2）Atheromatous plaque（atheroma）: Fibrous cap and Necrotic center.

Superficial fibrous cap: smooth muscle cells, Lipid-laden macrophage（Foam cells）、macrophage、lymphocytes、collagen、elastin、proteoglycans.

Central necrotic core: dead cells, lipid、cholesterol clefts、lipid-laden foamy cells、calcification.

（3）Around the plaque : neovascularization may be seen.

2. Acute myocardial infarction

(1) Brief Descriptions:

Sequential changes in myocardial infarction(Tab.6-1)

Tab. 6-1   Sequential charges in myocardial infarction

Time	Gross features	light microscope
1~4 h	none	none
4~12 h	none	begin coagulative necrosis, neutrophil infiltrates; edema, hemorrhage
18~24 h	pallor	continuing coagulation necrosis marginal contraction band necrosis
24~72 h	pallor, sometimes hyperemia	loss of nuclei and striation heavy infiltration of neutrophils
3~7 days	hyperemic border central yellow-brown	disintegration of dead myofibers macrophages present onset of marginal fibrovascular response
10 days	red-brown and depressed yellow and soft vascularized margins	well-develop necrotic changes prominent fibrovascular reaction in margin
7th weeks	scarring	fibrotic

(2) Micro Findings: Necrosis and degenerated of muscle bundles with densely inflammatory infiltration.

3. Myocardial infarction

(1) Irregular fibrous bundles replaced the cardiac muscle as chronic myocardial infarction. Interrupted and separated cardiac muscle by fibrous tissue.

(2) Granulation tissue with a rich vascular network and early collagen deposition. Fibrous bundles arrange in a parallel fashion with capillaries and minimal inflammation; separated and interrupted cardiac muscles.

(3) Proliferation of capillary in the interstitium.

4. Endocardial fibroelastosis

(1) Endocardial thickening due to marked increase of collagenous and elastic fibers.

(2) Fibroelastic layer extends into the immediate subjacent myocardium.

(3) Patch of fibroelastic thickening of endocardium extending into myocardium.

5. Kidney of hypertension (primarily contracted kidney)

(1) Arteries and ateriples occur sclerosis show hyaline degeneration and decreased cellularity of the wall with oaminated,eosinophilic intimal thickening.

(2) The glomeruli show a thickening of the capillary basement membranes and hyalinization and atrophy. Glomerular capsules become thickened and hyalinized.

6. Nephrosclerosis with ending stage change, Kidney

(1) Thickening of the vessel wall and narrowing of the lumen of afferent glomerular arterioles with obsolescence of glomeruli.

(2) Glomeruli: ischemic wrinkling of the tuft & thickening of the Bowman's capsule,some glomeruli will be completely hyalinized, and fibrosis.

(3) Tubule: atrophy with thickening basement membrane and containing hyaline casts.

(4) Blood vessel: hyaline deposit in intima and media of arterioles; subendothelial fibrosis

and lipid deposit in large vessels; thinned media & dilated lumen in sclerotic interlobular vessels.

(5) Interstitial: fibrosis and patchy chronic inflammation.

Others:

(1) Hypertensive nephrosclerosis (arteriolar sclerosis)/Malignant phase (malignant hypertension):Retinal change in the presence of diastolic pressure in excess of 125mmHg. Fibrinoid necrosis of small arteries and arterioles especially at the branching point of an afferent arterioles and where it enters the glomerulus. Wrinkling and duplication of base membrane as well as fibrinoid necrosis. Proliferative (onion skin) endoarteritis and arteriolar necrosis.

(2) Mesengial cellular proliferation and crescent formation of glomeruli Bowman's Capsule, inflammation usually scanty.

(3) Marked atrophy of tubules with hemorrhage (hematuria).

7. Arterio-venous malformation(Cerebrum)

(1) Tangles of abnormal vessels of various diameter seperated by gliotic tissue in the absence of intervening capillary bed often with evidence of prior hemorrhage. Abnormal communication between arteries and veins.

(2) Some vessels have the thin collagenous walls of veins,whereas others the muscular and elastic laminae of arteries or structural hybrids.

Artery feeding a vein.

Arterialization of vein: abnormally thick-walled veins.

(3) Elastic stains identify arteries and focal loss or duplication of elastin.

(4) Crescents of mural calcification may outline the contours of some vessels.

(5) Variable gliosis or hemosiderin-stained interposed brain parenchyma.

(6) Congestion of the vessels、thrombi.

(7) Perivascular inflammation.

8. Dissecting aneurysm

(1) Dissection between middle and outer thirds of tunica media with the formation of two lumens (Medial splitting by hemorrhage;usually associated with elastic fragmentation and fibrosis).true lumen:endotheial-lining wall,smooth. false lumen: RBC-coating irregular wall.

(2) Detail of atherosclerotic change of wall with cholesterol-laden macrophages (foamy histiocytes).

9. Rheumatic heart disease (rheumatic granuloma)

(1) In the myocardium mucoid degeneration and fibrinoid necrotic foci beside small blood vessels around the proliferation of histiocytic cells (Aschoff cells),lymphocytes, plasma cells or even neutrophilic leukocytes.

(2) Aschoff cells are large, elongated irregular with multiple vesicular nuclei and granular basophilic cytoplasm.

10. Subacute bacterial endocarditis (SBE)

(1) The valve leaflet covered at its tip by pink staining vegetations containing small colonies of blue-purple staining bacteria.

(2) Vegetation: be composed of fibrin、inflammatory cells and organisms. No apparent bacterial destruction of the valve.note densely inflammatory infiltrate in the valve leaflet.Blue purple color of bacterial clumps (colonies) in vegetation.

11. Myocarditis   Inflammatory involved the heart muscle characterized by a leukocytic infil-

trate and resultant nonischemic necrosis or degeneration of myocytes, or evident abscess, or granuloma.

Study Questions

Choose Tests

Directions: Each of the numbered items or incomplete statements in this section is followed by answers or by completions of the statement. Select the one lettered answer or completion that is best in each case.

1. Which coronary artery most commonly supplies blood to the posterior portion of the interventricular septum?

   A. Left main coronary artery   B. Left anterior descending coronary artery

   C. Left circumflex coronary artery   D. Proximal marginal coronary artery

   E. Right coronary artery

2. Which coronary artery most commonly thrombosis in myocardia infarction?

   A. Left main coronary artery   B. Left anterior descending coronary artery

   C. Left circumflex coronary artery   D. Proximal marginal coronary artery

   E. Right coronary artery

3. Which statement about heart failure is true?

   A. Forward failure refers to the motion of the heart pushing against the chest wall when the ventricular chambers are dilated

   B. Dyspnea is a result of stasis of blood in the extremities

   C. Right-sided failure may result in hepatomegaly

   D. Cor pulmonale usually is due to severe pulmonic stenosis

   E. The clinical manifestations of heart failure most commonly reflect right-sided failure

4. Which statement about ventricular aneurysm following acute myocardial infarction is true?

   A. The cardiac silhouette on chest radiograph often appears to be reduced in size

   B. Renal infarction may result

   C. Mural thrombi rarely form

   D. Hemorrhagic pneumonia is a common complication

   E. The aneurysm wall consists of amyloid with little collagen

5. Which type of inflammation is most characteristic of acute rheumatic fever?

   A. Endocarditis   B. Myocarditis   C. Pericarditis

   D. Pancarditis   E. Vasculitis

6. The classic histologic lesion of acute rheumatic fever is the

   A. Mallory's body   B. Aschoff body   C. psammoma body

   D. Negri body   E. Anitschkow cell

7. All of the following statements about infective endocarditis are correct EXCEPT

   A. it is most commonly caused by gram-negative bacilli

   B. it most often involves a previously damaged valve

   C. valve perforation may occur

   D. it is fatal if not treated

   E. damage to the left-sided valves is more common in the general population

8. Histologic findings present in chronic ischemic heart disease include all of the following EXCEPT
    A. diffuse myocardial fibrosis   B. fibrocalcific valvular changes
    C. small patchy myocardial scars   D. endocardial fibroelastosis
    E. coronary artery atherosclerosis

9. Morphologic examination of a heart diseased by pericarditis may reveal all of the following EXCEPT
    A. fibrinous exudate   B. calcification   C. fibrosis
    D. malignant cells   E. hemochromatosis

10. All of the following agents contribute to the kidney's regulation of systemic blood pressure EXCEPT
    A. renin-angiotensin system   B. aldosterone   C. prostaglandins
    D. kallikrein-kinin system   E. lymphokines

Directions: The group of items in this section consists of lettered options followed by a set of numbered items. For each item, select the one lettered option that is most closely associated with it. Each lettered option may be selected once, more than once, or not at all.

Questions 11~15

Match each phrase describing a feature of inflammatory heart disease with the disease it characterizes.
    A. Acute rheumatic fever   B. Chronic rheumatic heart disease C. Acute endocarditis
    D. Subacute endocarditis   E. Libman-Sacks endocarditis

11. Fusion of the commissures

12. Infection by group A β-hemolytic streptococci

13. Infection by α-hemolytic (viridans) streptococci

14. Infection by Staphylococcus aureus

15. Warty vegetations on the undersurface of the mitral valve

Questions

1. What are the pathological and haemodynamic features of Fallot's Tetrad?

2. What is atherosclerosis?

3. What factors contribute to the development of atherosclerosis?

4. How does atherosclerosis cause symptomatic disease?

5. Which are the common sites of atherosclerosis?

6. Desribe the development of atherosclerosis.

7. What is chorea minor?

8. What is Monckeberg's sclerosis?

9. What are the causes of aortic incompetence?

10. What are the causes of aortic stenosis?

11. What are the causes of aneurysms?

12. What are valvular vegetations?

13. What are the causes of valvular heart disease.

14. What is the aetiology of rheumatic fever?

15. What part of the heart is affected in acute rheumatic fever?

16. List the organs and tissues affected by acute rheumatic fever.

17. What are the features and complications of chronic rheumatic heart disease?
18. What is an Aschoff body?
19. What is the histological appearance of an Aschoff body?
20. Compare acute with subacute bacterial endocarditis.
21. What is infective endocarditis?
22. What are the effects of coronary occlusion?
23. What is angina pectoris?
24. What are the sequelae of a myocardial infarct?
25. How long after a myocardial infarct would you expect to see gross or microscopic hanges in the myocardium?
26. What inflammatory conditions may affect the heart?
27. What is meant by the term 'cardiomyopathy'?
28. What are the chief causes and the main clinical and pathological features of heart failure?
29. What conditions cause heart failure?
30. What causes systemic hypertension?
31. What are the pathological results aroused vessels and organs from hypertension?
32. What are the renal lesions observed microscopically in malignant hypertension?
33. Which artery of the brain is particularly liable to thrombose and what are the consequences?
34. What is cardiac tamponade?

第七章　呼吸系统疾病

大体观察	镜下观察
1. 肺气肿	1. 慢性支气管炎
2. 大叶性肺炎	2. 肺气肿
3. 小叶性肺炎	3. 吸入性肺炎
4. 间质性肺炎	4. 大叶性肺炎
5. 硅肺	5. 小叶性肺炎(支气管肺炎)
6. 肺的鳞状细胞癌	6. 卡氏肺囊虫性肺炎和巨细胞病毒性肺炎
7. 肺腺癌	7. 肺的透明膜病
	8. 硅肺
	9. 鼻咽癌(泡状核细胞癌)
	10. 肺鳞状细胞癌
	11. 肺腺癌
	12. 细支气管肺泡癌
	13. 肺腺样囊腺癌
	14. 肺小细胞癌

一、大体观察

1. 肺气肿

(1) 简要说明

定义:远端到终末细支气管气道壁的破坏导致气道的异常而永久性扩张。

(2) 大体标本观察:肺异常扩张,苍白而柔软。

2. 大叶性肺炎

(1) 肺组织融合性渗出性病变,呈红或灰褐色,类似肝组织的外观。

(2) 重量增加(因为肺水肿或淤血),肺呈紫色,质硬。

3. 小叶性肺炎　肺下叶可见分散的病变,明显实变和化脓的区域灶性增加。这种损害导致肺部模糊的棕黄色的软化灶,坏死性糊状内容物位于中心伴恶臭。

4. 间质性肺炎　不规则的小叶淤血区,有或无肺的实变。

5. 硅肺

(1) 肺部可见弥漫分布,逐渐变大的显著的胶原结节。

(2) 病变融形成大范围的致密瘢痕。

(3) 由炭末引起的钙化和组织变黑常常出现。

6. 肺的鳞状细胞癌

（1）简要说明

1）发生于化生的支气管鳞状上皮。

2）超过80%的鳞状细胞癌发生在男性，与吸烟关系密切。

（2）大体标本观察：巨大的团块，中央的或周围的，中心常常可出现空洞和坏死，常伴有肺门淋巴结肿大。

7. 肺腺癌

（1）简要说明：

1）通常出现在肺的边缘。（小支气管、细支气管或肺泡）

2）女性多见。

（2）大体所见：癌结节呈浅灰色到黑色，边缘浸润，常常发生在肺的边缘。

二、镜 下 观 察

1. 慢性支气管炎

（1）支气管黏膜水肿，炎细胞浸润，黏液或脓性分泌物充满气道。

（2）黏液腺和杯状细胞肥大。

（3）支气管上皮纤毛缺失，发生鳞状上皮化生或不典型增生。

2. 肺气肿　肺泡壁变薄，萎缩，局部被破坏形成肺大泡或增大的气囊。在肺泡中有一些小的吞噬了色素的巨噬细胞。

3. 吸入性肺炎

（1）急性炎症细胞和嗜酸性无定形的渗出物在细支气管和肺泡腔内。

（2）泡沫细胞(吞噬了脂质的巨噬细胞)或异物巨细胞。

（3）水肿和炎症导致肺泡隔增厚。

4. 大叶性肺炎　肺泡隔毛细血管充血，一些肺泡腔有大量的红细胞，中性粒细胞而实变，纤维素性胸膜炎，一些肺泡腔充满纤维素，仅伴有大量的中性粒细胞。

5. 小叶性肺炎(支气管肺炎)

（1）急性化脓性渗出物(中性粒细胞)充满肺泡腔和气道。

（2）围绕在细支气管周围的多个病灶，伴有大量的中性粒细胞。

6. 卡氏肺囊虫性肺炎和巨细胞病毒性肺炎

（1）大多数肺泡腔充填着粉红色的内容物，因此肺泡腔闭塞，一瞥难以区分肺的结构。其他肺泡腔呈肺气肿的改变。

（2）卡氏肺囊虫性肺炎：肺泡腔充满嗜双色性，泡沫状，无定形物质类似蛋白性水肿液，由增生的寄生虫和细胞碎片组成。

甲苯胺蓝：原虫。

环六亚甲基四胺银：典型的杯状包囊，原虫位于其中。

杯状的卡氏肺囊虫可出现在痰中。

（3）巨细胞病毒性肺炎：间质性肺炎，在增大的肺泡隔细胞，毛细血管内皮细胞和肺巨噬细胞内有特征性的核内包含体，周围有透亮的空晕。

　　巨细胞病毒感染增大的上皮细胞有典型的蓝眼样外观,有大量的核内包含体,周围有透亮的空晕。

　　7. 肺的透明膜病

　　(1) 粉红色,富含纤维蛋白的透明膜被覆在小的,萎陷的肺泡腔,在呼吸性细支气管,肺泡管和未开放的肺泡内出现坏死细胞的碎屑。

　　(2) 透明膜:血浆渗出物和细胞碎片混合组成。

　　8. 硅肺

　　(1) 肺内可见清楚的胶原结节(透明变性的同心圆状),包括非常致密,无细胞的,透明样变的纤维组织。很少有血管出现。

　　(2) 褐色的色素是炭末,大量纤维化的二氧化硅的粉尘是无色的,看不见的。

　　(3) 周围组织呈肺气肿,伴轻微的炎症。

　　9. 鼻咽癌(泡状核细胞癌)　癌细胞呈大的泡状核,核仁明显,胞浆丰富,细胞境界不清,在肿瘤细胞之间有大量的淋巴细胞浸润。

　　10. 肺鳞状细胞癌　高分化的鳞癌有角化珠和细胞间桥,低分化的肿瘤仅有极少的鳞状细胞特征的残留和角化不全细胞。

　　其他描述:

　　(1) 发生在支气管的鳞状上皮化生处。

　　(2) 占所有肺癌的 25% ~35%。

　　(3) 超过80%的鳞状细胞癌发生在男性,与吸烟关系密切。

　　(4) 大多数是位于肺段支气管的中心。

　　11. 肺腺癌

　　(1) 瘤细胞通常呈立方形,排列呈柱状,常分泌黏蛋白,形成管状,腺泡或乳头状结构。

　　(2) 肿瘤性的腺体呈筛状形式,注意基质中有大量的肿瘤细胞侵袭。

　　其他描述:

　　(1) 大多是肺癌的基本类型。

　　(2) 常见于女性。

　　(3) 定位:通常在肺周围,胸膜下,伴胸膜增厚和皱褶。

　　(4) 肺癌中预后较好的一型。

　　12. 细支气管肺泡癌　柱状到立方形的上皮细胞沿肺泡隔排列,很多分支形成乳头状突起,突入肺泡腔,常包含丰富的黏蛋白分泌物,保留原有的肺泡间隔结构,大多数肿瘤细胞分化较好。

　　13. 肺腺样囊腺癌

　　(1) 由小细胞组成,细胞核暗而致密,胞浆较少。

　　(2) 有形成管状,团块或筛状模式的倾向。

　　14. 肺小细胞癌

　　(1) 成片或实体的圆形癌细胞,细胞核深染,胞浆较少。小的圆形的蓝色的细胞向周围浸润。

　　(2) 邻近的肺显示肺气肿的改变。

（3）高度恶性,广泛转移,常位于肺门或中央,与吸烟有着非常密切的关系。

三、思　考　题

（一）选择题

选一个字母代表的最合适答案。

1. 下列哪项指职业原因造成慢性吸入颗粒或气体而引起的一组肺疾病?

　A. 肉芽肿病　　　　　　　　B. 尘肺病　　　　　　C. 分支杆菌病

　D. 假性淋巴瘤　　　　　　　E. 支气管扩张

2. 煤矿工人的 X 线片显示大面积不规则密度影和明显的气液平面,这些最可能提示

　A. 慢性硅肺病伴蛋壳样钙化　　B. 并发肺结核　　　C. 煤矿工人常见的尘肺病

　D. 石棉肺　　　　　　　　　　E. 肺脓肿

3. 下列石棉相关疾病的最好描述是

　A. 石棉肺常见于间皮瘤病人　　　　　　B. 船员工作 6 周后可能患间皮瘤

　C. 纤维类型和形状并不重要　　　　　　D. 含铁元素不少见

　E. 接触石棉增加患结核的危险

4. 哪种感染是引起间质性肺炎最常见的因素?

　A. 革兰阳性菌　　　　　　　B. 革兰阴性菌　　　C. 病毒

　D. 霉菌　　　　　　　　　　E. 寄生虫

5. 以下肺癌中哪种属于胺前体摄入和脱羧(APUD)肿瘤?

　A. 错构瘤　　　　　　　　　B. 黏液表皮样癌　　C. 腺样囊腺癌

　D. 支气管类癌　　　　　　　E. 鳞癌(SCC)

6. 哪种肿瘤与工作中暴露于石棉中有关?

　A. 支气管肺泡癌　　　　　　B. 燕麦细胞癌　　　C. 间皮瘤

　D. 鳞癌(SCC)　　　　　　　E. 腺癌

7. 一个 65 岁女性患者有长期吸烟病史,形成肺门肿块和纵隔淋巴结肿大。从纵隔淋巴结的组织学活检中不可能区分小细胞癌和恶性淋巴癌。下一步合理的诊断步骤是

　A. 肺切除　　　　　　　　　　　　　B. 活检组织的电镜观察

　C. 骨髓穿刺组织学检查排除白细胞累及　D. 临床检查副肿瘤综合征

　E. 外周血细胞流式细胞仪检查

8. 以下哪种疾病是引起慢性阻塞性肺病(COPD)的常见因素?

　A. 尘肺症　　　　　　　　　B. 肺炎　　　　　　C. 间质性肺病

　D. 肺气肿　　　　　　　　　E. 囊性纤维化

9. 哪种肿瘤生长呈高分化细胞并排列于呼吸道,而不侵犯肺泡间质?

　A. 鳞状细胞癌　　　　　　　B. 未分化细胞癌　　C. 大细胞癌

　D. 小细胞癌　　　　　　　　E. 支气管肺泡癌

10. 淋巴上皮瘤是鼻咽的肿瘤,除了下列哪项都是其特点

　A. 在年轻的亚洲人高发　　　B. 生长迅速　　　　C. 包含有淋巴和上皮成分

D. 手术切除后治愈的可能性大   E. 一些与 EB. V 感染有关

给每一题选出最接近的答案。每个选项可选一次,多次或不选。

11~15. 对每个病理反应,选择最可能相关的疾病

    A. 硅肺病　　　　　　　　B. 石棉肺　　　　C. 结核

    D. 慢性铍中毒　　　　　　E. 煤矿工人肺尘症

11. 干酪样肉芽肿

12. 中央型肺气肿

13. 非干酪样肉芽肿

14. 胸膜钙化

15. 有极性的斑块结节

（二）问答题

1. 肺不张和肺萎陷是同一概念吗?

2. 大叶性肺炎的分期?

3. 大叶性肺炎的并发症有哪些?

4. 比较大叶性肺炎和小叶性肺炎。

5. 吸入石棉纤维有什么危害?

6. 肺气肿与肺膨胀过度之间的区别有哪些?

7. 肺气肿有哪些类型?

8. 简述慢性支气管炎的病理学特征。

9. 什么是肺源性心脏病?

10. 什么是新生儿透明膜病?

11. 肺癌(支气管源性)的诱发因素有哪些?

12. 简述肺癌的分类。

13. 燕麦细胞癌的组织发生是什么?

Chapter 7 Diseases of the Respiratory System

Gross Findings	Micro Findings
1. Emphysema	1. Chronic bronchitis
2. Lobar pneumonia	2. Emphysema, Lung
3. Lobular pneumonia	3. Aspiration pneumonia
4. Interstitial pneumonia	4. Lobar pneumonia
5. Silicosis	5. Lobular pneumonia (Bronchopneumonia)
6. Squamous cell carcinoma of lung	6. Pneumocystis carinii pneumonia and Cytomegalovirus (CMV)
7. Adenocarcinoma of Lung	pneumonitis
	7. Hyaline membrane disease, Lung
	8. Silicosis (lung)
	9. Nasopharyngeal carcinoma (vesicular nucleus cell carcinoma)
	10. Squamous cell carcinoma, Lung
	11. Adenocarcinoma, Lung
	12. Bronchiolo-alveolar carcinoma, Lung
	13. Adenoid cystic carcinoma, Lung
	14. Small cell carcinoma, Lung

Gross Findings

1. Emphysema

(1) Brief Descriptions

Definition: abnormal permanent enlargement of air spaces distal to the terminal bronchioles with destruction of the air space wall.

(2) Gross Findings: abnormal enlargement of lung, pale and soft.

2. Lobar pneumonia

(1) The lung tissue with confluent exudation giving a red or gray-brown color show liver like gross appearance.

(2) Heavy (because of pulmonary edema, congestion), purple and solid appearance of lung.

3. Lobular pneumonia The lesions found in lower lobes of lung show dispersed, elevated focal area of palpable consolidation and suppuration. The lesion causing ill-defined brownish-yellow areas of softening in the lung, and necrotic slimy contents in the centers with malodor.

4. Interstitial pneumonia Patchy of lobar areas of congestion with or without the consolidation of lung.

5. Silicosis

(1) Distinct collagenous nodules are larger and more diffuse in the lung.

(2) Coalescence of lesions forms large areas of dense scar.

(3) Calcification of concomitant blackening by coal dust is often present.

6. Squamous cell carcinoma of lung

（1）Brief Descriptions

1）Arises in metaplastic squamous epithelium of bronchi.

2）Over 80% of squamous cell carcinomas occur in males and is strongly associated with cigarette smoking.

（2）Gross Findings：bulky mass, central or peripheral; central cavitation and necrosis is common, hilar lymphopathy.

7. Adenocarcinoma of Lung

（1）Brief Descriptions

1）Usually arise in the periphery of the lung（small bronchus, a bronchiole or the alveoli）.

2）Women appear to have propensity to develop adenocarcinoma.

（2）Gross Findings：Carcinoma nodules with grayish to tan in color; with infiltrating border occur in the periphery of the lung.

Micro Findings

1. Chronic bronchitis

（1）Hyperemia,edema and inflammatory cells infiltrite in the bronchial mucous membranes, mucous secretions or purulent casts filling airways.

（2）Hypertrophy of mucous glands and goblet cells.

（3）Squamous metaplasia or dysplasia with loss of cilia of bronchial epithelium.

2. Emphysema, Lung   The alveolar walls are thin and atrophic and in places have broken down to form bullae or enlarged air spaces, There are a few small collections of pigment laden macrophages in the alveoli.

3. Aspiration pneumonia

（1）Acute inflammatory cells and eosinophilic amorphous exudate in the bronchioles and alveolar space.

（2）Foamy cells（lipid-laden macrophages）or foreign body giant cells.

（3）Thickening alveolar septum due to edema and inflammation.

4. Lobar pneumonia   Interalveolar capillary congestion, the some alveolar spaces. consolidation with large number of red cells and neutrophilic leukocytes,fibrinous pleuritis,and some alveolar spaces.chumping of fibrin with only large amount of neutrophilic leukocytes.

5. Lobular pneumonia（Bronchopneumonia）

（1）An acute suppurative exudates(neutrophilic) filling air spaces and airways.

（2）Multifold lesions around bronchioles with large amount of neutrophilic leukocytes.

6. Pneumocystis carinii pneumonia and Cytomegalovirus（CMV）pneumonitis

（1）A high proportion of alveolar space is filled with pinkish substance, so the airspace is obliterated, and the architecture of lung is hard to identified at a glance.

The non-involved alveoli show emphysematous change

（2）Pneumocystis carinii pneumonia：The alveolar spaces filled by an amphophilic, foamy, amorphous material resembling proteinaceous edema fluid composed of proliferating parasites and cell debris.

Toluidine blue: trophozoites.

Methenamine-silver: typical cup-shaped cyst with trophozoites in the cyst.

The cup-shaped Pneumocystis carinii organisms within a sputum sample.

（3）Cytomegalovirus（CMV）pneumonitis：Interstitial pneumonitis by the characteristic intranuclear inclusion body surrounded by a clear halo in the enlarged alveolar lining cells, endothelial cells of septal capillaries and alveolar macrophages.

A CMV-infected enlarged epithelial cell with typical bull-eye appearance with large intranuclear inclusion body surrounded by a clear halo.

7. Hyaline membrane disease, Lung

（1）Pink, fibrin-rich hyaline membranes lining small and collapsed alveolar spaces and necrotic debris mainly within the respiratory bronchioles, alveolar ducts and unopened alveoli.

（2）Hyaline membrane: compacted plasma exudates and cellular debris.

8. Silicosis（lung）

（1）Distinct collagenous nodules（hyaline change whorls）in the lung. It consists of extremely dense, virtually acellular, hyalined fibrous tissue. Very few blood vessels are present.

（2）The brown pigment is coal dust, the highly fibrogenic silica dust being colourless and invisible.

（3）Adjecent tissues are emphysema with scant inflammation.

9. Nasopharyngeal carcinoma（vesicular nucleus cell carcinoma）   Carcinoma cells show large vesicular nuclei with prominent nucleoli, abundant cytoplasm and indistinct cell border,with numerous lymphocytes infiltrate among the tumor cells.

10. Squamous cell carcinoma, Lung   Range from well-differentiated SCC showing keratin pearls and intercellular bridge to poor-differentiated neoplasm having only minimal residual squamous features and dyskeratocytes.

Others:

（1）Arises in metaplastic squamous epithelium of bronchi.

（2）Accounts for 25% ~ 35% of all lung cancers.

（3）Over 80% of squamous cell carcinomas occur in males, and is strongly associated with cigarette smoking.

（4）Most cases are centered in segmental bronchi.

11. Adenocarcinoma, Lung

（1）Neoplastic cells are generally cuboid to columnar, frequently secrete mucin and form tubular, acinar or papillary structure.

（2）Neoplastic glands with cribriform pattern; note stroma invasion with severe desmplasia.

Others:

（1）Most common of primary lung cancer

（2）Most common in female

（3）Location: usually in peripheral, subpleural lung with pleural thickening and puckering

（4）Best prognosis of lung cancer

12. Bronchiolo-alveolar carcinoma, Lung   Columnar to cuboid epithelial cells lining up along the alveolar septa and projecting into the alveolar spaces in numerous branching papillary formations, often containing abundant mucinous secretions, preserving the native septal wall architecture, and well-differentiated in most tumors.

13. Adenoid cystic carcinoma, Lung

（1）Composed of small cells having dark, compact nuclei and scant cytoplasm.

（2）They tend to be disposed in tubular, solid or cribriform patterns.

14. Small cell carcinoma, Lung

（1）Sheets or solid pattern of the cancer cells with round-shaped, hyperchromatic nuclei and scanty cytolasm.Small round blue cell with infiltrating borders.

（2）The adjacent lung showing emphysematous chang.

（3）Highly malignant, extensively metastasis, usually hilar or centrally located.

（4）It has a strong relationship to cigarette smoking.

Study Questions

Choose Tests

Directions：**Each of the numbered items or incomplete statements in this section is followed by answers or by completions of the statement. Select the one lettered answer or completion that is best in each case.**

1. What is the term given to the group of lung diseases that result from the chronic inhalation of particulate or gaseous agents as a result of occupational exposure?

    A. Granulomatous disease   B. Pneumoconiosis   C. Mycobacteriosis

    D. Pseudolymphoma   E. Bronchiectasis

2. Large irregular densities and apparent cavitation with air-fluid levels are noted on the chest X-ray of a coal miner. These findings are most suggestive of

    A. chronic silicosis with eggshell Calcifications   B. superimposed tuberculosis

    C. simple coal worker's pneumoconiosis（CWP）   D. asbestosis

    E. lung abscese

3. Asbestos-related disease is best characterized by which statement?

    A. Asbestosis is often seen in patients with mesothelioma

    B. Mesothelioma may occur years after holding a job for 6 weeks as a ship worker

    C. Fiber type and shape are not Significant

    D. Ferruginous bodies are nonspecific findings

    E. Asbestos exposure increases the risk of tuberculosis

4. Which infection is often the cause of interstitial pneumonia?

    A. Gram-positive bacterial   B. Gram-negative bacterial   C. Viral

    D. Fungal   E. Parasitic

5. Of the lung tumors listed, which type belongs to the amine precursor uptake and decarboxylation（APUD）group of tumors?

    A. Hamartoma   B. Mucoepidermoid carcinoma

    C. Adenoid cystic carcinoma   D. Bronchial carcinoid

    E. Squamous cell carcinoma（SCC）

6. Which tumor is associated mainly with occupational exposure to asbestos?

    A. Bronchioalveolar carcinoma   B. Oat cell carcinoma

    C. Mesothelioma   D. Squamous cell carcinoma（SCC）

    E. Adenocarcinoma

7. A 65-year-old woman with a long history of smoking develops a hilar lung mass and mediastihal lymphadenopathy. From the histology of a biopsy of a mediastinal lymph node, it is impossible to distinguish between small cell cancer and malignant lymphoma. A logical next step to make the diagnosis would be

A. lung resection.

B. electron microscopy of biopsy material.

C. a bone marrow biopsy to rule out leukemic involvement.

D. a medical workup for paraneoplastic conditions.

E. flow cytometry of peripheral blood.

8. Which disorder is a common cause of chronic obstructive pulmonary disease (COPD) in the United States?

A. Pneumoconiosis　　　　　B. Pneumonia　　　　　　　C. Interstitial lung diseases

D. Emphysema　　　　　　　E. Cystic fibrosis

9. Which carcinoma grows as well-differentiated cells that line the respiratory airspaces without invading the stroma of the lung?

A. Squamous cell　　　　　　B. Anaplastic　　　　　　　C. Large cell

D. Small cell　　　　　　　　E. Bronchioalveolar

10. Lymphoepithelioma is a malignant neoplasm of the nasopharynx characterized by all of the following EXCEPT

A. high incidence in young Asians　　　B. rapid growth

C. lymphoid and epithelial elements　　D. high rate of cure with surgical resection

E. some association with Epstein-Barr virus (EBV) infection

Directions: Each group of items in this section consists of lettered options followed by a set of numbered items. For each item, select the one lettered option that is most closely associated with it. Each lettered option may be selected once, more than once, or not at all.

Questions 11~15

For each pathologic response, select the disease with which it is most.likely to be associated.

A. Silicosis　　　　　　　　B. Asbestosis　　　　　　　C. Tuberculosis

D. Chronic berylliosis　　　E. Coal worker's pneumoconiosis (CWP)

11. Caseating granulomas

12. Centrilobular emphysema

13. Noncaseating granulomas

14. Pleural calcifications

15. Polarizable flecks in nodules

Questions

1. Are atelectasis and collapse of the lung the same thing?

2. What are the stages of lobar pneumonia?

3. What are the complications of lobar pneumonia?

4. Compare lobar pneumonia with lobular pneumonia.

5. What are the dangers of inhaling asbestos fibres?

6. What is the difference between emphysema and overinflation of the lung?

7. What varieties of emphysema are recognised?

8. What are the pathognomonic features of chronic bronchitis?

9. What is cor pulmonale?

10. What is hyaline membrane disease?

11. What known actors predispose to the development of lung (bronchogenic) cancer?

12. Classify lung cancers.

13. What is the histogenesis of oat-cell carcinoma?

第八章 消化系统疾病

一、大体观察

1. 慢性萎缩性胃炎　黏膜变薄,皱襞变平,黏膜下血管明显。

2. 慢性胃溃疡

(1) 简要说明:原因:黏膜防御机制和损害因素(胃酸,胃蛋白酶,幽门螺杆菌)之间失衡。

(2) 大体所见:溃疡的边缘非常清楚,溃疡底部为肉芽组织。

3. 十二指肠溃疡　十二指肠溃疡小而表浅,多灶。其他特征和胃溃疡一样。

4. 食管鳞状细胞癌

(1) 简要说明

1) 多发于50岁以上。

2) 男女比:2∶1 到 20∶1。

3) 危险因素:饮食,食管疾病,遗传素质。

(2) 大体所见:大体类型包括髓质型,蕈伞型,溃疡型和缩窄型。切面呈灰白色。

5. 胃腺癌(早期胃癌)

(1) 简要说明

1）肿瘤局限于黏膜层或黏膜下层,与淋巴结是否发生转移无关。

2）两种类型:黏膜内和黏膜下。

3）与原位癌不同义。

（2）大体所见:早期胃癌,肿瘤局限在黏膜和黏膜下,可稍隆起,平坦或凹陷或挖开。

6. 胃类癌

（1）简要说明

1）胃肠道的黏膜有分散的内分泌细胞,合成,储存,释放生物胺或肽类参与胃肠功能的调节。来源于这些细胞的肿瘤称为类癌。

2）阑尾是发生胃肠类癌最常见的部位,其次是小肠,直肠,胃和回肠。

3）类癌是潜在恶性的肿瘤,恶性行为的倾向与起源的位置,局部穿透的深度和肿瘤的大小有关。

（2）大体所见

1）肿瘤位于消化管壁内或黏膜下呈团块状,形成小的息肉状或似高丘样的隆起,直径很少超过3cm。

2）受压的黏膜可以是完整的或形成溃疡。

7. 结肠腺癌

（1）简要说明

1）结肠恶性上皮肿瘤。

2）大多数肿瘤发生于乙状结肠和直肠。

3）大体类型包括溃疡型,隆起型,浸润型。

4）肿瘤显示腺样结构的百分比可被用来进行分级:

高分化:大于95%的腺样结构;中分化:50%~95%的腺样结构;低分化:5%~50%的腺样结构。

未分化:小于5%的腺样结构。

（2）大体所见:息肉样,外生型或溃疡型肿块。

8. 重症肝炎

（1）简要说明:从肝功能不全开始到肝性脑病症状出现在2~3周内。肝炎病毒是主要原因。

（2）大体所见:急性大块坏死或急性亚大块坏死。

9. 脂肪肝　肝脏体积增大到4~6kg,切面柔软,油腻,黄色。

10. 门脉性肝硬化

（1）简要说明:主要来源于慢性病毒性肝炎。

（2）大体所见:结节大小较规则(小结节),伴纤维化和再生的结节。

11. 坏死后性肝硬化

（1）简要说明:原因:滥用酒精,慢性肝炎,胆道疾病和铁超负荷。肝实质进行性纤维化。通常是不可逆的。

（2）大体所见:大结节型肝硬化,结节的大小和形状有明显的变化(3~10mm或更大)。

12. 胆汁性肝硬化　肝脏呈黄绿色,有细小结节。

13. 食管静脉曲张

（1）简要说明：食管和胃静脉曲张出血是门脉高压和肝硬化的最重要的并发症，它与约50%的死亡率有关。

（2）大体所见：食管黏膜下的静脉腔扩张，通过胃冠状静脉和食管静脉与门静脉相通。

14. 脾肿大

（1）淤血性脾肿大是门脉高压的重要征象。

（2）脾的重量可增加到1kg，脾功能亢进，外周血成分减少，导致血细胞减少症，与反应性骨髓增生相关。

15. 肝细胞肝癌

（1）简要说明：与乙型肝炎病毒感染有明显的联系。

（2）大体所见

1）肿瘤境界清楚，切面见坏死，出血，胆汁染色，软化。

2）通常比周围的肝组织苍白。

3）肉眼类型包括巨块型，结节性和弥漫型。

二、镜 下 观 察

1. 慢性萎缩性胃炎

（1）腺体萎缩表现为数量和大小的减小（部分或全部），伴腺腔扩张，黏膜萎缩。

（2）慢性炎症细胞浸润包括黏膜和黏膜下层弥散的集合淋巴小结。

（3）化生包括胃体的幽门腺化生，胃窦的肠上皮化生。

（4）部分黏膜显示不典型增生或异型增生。

2. 胃溃疡

（1）溃疡延伸至少到黏膜下层，常达到固有肌层。

（2）溃疡结构包括炎性渗出层，坏死层，肉芽组织层和瘢痕层。

（3）溃疡口边缘黏膜炎症、变性和再生。

3. 食管鳞状细胞癌

（1）癌细胞巢浸润入食管全层。

（2）低分化的癌细胞巢与周围的间质区分不清。

（3）高分化的细胞有细胞间桥和角化珠形成，成片的部分角化的细胞。

4. 胃腺癌（早期胃癌，溃疡恶变）

（1）溃疡边缘的肿瘤性腺体有纤维素性及脓性渗出，溃疡的基底层有坏死的碎屑。

（2）溃疡边缘的癌细胞排列不规则（复杂的腺样结构，筛状的腺体形成），呈现多形性，深染的核，核仁清楚。

（3）肿瘤性的腺体位于溃疡边缘，向黏膜下层延伸。

5. 胃印戒细胞癌

（1）胞浆内的黏液形成典型的印戒样的外观。

（2）癌细胞浸润穿过全层，有时形成腺样结构或黏液湖。

（3）广泛的纤维化（促结缔组织生成），致密的炎症性浸润。

（4）深染的癌细胞漂浮在黏液湖中。肿瘤侵犯到浆膜下层。印戒样细胞胞质内黏液聚集，把核挤向周边。

6. 胃类癌

（1）单一形态的细胞排列成小梁状，实体的，岛状的，花彩样（带状的）或管状结构，一些小的腺体呈玫瑰花样的外观。

（2）肿瘤细胞有一致的圆形到椭圆形的核，中等量颗粒状胞浆。核居中，伴有明显的核仁和细染色质（盐粉状）。

（3）丰富的血管和显著的纤维间质。

7. 结肠腺癌

（1）不同大小和形状的腺体。

（2）大的多层高染色质的细胞，核浆比和有丝分裂数增高。肿瘤细胞多形性，空泡状核，显著的核仁。核分裂象可见。

（3）肿瘤起源于黏膜上皮，向周围的脂肪组织扩展。

（4）可见灶性的坏死。

8. 重症肝炎

（1）坏死导致广泛的肝细胞减少。破坏的肝实质区融合。正常的肝结构几乎完全被破坏。

（2）残余的肝细胞再生活跃，显示围绕门管区的导管样结构的新生血管是部分胆管和部分肝细胞起源。

（3）炎症细胞浸润。

（4）网状支架塌陷。

9. 肝硬化

（1）纤维化，全部肝实质被分成大小不一的结节，再生的结节其血管微解剖结构完全变形。

（2）假小叶，有多个中央静脉，门管区结构有或无，可见再生的非典型的肝细胞（多核，深染）。

（3）形成的纤维间隔延伸，穿过肝窦从中央到门管区，从门管区到门管区。厚薄不一的纤维间隔中有短路的静脉，炎细胞，胆管，血管和动脉，没有正常的门管结构。纤维间隔中致密的炎症浸润分隔肝实质。

（4）肝细胞脂肪变性可以见到。

10. 肝细胞肝癌

（1）肿瘤细胞有嗜酸性胞浆，圆形的泡状核，核仁清楚。

（2）排列成盘状或小梁状，或排列成腺泡状和实性条索，通常几层细胞厚度，被有内皮，缺少网状纤维的窦状隙分隔，但没有 Kupffer 细胞。

（3）肿瘤细胞显示颗粒状或透亮的胞浆（胞浆内有糖原）。有时可见多形性或多核瘤巨细胞。

（4）血管侵润。

其他：AFP 有很大的诊断价值。

三、思 考 题

（一）选择题

选一个字母代表的最合适答案。

1. 以下哪种是最常见的食管炎？

　　A. 反流性　　　　　　　　B. 病毒性　　　　　　　　C. 真菌性

　　D. 急性腐蚀性　　　　　　E. 慢性肉芽肿性

2. 在许多引起慢性非特殊性胃炎和消化道溃疡的疾病中，哪种微生物被发现可能是致病因素？

　　A. 大肠杆菌　　　　　　　B. 埃希氏菌　　　　　　　C. 幽门螺杆菌

　　D. 克雷伯杆菌　　　　　　E. 佛氏枸橼酸菌

3. 先天性巨结肠病常由于哪一节大肠内先天性缺乏神经节细胞？

　　A. 盲肠　　　B. 升结肠　　　C. 横结肠　　　D. 降结肠　　　E. 直肠

4. 最常见发生消化道类癌的部位是

　　A. 小肠　　　B. 结肠　　　C. 阑尾　　　D. 食道　　　E. 胃

5. 反流性食管炎以哪一项为特征？

　　A. 下段食管括约肌的压力不适当的增加

　　B. 在慢性病变中出现 Barrett 上皮

　　C. 鳞癌多于腺癌

　　D. 缺乏结肠发育的潜能

　　E. 和急性食管炎密切相关

6. Menetrier 病以什么为特征？

　　A. 胃皱壁增厚，黏膜细胞增生，血液蛋白不足和蛋白缺乏性肠下垂

　　B. 胃皱壁增厚与淋巴浸润相关

　　C. 出现大量幽门螺杆菌

　　D. 胃皱壁增厚与印戒细胞癌有关

　　E. 胃皱壁变薄与慢性萎缩性胃炎有关

7. 哪一种直肠结肠息肉被认为是非肿瘤性的？

　　A. 管状绒毛状腺瘤　　　　B. 绒毛腺瘤　　　　C. 家族性多发性息肉病（FAP）

　　D. 增生性息肉　　　　　　E. 平滑肌瘤

8. 哪项关于假膜性结肠炎的描述是正确的？

　　A. 由肠毒素引起　　　　　B. 引起便秘

　　C. 常与近期使用抗生素有关，肠壁上可形成溃疡

　　D. 组织学上以透壁的慢性炎症为特征

　　E. 是一个不常见的增生性结肠炎

9. 早期胃癌（EGC）的定义是

　　A. 直径小于 2cm 的肿瘤　　　　B. 病人出现症状少于 2 年

　　C. 没有淋巴结浸润　　　　　　D. 肿瘤的浸润不超过黏膜下层

E. 镜下可发现肿瘤

10. 患者胃溃疡活检发现为腺癌,行胃部分切除术,发现癌细胞中度分化,浸润不超过黏膜下层。在 1/5 个局部淋巴结中出现腺癌的转移,以下关于腺癌的描述哪一个是正确的?

A. 这个病例很少见,因为鳞癌是胃癌最常见的组织学类型

B. 患者将可能在 5 年内死亡

C. 根据定义,病人为进展期(中晚期)胃癌

D. 胃癌的大小比黏膜的浸润程度对判断患者的预后更重要

E. 患者为早期胃癌

11. 结肠腺瘤的特征与以下癌肿危险性增加有关,除了

A. 严重的间变　　　　　　B. 绒毛结构　　　　C. 大小超过 2cm

D. 显著炎症　　　　　　　E. 多发性腺瘤

12. 以下对结、直肠癌的描述是正确的除了

A. 是现在引起癌肿死亡的主要原因

B. 患此病的高峰年龄是 70 岁

C. 腺癌的发生率高于鳞癌

D. 只有少数的结、直肠癌出现肠管的炎症性疾病

E. 在结、直肠癌中偶尔有染色体异常

13. 以下描述是关于慢性消化性溃疡的除了

A. 结肠憩室　　　　　　　　　　B. O 型血人群

C. 幽门螺杆菌的感染　　　　　　D. 在卓艾综合征中,胃泌素过多

E. 非类固醇类抗感染药物的使用

14. 以下关于胃溃疡的描述是正确的除了

A. 在大部分病人中,幽门螺杆菌的发现与慢性胃溃疡有关

B. 在许多胃溃疡发病中,非类固醇类抗感染药物是重要病因

C. 慢性胃炎与慢性消化道溃疡有很大关系

D. 通过内镜检查可容易区分癌和消化道溃疡

E. 出血、穿孔是消化道溃疡的并发症

15. 下列哪种玻璃样团块存在于酒精性肝炎病人的肝实质细胞胞质中

A. Councilman 小体　　　　B. Negri 小体　　　C. Mallory 小体

D. Achoff 小体　　　　　　E. Lupus 小体

16. 缩窄性心包炎最可能引起肝的哪种组织学表现

A. 大结节性肝硬化　　　　B. 门管区淋巴细胞浸润　　　C. 胆管增生

D. 窦状隙的扩大　　　　　E. Mallory 小体

17. 下面哪种关于慢性肝炎的说法是正确的?

A. 急性肝炎有 5% ~ 10% 可发展为慢性肝炎

B. 急性肝炎组织学上的特点是有碎片状坏死

C. 慢性肝炎组织学上的特点是完整的肝小叶界板

　　　D. 药物所致的慢性肝炎在部分病人体内可在血浆出现自身抗体

　　　E. 慢性肝炎病毒携带者发展为肝硬化

18. 哪种肝肿瘤与使用口服避孕药有关

　　　A. 胆管的腺瘤　　　　　　B. 胆管的错构瘤　　　　　C. 局灶结节性增生

　　　D. 肝细胞癌　　　　　　　E. 肝细胞腺瘤

19. 酒精性肝损伤的病人组织学上最典型的特征性是

　　　A. 小叶中肝细胞大量坏死伴有大量的 Councilman 小体

　　　B. 门管区明显的慢性炎症并有肝小叶的轻度损伤

　　　C. 脂肪变性、Mallory 透明小体、小叶中央纤维化、伴显著的中性粒细胞的小叶炎性
　　　　　细胞浸润

　　　D. Mallory 透明小体、含丰富嗜酸细胞的炎性渗出、并有大量 Councilman 小体

　　　E. 肝静脉血栓形成导致静脉流出受阻

20. 下列哪种说法准确地描述了不同的病毒性肝炎的主要的感染或传染途径

　　　A. A 型肝炎是通过非肠道传播　　　　B. B 型肝炎是通过非肠道传播

　　　C. C 型肝炎是通过消化道传播　　　　D. D 型肝炎是通过消化道传播

　　　E. E 型肝炎是通过非肠道传播

21. 发展为肝细胞癌风险增加的因素下列除了哪项

　　　A. 酒精相关性硬化　　　　　　　　　B. HBV 相关性硬化

　　　C. 遗传性血色素沉着病相关性硬化　　D. 原发性胆汁性硬化

　　　E. HCV 相关性硬化

22. 在慢性肝炎中可见下列组织病理学特点除了哪项

　　　A. 门管区的炎症　　　　　　B. 桥接坏死　　　　C. 纤维组织间隔

　　　D. 碎片状坏死　　　　　　　E. 肝静脉的血栓形成

（二）问答题

1. 什么是食管静脉曲张？

2. 什么是 Barrett 食管？

3. 什么可以引起食管梗阻？

4. 食管可以发生什么样的恶性上皮性肿瘤？

5. 描述肉眼及镜下食管鳞状上皮肿瘤的特征。

6. 食管鳞癌的好发部位是哪里？

7. 描述食管癌的扩散方式。

8. 胃糜烂和胃溃疡的区别是什么？

9. 描述消化道溃疡的镜下表现。

10. 胃和十二指肠溃疡的并发症有哪些？

11. 影响胃癌的发病率的因素有哪些？

12. 什么是早期胃癌？

13. 胃癌的好发部位是什么？

14. 胃癌是怎样扩散的？

15. 什么叫类癌？

16. 什么是结肠息肉？

17. 什么是结直肠癌的 Duke 分期？

18. 癌胚抗原与结肠癌有什么关系？

19. 哪些因素可诱发消化性溃疡？

20. 慢性胃炎的类型有哪些？

21. 幽门螺旋杆菌引起消化性溃疡的机制是什么？

22. 慢性肝炎的病理学特征？

23. 解释并描述肝硬化.

24. 发生在肝细胞的坏死类型有哪些？

25. 什么是原发性胆汁性肝硬化？其病理特点是什么？

26. 肝脏可能会发生哪些肿瘤？

27. 请描述 Zollinger-Ellison 综合征。

Chapter 8　Diseases of the Digestive System

<table>
<tr><td>

Gross Findings
1. Chronic atrophic gastritis
2. Chronic gastric ulcer
3. Duodenal ulcer
4. Squamous Cell Carcinoma of esophagus
5. Adenocarcinoma (early gastric cancer)
6. Carcinoid tumor, Stomach
7. Adenocarcinoma of colon
8. Fulminant hepatitis
9. Fatty liver
10. Portal cirrhosis
11. Postnecrotic Cirrhosis
12. Biliary cirrhosis
13. Esophageal varices
14. Splenomegaly
15. Hepatocellular carcinoma

</td><td>

Micro Findings
1. Chronic atrophic gastritis
2. Gastric ulcer
3. Squamous Cell Carcinoma, Esophagus
4. Adenocarcinoma (early gastric cancer, ulcer malignant change) of Stomach
5. Signet ring cell carcinoma, Stomach
6. Carcinoid tumor, Stomach
7. Adenocarcinoma, Colon
8. Fulminant hepatitis
9. Liver cirrhosis
10. Hepatocellular carcinoma

</td></tr>
</table>

Gross Findings

1. Chronic atrophic gastritis　The mucosa thinned and rugal folds flattened the blood vessels distincted under mucosa.

2. Chronic gastric ulcer

(1) Brief Descriptions：Cause: imbalance between the mucosal defense mechanisms and the damaging forces (gastric acid and pepsin; H. pylori).

(2) Gross Findings：Sharply demarcated ulcer edges with granulation tissue in ulcer base.

3. Duodenal ulcer　Duodenal ulcer is smaller and superficial, or multiulcer. Other characteristics are same as gastric ulcer.

4. Squamous Cell Carcinoma of esophagus

(1) Brief Descriptions

1) Occur in adults over age 50.

2) Male-female ratio: 2 :1 to 20 :1.

3) Risk factors: dietary, lifestyle, esophageal disorders, genetic predisposition.

(2) Gross Findings：Gross types including medullary form, fungoid form, ulcerating form, and constrictive form.

Grayish white in cut surface.

5. Adenocarcinoma (early gastric cancer)

(1) Brief Descriptions

1) A carcinoma limited to the mucosa or to the mucosa and submucosa only, irrespective of whether or not metastasis to lymph nodes has occurred.

2) Two groups: intramucosal and submucosal.

3) Not synonymous with carcinoma in situ.

(2) Gross Findings: In early gastric carcinoma, tumor in confined to the mucosa and submucosa and may exhibit an exophytic, flat or depressed, or excavated conformation.

6. Carcinoid tumor, Stomach

(1) Brief Descriptions

1) In the mucosa of the G-I tract, there are scattered endocrine cells which synthesize, store, and secret biogenic amines or peptides participating in coordinate gut function. The tumor arise from these cells are designated as carcinoid tumor.

2) The appendix is the most common site of gut carcinoid tumor, followed by the small intestine, rectum, stomach and ileum.

3) Carcinoid tumor are potentially malignant and the tendency of malignant behavior correlate with the site of origin, the depth of local penetration and the size of the tumor.

(2) Gross Findings

1) The tumor appear as intramural or submucosal masses that creat small, polypod or plateau-like elevations rarely more than 3 cm in diameter.

2) The overlying mucosa may be intact or ulcerated.

7. Adenocarcinoma of colon

(1) Brief Descriptions

1) Malignant epithelial tumor of colon.

2) Most colorectal carcinomas are located in sigmoid colon and rectum.

3) Gross types including ulcerating form, projection form, infiltrating form.

4) The percentage of the tumor showing formation of gland-like structure can be used to be defined the grade:

Well-differentiated: > 95% gland-like structure. Moderate-differentiated: 50% ~ 95% gland-like structure. Poor-differentiated: 5% ~ 50% gland-like structure. Undifferentiated: < 5% gland-like structure.

(2) Gross Findings: Polypoid, exophytic or ulcerated tumor masses.

8. Fulminant hepatitis

(1) Brief Descriptions: From onset of hepatic insufficiency to the symptom of hepatic encephalopathy within 2 to 3 weeks.

Hepatitic Viral hepatitis is the main causes.

(2) Gross Findings: Acute massive necrosis or acute submassive necrosis.

9. Fatty liver　The liver is enlargment to 4 ~ 6kg with a soft, greasy, yellow cut surface.

10. Portal cirrhosis

(1) Brief Descriptions: Mainly due to chronic viral hepatitis.

(2) Gross Findings: The size of nodules is more small and regular (micronodular) with fibrosis and regenerated nodules.

11. Postnecrotic Cirrhosis

(1) Brief Descriptions: Cause: alcohol abuse, chronic hepatitis, biliary disease and iron overload. Progressive fibrosis of liver parenchyma. It is generally irreversible.

(2) Gross Findings:Macronodular cirrhosis with marked variation in size and shape of the nodules (3~10mm or larger).

12. Biliary cirrhosis   The liver color is in yellow-green with micronodules.

13. Esophageal varices

(1) Brief Descriptions:Bleeding from esophageal and gastric varices is the most important complication of portal hypertension and cirrhosis; it is associated with a mortality rate of about 50%.

(2) Gross Findings: Under esophageal mucosa dilated venous channels arise as the portal vein communicates with the gastric coronary vein and the esophageal veins.

14. Splenomegaly

(1) Congestive splenomegaly serves as a key sign of portal hypertension.

(2) Spleen weight may increase up to 1000g. Hypersplenism-sequestration of a peripheral blood element decrease and cause cytopenia, with associated reactive bone marrow hyperplasia.

15. Hepatocellular carcinoma

(1) Brief Descriptions:Strongly linked to prevalence of HBV infection.

(2) Gross Findings

1) Well demarcated nodules with necrosis, hemorrhage and bile stained; soft bulging cut surface.

2) Usually paler than the surrounding liver substance.

3) Gross types include massive type, nodular type,and diffuse type.

Micro Findings

1. Chronic atrophic gastritis

(1) Glandular atrophy show the number and size is decreased (partial or complete) with cystical dilatation of glands. Some mucosal flattening.

(2) Chronic inflammatory infiltration include scattered lymphoid aggregates in the mucosa and submucosa.

(3) Metaplasia include in corpus region with pyloric gland metaplasia,in antrum region with intestinal metaplasia.

(4) Partial mucosa display atypical hyperplasia or dysplasia.

2. Gastric ulcer

(1) The ulcer extend at least into the submucosa and often into the muscularis propria.

(2) The ulcer structure including inflammationand exudation,necrosis, granulation and scarring layers

(3) Ulcer crater with inflamed, degenerated and regenerated mucosa at the edge.

3. Squamous Cell Carcinoma, Esophagus

(1) Infiltration of cancer cell nests through whole layers.

(2) Poorly demarcated cell nests from the surrounding stroma.

(3) Well differentiated cells with intercellular bridge and keratin pearl formation and sheets of partially keratinized cells.

4. Adenocarcinoma (early gastric cancer, ulcer malignant change)of Stomach

(1) Neoplastic glands in the edge of the ulcer with fibrinopurulent exudate and necrotic

debris in the ulcer base.

(2) Cancer cells in the edge of the ulcer with irregular arrangement (complicated glandular structure,cribriform gland formation) and exhibiting pleomorphous, hyperchromatic nuclei with some distinct nucleoli.

(3) The neoplastic glands locate in the edge of ulcer and extending to the submucosa

5. Signet ring cell carcinoma, Stomach

(1) Intracytoplasmic mucin resulting in the typical signet ring appearance.

(2) Infiltration of cancer cells through whole layers with occasional glandular formation and mucin pooling.

(3) Extensive fibrosis (desmoplasia) and dense inflammatory infiltration.

(4) Hyperchromatic cancer cells floating in the mucin pools. Tumor invaded into subserosal layer. Signet-ring-like cells with intracytoplasmic mucin pooling and pushing the nuclei to the periphery.

6. Carcinoid tumor, Stomach

(1) Monomorphic cells in trabecular, solid, insular, festoon (ribbon-like), or tubular structures, some small glands with a rosette-like appearance.

(2) Tumor cells have uniform round to oval nuclei and scant to moderate amount of finely granular cytoplasm. Central located nuclei with prominent nucleoli and fine chromatin (salt and pepper).

(3) Rich of vascularity and prominent fibrous stroma.

7. Adenocarcinoma, Colon

(1) Gland-forming with variability in size and configuration.

(2) Large, stratified, hyperchromatic cells with high nuclear/ cytoplasm ratio and mitotic counts. The tumor cells have pleomorphic, vesicular nuclei with some distinct nucleoli. Mitotic figures are noticed.

(3) The tumor arise from epithelial mucosa and extending to the peripheral fatty tissue.

(4) Focal necrosis is noticed.

8. Fulminant hepatitis

(1) Panacinar necrosis by extensive hepatocytes loss. Confluent area of destructed hepatic parenchyma. The normal hepatic architecture is nearly totally destructed.

(2) Regenerative activity of remainder hepatocytes showing neocholangioles with ductile-like structure around portal tracts, partly of bile-duct and partly of hepatocellular origin.

(3) Inflammatory-cell infiltration.

(4) Collapse of the reticular framework.

9. Liver cirrhosis

(1) Fibrosis, The entire liver parenchyma is divided into nodules of variable size. regenerated nodules and complete vascular/microanatomical distortion.

(2) Pseudolobule, in which there are more central veins, portal tract structure or not present, showing regenerating atypia of hepatocytes (multinucleation and hyperchromatism).

(3) The developing fibrous septa are extend through sinusoids from central to portal regions as well as from portal tract to portal tract. Thick or thin fibrous septi with venous radicals, inflammatory cells, bile ducts, vessels, and arteries without normal portal tracts. Dense inflammatory infiltrate in the fibrous septae segregated liver parenchyma.

（4）Areas of fatty change of hepatocytes are also seen.

10. Hepatocellular carcinoma

（1）Tumor cells have eosinophilic cytoplasm and round, vesicular nuclei with distinct nucleoli.

（2）Arranged in plates or trabeculae, Or arranged in acinar pattern and solid pattern usually several cell thick, and separated by sinusoidal channels which have an endothelial and very scanty reticulin, but no Kupffer cells.

（3）Tumor cell showing granular or clear cytoplasm（glycogen in cytoplasm）. Sometimes pleomorphic or multinucleated giant tumor cells.

（4）Vascular invasion.

Others:Alfa-fetoprotein is of great diagnostic value.

Study Questions

Choose Tests

Directions：**Each of the numbered items or incomplete statements in this section is followed by answers or by completions of the statement. Select the one lettered answer or completion that is best in each case.**

1. Which type of esophagitis is the most common?
   A. Reflux   B. Viral   C. Fungal
   D. Acute corrosive   E. Chronic granulomatous

2. An organism that is discovered（and appears to play a causative role）in many cases of chronic nonspecific gastritis and chronic peptic ulcer disease is
   A. Enterobacter cloacae   B. Escherichia coil   C. Helicobacter pylori
   D. Klebsiella pneurnoniae   E. Citrobacter freundii

3. Hirschsprung's disease usually is caused by the congenital absence of ganglion cells in which segment of the large intestine?
   A. Cecum   B. Ascending colon   C. Transverse colon
   D. Descending colon   E. Rectum

4. The most common site of gastrointestinal carcinoid tumors is
   A. small bowel   B. colon   C. appendix
   D. esophagus   E. stomach

5. Reflux esophagitis is characterized by
   A. inappropriately increased lower esophageal sphincter pressure.
   B. the development of Barrett's epithelium in some chronic cases.
   C. more frequent development of squamous cell carcinoma（SCC）rather than adenocarcinoma.
   D. the lack of potential for stricture development.
   E. a high frequency of associated acute esophagitis.

6. Ménétrier's disease is characterized by
   A. thickened gastric folds, mucous cell hyperplasia, hypoproteinemia and protein-losing enteropathy
   B. thickened gastric folds related to infiltration by lymphoma
   C. the presence of numerous Helicobacter pyloriorganisms

    D. thickened gastric folds related to signet-ring cell adenocarcinoma

    E. loss of gastric folds related to chronic atrophic gastritis

7. Which colorectal polyp is considered to be nonneoplastic?

    A. Tubulovillous adenoma   B. Villous adenoma

    C. The polyps of familial adenomatous polyposis(FAP)

    D. Hyperplastic polyp   E. Leiomyoma

8. Which statement about pseudomembranous enterocolitis is true? It

    A. is caused by the enterotoxin of Clostridium perfringens.

    B. causes constipation.

    C. is usually associated with a recent history of antibiotic use and ulceration in bowel wall.

    D. is characterized histologically by transmural chronic inflammation.

    E. is an uncommon proliferative colitis.

9. The definition of early gastric cancer (EGC) requires

    A. a tumor smaller than 2cm in diameter

    B. a patient with symptoms for less than 2 years

    C. no lymph node involvement

    D. tumor invasion no further than the submucosa

    E. a tumor with a raised macroscopic appearance

10. A biopsy performed on a gastric ulcer reveals adenocarcinoma. When a partial gastrecto-my is performed, it reveals invasive, moderately differentiated adenocarcinoma extending into, but not beyond, the submucosa. One of five regional lymph nodes is positive for metastatic adenocarcinoma. Which statement about adenocarcinoma is true?

    A. This case is unusual because squamous cell carcinoma (SCC) is the most common histologic type of gastric carcinoma.

    B. This patient will most likely die of her disease within 5 years.

    C. By definition, this patient has advanced gastric carcinoma (AGC).

    D. The size of the gastric carcinoma, rather than the degree of mural invasion, is the most important factor pertaining to patient prognosis.

    E. This patient has early gastric carcinoma.

11. Features of colonic adenomas that are associated with an increased risk for carcinoma in-clude all of the following EXCEPT

    A. severe dysplasia   B. villous architecture   C. size exceeding 2cm

    D. marked inflammation   E. multiple adenomas

12. All of the following statements about colorectal carcinoma are true EXCEPT

    A. it is the major common cause of cancer deaths in the nowadays.

    B. the peak incidence is in the seventh decade.

    C. adenocarcinoma is more common than squamous cell carcinoma (SCC).

    D. only a minority of colorectal carcinomas arise in the setting of inflammatory bowel disease(IBD).

    E. chromosomal abnormalities are rarely encountered in colorectal carcinoma.

13. All of the following factors appear to predispose to chronic peptic ulcers EXCEPT

    A. colonic diverticula   B. blood group O

    C. Helicobacter pylori infection

    D. excessive gastrin secretion in the Zollinger-Ellison syndrome

    E. nonsteroidal antiinflammatory drugs (NSAIDs)

14. All of the following statements about gastric ulcers are true EXCEPT

    A. Helicobacter pylori is found in association with chronic peptic ulcers of the stomach in the majority of patients.

    B. nonsteroidal antiinflammatory drugs (NSAIDs) appear to be important in the pathogenesis of many gastric ulcers.

    C. chronic gastritis is often found in association with chronic peptic ulcers.

    D. carcinoma is easily distinguished from benign peptic ulcers on macroscopic (endoscopic) inspection.

    E. bleeding and perforation are all potential complications of peptic ulcer disease.

15. Which hyaline masses are often seen in the cytoplasm of hepatocytes in patients with alcoholic hepatitis?

    A. Councilman bodies   B. Negri bodies   C. Mallory's bodies

    D. Achoff's bodies   E. Lupu's bodies

16. Constrictive pericarditis is most likely to proce which histologic finding in the liver?

    A. Macronodular cirrhosis   B. Portal lymphocytic infiltrate

    C. Bile duct proliferation   D. Sinusoidal dilatation

    E. Mallory's body

17. Which statement regarding chronic hepatitis is correct?

    A. Hepatitis A progresses to chronic hepatitis in 5% ~ 10% of cases.

    B. Chronic persistent hepatitis is characterized histologically by the presence of piecemeal necrosis.

    C. Chronic active hepatitis is characterized histologically by an intact limiting plate.

    D. Autoantibodies are detected in the serum of some patients with drug-induced chronic hepatitis.

    E. Chronic viral hepatitis virus carriers often progresses to cirrhosis.

18. Which liver tumor is most commonly associated with the use of oral contraceptives?

    A. Bile duct adenoma   B. Bile duct hamartoma

    C. Focal nodular hyperplasia   D. Hepatocellular carcinoma

    E. Hepatocellular adenoma

19. Which histologic description is most typically seen in patients with alcoholic liver injury?

    A. Massive centrilobular hepatocyte necrosis with numerous Councilman bodies.

    B. Prominent portal chronic inflammation with minimal damage to the hepatic lobule.

    C. Steatosis, Mallory's hyalin, centrilobular fibrosis, and a lobular inflammatory infiltrate with a conspicuous component of neutrophils.

    D. Mallory's hyalin, an inflammatory infiltrate rich in eosinophils, and many Councilman bodies.

    E. Thrombosis of the hepatic veins causing venous outflow obstruction.

20. Which statement accurately describes the primary route of transmission of the various forms of acute viral hepatitis?

    A. Hepatitis A is transmitted by the parenteral route.

    B. Hepatitis B is transmitted by the parenteral route.

C. Hepatitis C is transmitted by the fecal-oral route.

D. Hepatitis D is transmitted by the fecal-oral route.

E. Hepatitis E is transmitted by the parenteral route.

21. Conditions that are viewed as significantly increasing the risk for developing hepatocellular carcinoma include all of the following Except

A. alcohol-related cirrhosis

B. hepatitis B virus (HBV)-related cirrhosis

C. genetic hemochromatosis-related cirrhosis

D. primary biliary cirrhosis

E. hepatitis C virus (HCV)-related cirrhosis

22. Histopathologic features that are often found in chronic active hepatitis include all of the following EXCEPT

A. portal inflammation   B. bridging necrosis   C. fibrous tissue septa

D. piecemeal necrosis   E. hepatic vein thrombosis

Questions

1. What are oesophageal varices?

2. What are Barrett's oesophagus?

3. What are the causes of oesophageal obstruction?

4. What types of malignant epithelial tumour occur in the oesophagus?

5. Describe the macroscopic and microscopic appearances of squamous cell turnouts of the oesophagus.

6. Which are the most common sites of origin of squamous carcinomata of the oesophagus?

7. Describe the spread of carcinoma of the oesophagus.

8. What is the difference between a gastric erosion and a gastric ulcer?

9. Describe the microscopic appearance of a chronic peptic ulcer.

10. What are the complications of chronic gastric and duodenal ulceration ?

11. What factors appear to influence the occurrence of gastric cancer?.

12. What is meant by the term early gastric cancer?

13. From which common sites do gastric carcinoma arise?

14. How does gastric cancer spreads?

15. What is a carcinoid tumour?

16. Define a colonic polyp.

17. What is meant by Duke's classification of colorectal cancers?

18. What is the relation of carcinoembryonic antigen to carcinoma of the colon?

19. What factors predispose to the development of chronic peptic ulceration?

20. What types of chronic gastritis are recognised?

21. What is the mechanism by which H. pylori causes peptic ulceration?

22. What is the pathology of chronic hepatitis?

23. Define and describe cirrhosis of the liver.

24. What patterns of necrosis occur in the hepatocyte?

25. What is primary biliary cirrhosis and what are its pathological features?

26. What tumours may be found in the liver?

27. Describe the Zollinger-Ellison syndrome.

第九章 造血及淋巴系统疾病

大体观察

1. 霍奇金淋巴瘤,淋巴结
2. 恶性淋巴瘤
3. 慢性白血病

镜下观察

1. 霍奇金淋巴瘤,淋巴结
2. 滤泡性淋巴瘤
3. 弥漫性大 B 细胞淋巴瘤
4. 伯基特淋巴瘤
5. 恶性淋巴瘤(间变性大细胞性),胃
6. 郎格罕细胞组织细胞增生症,软组织

一、大体观察

1. 霍奇金淋巴瘤,淋巴结

(1) 简要说明

1) 霍奇金淋巴瘤的形态学特征是出现与众不同的肿瘤性巨细胞,R-S 细胞,引起反应性淋巴细胞,组织细胞和粒细胞的积聚。

2) 分类:结节型淋巴细胞为主型和经典型,后者又分为结节硬化型,混合细胞型,淋巴细胞为主型,淋巴细胞减少型。

(2) 大体所见:增大的和有包膜的淋巴结切面均质呈新鲜鱼肉状。

2. 恶性淋巴瘤　淋巴结肿大,切面为均质状鱼肉状,多个淋巴结融合。

3. 慢性白血病　肝脏增大,变硬,包膜增厚。切面呈暗红色,结构紊乱,可见不规则的梗死灶。

二、镜下观察

1. 霍奇金淋巴瘤,淋巴结

(1) 结构消失,被异源性细胞浸润。

(2) 中等量的 R-S 细胞,霍奇金细胞,陷窝细胞,干尸样的细胞。

(3) 背景:良性的小淋巴细胞,组织细胞。

(4) 轻度间质纤维化和一些胶原带(尤其沿着血管分布)。

(5) R-S 细胞

1) 典型的 R-S 细胞

体积大(直径 15~45μm),双核或分叶状核,双核细胞常呈镜影样。

核:双核或多核,有大的,包涵体样的,枭眼样的核仁,大约有小淋巴细胞样大小(5~7μm),周围常有透亮的空晕。胞浆:丰富,嗜双色性。

2）变异的 R-S 细胞

a. 单核变异的霍奇金细胞　单个圆形或椭圆形核,有大的包涵体样的核仁。

b. 陷窝细胞　皱褶或分叶状的核,周围有丰富、淡染的胞浆,在切片制作中胞浆收缩,使细胞好像位于一个空腔中,多见于结节硬化型。

c. 变异的淋巴细胞和组织细胞(LH 细胞)　息肉样的核类似爆米花,核仁不明显,适度的丰富的胞浆。常见于淋巴细胞为主型。

d. 干尸样细胞　LH 细胞或 R-S 细胞的退化。细胞体积大,深染的嗜酸性胞浆,致密的固缩核。

2. 滤泡性淋巴瘤

(1) 滤泡结构,其中为中心细胞和中心母细胞。

(2) 肿瘤性 B 细胞比正常的淋巴细胞大,有不规则的裂隙状核,以明显的核皱褶为特征。核染色质粗糙,浓染,核仁明显。核分裂象少。

3. 弥漫性大 B 细胞淋巴瘤

(1) 肿瘤细胞包括中心母细胞,免疫母细胞,浆母细胞和中心细胞。

(2) 弥漫生长不形成滤泡结构。

4. 伯基特淋巴瘤

(1)"星空样"细胞弥漫浸润。大量良性的巨噬细胞摄取凋亡的肿瘤细胞形成"星空状"。

(2) 中等大小的淋巴细胞:圆形或卵圆形的核,染色质粗糙,多个核仁,中等量的嗜碱性胞浆。

(3) 大量核分裂象。

5. 恶性淋巴瘤(间变性大细胞性),胃

(1) 黏膜层和黏膜下层被淋巴瘤细胞弥漫浸润。

(2) 多形性大的淋巴瘤细胞。

1) 核的外形有很大的变异,可见一些多核的瘤巨细胞。马蹄形或肾形或类似多核的 R-S 细胞。

2) 分散的染色质,多个明显的核仁,丰富的胞浆。

(3) 非典型性有丝分裂象多见。

(4) 定义:间变性大细胞淋巴瘤是一种 T 细胞淋巴瘤,包括淋巴样细胞。

(5) 肿瘤细胞的细胞膜和高尔基区 CD30 和 EMA 阳性。

(6) 中度侵袭性肿瘤。

6. 朗汉斯细胞组织细胞增生症,软组织

(1) 增生的朗汉斯细胞直径 10~15μm,核凹陷、皱褶、分叶状(肾形)。染色质细腻,核仁不明显,核膜薄。中等量丰富的胞浆,轻微的嗜酸性。

(2) 背景:嗜酸粒细胞,组织细胞,中性粒细胞,淋巴细胞。可见嗜酸性微脓肿形成。

(3) 灶性坏死和水肿。坏死和微脓肿形成,嗜酸粒细胞显著浸润。

(4) 定义:朗汉斯细胞组织细胞增生症是朗汉斯细胞的肿瘤性增殖,表达 CD1a, S-100 蛋白,超微结构检查存在伯贝克(Birbeck)颗粒。

（5）同义词：组织细胞增生症 X，朗汉斯细胞肉芽肿。

（6）临床类型：莱特勒－西韦病（Letterer-Siwedisease），汉－许－克病（Hand-Schuller-Christian-disease），孤立的嗜酸性肉芽肿。

三、思 考 题

（一）选择题

选一个字母代表的最合适答案。

1．一名 36 岁男病人诉，2 周来有紫癜和牙龈出血。体检：苍白，体温 39℃。这个临床表现与哪种疾病一致

    A．慢性淋巴细胞白血病   B．急性淋巴细胞白血病   C．慢性骨髓白血病

    D．急性骨髓白血病   E．感染性单核细胞增多症

2．下列有关人类急性白血病的病因都正确除了

    A．病毒   B．射线辐射   C．抗生素   D．抗肿瘤药   E．苯化合物

（二）问答题

1．什么情况会引起血液中嗜酸粒细胞增多？

2．什么是组织细胞增生症？

3．怎么理解淋巴瘤？

4．非霍奇金淋巴瘤（NHL）如何分类？

5．请描述 R-S 细胞。

6．霍奇金淋巴瘤如何分期？有什么意义？

7．霍奇金淋巴瘤如何分型？

8．请描述蕈样霉菌病。

Chapter 9　Disorders of Hematopoietic and Lymphoid System

<table>
<tr><td>

Gross Findings

1. Hodgkin lymphoma, Lymph node
2. Malignant lymphoma
3. Chronic leukemia

</td><td>

Micro Findings

1. Hodgkin lymphoma, Lymph node
2. Follicular lymphoma
3. Diffuse large B cell lymphoma
4. Burkitt lymphoma
5. Malignant lymphoma (anaplastic large cell), Stomach
6. Langerhans cell histiocytosis, Soft tissue

</td></tr>
</table>

Gross Findings

1. Hodgkin lymphoma, Lymph node

(1) Brief Descriptions

1) Hokgdin lymphoma is characterized morphologically by the presence of distinctive neoplastic giant cells, RS cells, which induce the accumulation of reactive lymphocytes, histiocytes, and granulocytes.

2) Classification: Nodular lymphocyte redominant Hodgkin lymphoma and Hodgkin lymphoma, the latter including Nodular sclerosis, Mixed cellularity, Lymphocyte predominance, Lymphocyte depletion.

(2) Gross Findings: Enlarged and encapsulated lymph noeds with homogeneous fish flesh cut surface.

2. Malignant lymphoma　Lymphadenopathy, homogeneous fish flesh on cut surface, multinodular confluent.

3. Chronic leukemia　Liver is enlarged and firm with cupsule thicken. Cut surface shows dark red with the structure disorder and irregular infarct lesions.

Micro Findings

1. Hodgkin lymphoma, Lymph node

(1) Diffuse effacement of lymph nodes by a heterogeneous cellular infiltrate.

(2) Moderate amount of RS cells, hodgkin cells, lacunar cells, mummified cells.

(3) Background: benign-looking small lymphocytes, histiocytes.

(4) Mild interstitial fibrosis and a few bands of collagen (especially along vessels).

(5) Reed-Sternberg cell (RS cell).

1) Classic RS cell : Large (15~45μm), binucleate or bilobed, with the two halves often appearing as "mirror-image" of each other. Nucleus: may be multiple or multilobate, contains large,

inclusion-like, owl-eyed nucleoli, generally surrounded by a clear halo, that are about the size of a small lymphocyte ($5 \sim 7 \mu m$). Cytoplasm: abundant amphophilic.

2）Variants of RS cells

a. Mononuclear variants Hodgkin cells. A single round or oblong nucleus with a large inclusion-like nucleolus.

b. Lacunar variants ：Folded or multilobate nuclei surrounded by abundant pale cytoplasm which distrupted during the cutting of sections, leaving the nucleus sitting in an empty hole. Predominant in nodular sclerosis type.

c. Lymphocytic and histiocytic variants (L H cells).

Polypoid nuclei resembling popcorn kernels, inconspicuous nucleoli, and moderately abundant cytoplasm. Specific to the lymphocyte predominance subtype.

d. Mummified cells：Degenerate L+H cells or RS cells. Large cell with darkly staining eosinophilic cytoplasm and a dense pyknotic nucleus.

2. Follicular lymphoma

（1）Follicular structure with centercyte and centerblast.

（2）The neoplastic B cells are large than normal lymphocytes with a irregular cleaved nuclear contour,characterized by prominent nuclear infoldings. Nuclear chromatin is coarse and condensed and nucleoli are instinct. Mitosis are infrequent.

3. Diffuse large B cell lymphoma

（1）tumor cells include centroblast and immunoblast plasmablast and centercyte.

（2）Diffuse grow without follicular structure.

4. Burkitt lymphoma

（1）Diffuse monotonous infiltration with a "starry sky" pattern. Numerous benign macrophages that have ingested apoptotic tumor cell→"stars".

（2）Intermediate-sized lymphoid cells: round or oval nuclei with coarse chromatin, several nucleoli, and a moderate amount of basophilic cytoplasm.

（3）Mitotic figures are numerous.

5. Malignant lymphoma (anaplastic large cell), Stomach

（1）Gastric mucosa and submucosa are diffusely infiltrated by lymphoma cells.

（2）Pleomorphism large lymphoma cells:

1) Great variability in nuclear appearance. Some multinucleated tumor giant cells are found. horseshoe-or kidney-shaped (hallmark cells) or are multinucleated resembling RS cells.

2) Dispersed chromatin, multiple prominent nucleoli, abundant cytoplasm.

（3）Atypical mitotic figures are numerous.

（4）Definition: Anaplastic large cell lymphoma is a T-cell lymphoma consisting of lymphoid cells.

（5）The tumor cells are positive for CD30 and EMA on the cell membrane and in the Golgi region.

（6）Moderately aggressive tumor.

6. Langerhans cell histiocytosis, Soft tissue

（1）Proliferation of Langerhans cells $10 \sim 15m$, grooved, folded, indented, or lobulated nuclei (kidney-shaped). Fine chromatin, inconspicuous nucleoli and thin nuclear membranes. Cytoplasm: moderately abundant and slightly eosinophilic.

(2) Background: eosinophils, histiocytes, neutrophils, lymphocytes. Eosinophilic microabscess formation is noticed.

(3) Focal necrosis and edema.

Necrosis and microabscess formation with predominant eosinophils infiltrates

(4) Definition: Langernans cell histiocytosis is a neoplastic proliferaion of Langerhans cells, with expresion of CD1a, S-100-protein, and the presence of Birbeck granules by ultrastructural examination.

(5) Synonymys: Histiocytosis X, Langerhans cell granulomatosis.

(6) Clinical variants: Letterer-Siwe disease, Hand-Schuller-Christian disease, and solitary e-osinophilic granuloma.

Study Questions

Choose Tests

Directions: Each of the numbered items or incomplete statements in this section is followed by answers or by completions of the statement. Select the one lettered answer or completion that is best in each case.

1. For 2 weeks, a 36-year-old man has complained of purpura bleeding of the gnms. On examination he is pale and his temperature is 39℃. This clinical picture is compatible with
   A. Chronic lymphocytic leukemia (CLL)   B. Acute lymphocytic leukemia (ALL)
   C. Chronic myelogenous leukemia (CML)   D. Acute myelogenous leukemia (AML)
   E. infectious mononucleosis

2. All of the following etiologic associations with human acute leukemia have been proved valid EXCEPT
   A. viruses   B. irradiation   C. antibiotics
   D. antineoplastic drugs   E. benzene compounds

Questions

1. What conditions are associated with blood eosinophilia?
2. What is Histiocytosis X (or the histocytoses)?
3. What do you understand by lymphoma?
4. How are non-Hodgkin's lymphomata(NHL) classified?
5. Describe the Reed-Sternberg cell.
6. How is Hodgkin's lymphoma (HL) staged and what is the significance?
7. How is Hodgkin's lymphoma classified?
8. Describe mycosis fungoides.

第十章 免疫性疾病

大体观察	镜下观察
Kaposis 肉瘤,皮肤	1. 狼疮性肾小球肾炎
	2. 硬皮病
	3. Kaposis 肉瘤,皮肤
	4. 放线菌病,舌
	5. 巨细胞病毒感染肾
	6. 脑念珠菌病
	7. 肺曲菌病

一、大 体 观 察

Kaposis 肉瘤,皮肤

(1) 简要说明:慢性淋巴结病,移植相关,艾滋病相关。

(2) 大体所见

1) 多个红紫色的皮肤斑块或结节。

2) 无症状的,局限在皮肤和皮下组织。

二、镜 下 观 察

1. 狼疮性肾小球肾炎 肾小球局灶性和节段性内皮细胞肿胀,系膜细胞增生,中性粒细胞浸润,纤维蛋白沉积,毛细血管血栓,免疫复合物沉积在内皮下。

2. 硬皮病,皮肤 血管周围淋巴细胞浸润,毛细血管和小动脉受损,部分阻塞,水肿,胶原纤维变性。进行性皮肤纤维化,血管透明变性增厚。

3. Kaposis 肉瘤,皮肤

(1) 肿瘤中有淋巴细胞和扩张的血管。

(2) 肿瘤细胞呈相对温和的梭形细胞,排列成不明显的束状。

(3) 细胞被含有血细胞的裂隙样血管分隔。

4. 放线菌病,舌

(1) 化脓性炎症,脓肿形成,有一个或多个颗粒(丝状聚集物),直径 30~3000um,其边缘有嗜酸性的棒状丝(Sendore-Hoeppli 物质)。一个巨大的粉红-紫色的颗粒位于脓肿区域。粉红-紫色颗粒(硫磺样颗粒)由周围排列成放射状的丝状的放线菌组成,边缘围绕着淋巴细胞。

(2) 细菌染色显示颗粒由微小的分支状的革兰阳性菌丝组成,直径 1um,随意地排列成无定形的基质中。

5. 巨细胞病毒感染肾

（1）巨细胞病毒感染的肾小管上皮细胞呈典型的牛眼样外观。胞质内或核内包涵体在小管中。

（2）嗜碱性包涵体周围是透亮的空晕——牛眼样外观。

（3）间质可出现炎症。在肾实质中有灶性集中的炎症性浸润。

其他：机会性感染：唾液腺，肾，肝，肺，胰腺，甲状腺，肾上腺，脑可经常发生。

6. 脑念珠菌病

（1）脓肿形成，边缘有增生的神经胶质细胞围绕。一些结节结构在脑实质中。

（2）念珠菌可见于脓肿壁附近的急性和慢性炎细胞中。结节结构由坏死碎屑和炎症细胞组成。

（3）有许多酵母菌形状和丝状的真菌位于坏死区域。芽孢型酵母菌型的真菌单行排列，彼此相邻，类似（假性菌丝）。

7. 肺曲菌病

（1）真菌的菌丝呈球状聚积在破坏的肺实质中。

（2）肺泡腔内有大量的炎症细胞浸润。

（3）真菌的菌丝：狭窄（3~5mm），分离的，分支状，锐角分支。

（4）中心出血，周围有坏死的碎屑。坏死的碎屑中能发现真菌的成分。

其他描述：

（1）特殊染色：GMS 或 PASD。

（2）感染导致许多不同形式的疾病，取决于组织和宿主的反应程度。

三、思 考 题

（一）选择题

选一个字母代表的最合适答案。

1. 下列哪种自身抗体在硬皮病中最特异？

　A. 抗核因子抗体　　　　　B. 抗多种胶原抗体　　　　　C. 双股 DNA 抗体

　D. 组蛋白抗体　　　　　　E. 元素钐的抗体

2. 人类免疫缺陷病毒（HIV）与哪种细胞感染关系密切？

　A. $CD8^+$ T 细胞　　　　　B. $CD4^+$ T 细胞　　　　　C. 自然杀伤细胞

　D. 树突状细胞　　　　　　E. B 细胞

3. 下列哪项是描述系统性红斑狼疮？

　A. 器官损害主要由自然杀伤细胞介导

　B. 自身抗体受自身双链 DNA 抗体的限制

　C. 病情与补体 C2 和 C4 的缺陷有关

　D. 免疫复合物沉积较少

　E. 临床疾病的形式有限

4. 哪个自身抗体对干燥（Sjögren）综合征有特异性？

A. 抗核抗体　　　　B. 抗-Scl-70　　　　C. 抗 SS-B　　　　D. 抗 JO-1　　　　E. 抗 Sm

5. 着丝粒抗体与哪项有关
　　A. 系统性红斑狼疮　　　　B. 干燥(Sjögren)综合征　　　　C. 渐进性硬皮病
　　D. 多肌炎　　　　E. CREST 综合征

6. 先天性胸腺发育不全(DiGeorge)综合征包括以下特征除了
　　A. 低钙血症　　　　B. 手足抽搐　　　　C. 无胸腺
　　D. 无浆细胞　　　　E. 无甲状旁腺

7. 移植肾的活检显示血管有纤维化坏死。是由于下列哪项免疫机制引起?
　　A. 细胞介导的细胞毒性　　　　B. 抗体-补体介导的损伤　　　　C. CD8 介导的损伤
　　D. 自然杀伤细胞介导的细胞毒性　　　　E. Ⅳ型超敏反应

8. 肝移植中,损伤引起淋巴细胞性炎症直接针对
　　A. 胆管和微血管　　　　B. 肝细胞　　　　C. Kupffer 细胞
　　D. Ito 细胞　　　　E. 窦状小管

9. 接受肾移植的患者在术后 48 小时无尿。进行活检,发现小管内无刷状缘,细胞核缺失,管形形成。没有其他改变。病人这种情况最可能的病因是什么?
　　A. 急性细胞排斥　　　　B. 过急性排斥　　　　C. 慢性排斥
　　D. 急性小管坏死　　　　E. 疾病复发

10. 肾活组织切片的标本显示肾小球的内皮下有电子致密物的沉积是下列哪种病变的特点
　　A. 快速进行性肾小球肾炎　　　　B. 链球菌感染后肾小球肾炎
　　C. 膜性肾小球肾炎　　　　D. 系统性红斑狼疮
　　E. Goodpasture 综合征

11. 除了哪项都是 Sjögren 综合征的特点
　　A. 泪腺和唾液腺增大　　　　B. 形成肌上皮岛　　　　C. 与风湿性关节炎有关
　　D. 转移至局部淋巴结　　　　E. 可发展为恶性淋巴瘤

(二) 问答题
1. 什么是机会性感染?
2. 什么是 Kaposis 肉瘤?
3. HIV 病毒感染的特点和结果是什么?
4. 艾滋病患者可能发生哪些肿瘤?
5. 移植物抗宿主反应的机制是什么?
6. 移植排斥反应如何影响移植肾?
7. 请描述与慢性排斥反应有关的供体肾的组织学改变。
8. Down 综合征的原因是什么?
9. 巨细胞病毒感染的基本特点是什么?
10. 什么是 Sjögren 综合征?

Chapter 10　Diseases of Immunity

Gross Findings	Micro Findings
Kaposis sarcoma, Skin	1. Lupus glomerulonephritis
	2. Scleroderma
	3. Kaposis sarcoma, Skin
	4. Actinomycosis, Tongue
	5. Cytomegalovirus (CMV) infection, Kidney
	6. Candidasis, Brain
	7. Aspergillosis, Lung

Gross Findings

Kaposis sarcoma, Skin
(1) Brief Descriptions
Chronic, lymphadenopathic, transplant-associated, AIDS-associated.
(2) Gross Findings
1) Multiple red-to-purple skin plaques or nodules.
2) Asymptomatic and localized to the skin and subcutaneous tissues.

Micro Findings

1. Lupus glomerulonephritis　Focal and segmental glomerular swelling with endothelial and mesangial proliferation neutrophil infiltration, fibrinoid deposits, capillary thromb and i immune complex substances deposit in subendothelial.

2. Scleroderma　There are perivascular lymphocytic infiltrates with capillary and arteriolat injury and partial occlusion, edema and collagen fiber degeneration. Progressive dermal fibrosis and vascular hyaline thickening.

3. Kaposis sarcoma, Skin
(1) Circumscribed by lymphocytes and ectatic vessels.
(2) Tumor cells are relatively bland spindle cells arranged in ill-defined fascicles..
(3) Cells are separated by slit-like vessels containing erythrocytes.

4. Actinomycosis, Tongue
(1) Suppurative inflammation with abscess formation that contain one or more granules (organized aggregates of filaments), 30 to 3000 um in diameter, that are bordered by eosinophilic, club-like (Sendore-Hoeppli materials) filaments. A large, pink-purple granule within abscess area The pink-purple granule (sulfur granule) is composed of filamentous Actinomycetes with radial arrangement at periphery and surrounded by a rim of lymphocytes.
(2) Bacterial stain reveal that the granules are composed of delicate, branched, Gram-posi-

tive filaments, 1. um diameter, haphazardly arranged in an amorphous matrix.

5. Cytomegalovirus (CMV) infection, Kidney

(1) CMV-infected renal tubular epithelial cell with typical bull-eye appearance. Intracytoplasmic or intranuclear inclusion in tubule.

(2) Basophilic inclusion surrounded by a clear halo—bull eye appearance.

(3) Interstitial inflammation may present. There are foci of concentrated inflammatory infiltrate in renal parenchyma.

Others: Opportunistic infection. Salivary gland, kidney, liver, lung, pancreas, thyroid, adrenal gland, brain are frequently affected.

6. Candidasis, Brain

(1) Abscess formation surrounded by a rim of gliosis. Several nodular structures within brain parenchyma.

(2) Candida are seen among acute and chronic inflammatory cells near the abscess wall. The nodular structures are composed of necrotic debris and inflammatory cells.

(3) There are many yeast-form and filamentous-form fungal organisms within necrotic area. The sprouting yeast-form fungi aligned in single array side-by-side resembling filemantous structure with hyphae (pseudohyphae).

7. Aspergillosis, Lung

(1) Accumulation of fungal hyphae as a fungal ball in the destructed lung parenchyma.

(2) Cavitation with densely inflammatory infiltration.

(3) Fungal hyphae: narrow (3~5mm), separated, dichotomous, acute branching angle.

(4) Hemorrhagic center surround by necrotic debris. Fungal element can be found in necrotic debris.

Others:

(1) Special stains: GMS. or PASD.

(2) Infection produces several different pattern of disease, depending on the degree of tissue reaction and host reaction.

Study Questions

Choose Tests

Directions: Each of the numbered items or incomplete statements in this section is followed by answers or by completions of the statement. Select the one lettered answer or completion that is best in each case.

1. Which autoantibody is most specific for scleroderma?

    A. Antinuclear antibody   B. Antibodies to various collagens

    C. Antibody to double-stranded DNA   D. Antibody to histone

    E. Antibody to Sm

2. Human immunodeficiency virus (HIV) has a special affinity for infecting which type of cell?

    A. CD8$^+$ T cell   B. CD4$^+$ T cell   C. Natural killer (NK) cell

    D. Dendritic cell   E. B cell

3. Which statement describes systemic lupus erythematosus (SLE)?

    A. Organ damage is predominantly mediated by natural killer (NK) cells.

    B. Autoantibodies are restricted to antibodies, against native double-stranded DNA.

    C. The condition is associated with deficiencies of complement components C2 and C4.

    D. Immune complex deposition is sparse.

    E. The patterns of clinical disease are very limited.

4. Which autoantibody is highly specific for Sjögren's syndrome?

    A. Antinuclear antibody (ANA)   B. Anti-Scl-70   C. Anti-SS-B

    D. Anti-JO-1   E. Anti-Sm

5. Antibody to centromere is associated with

    A. systemic lupus erythematosus (SLE)   B. Sjögren's syndrome

    C. progressive scleroderma   D. polymyositis

    E. CREST syndrome

6. DiGeorge syndrome involves all of the following features EXCEPT

    A. hypocalcemia   B. tetany   C. absent thymus

    D. absent plasma cells   E. absent parathyroid glands

7. A biopsy of a renal allograft shows fibrinoid necrosis of small vessels. Which one of the following immune mechanisms is most likely at work?

    A. Cell mediated cytotoxicity

    B. Antibody and complement mediated damage

    C. CD8 mediated damage

    D. Natural killer cell mediated cytotoxicity

    E. Type Ⅳ hypersensitivity

8. In hepatic allografts, the damaging lymphocytic inflammation is directed against

    A. bile ducts   B. hepatocytes   C. Kupffer cells   D. Ito cells   E. sinusoids

9. A renal allograft recipient fails to produce urine after 48. hours. A biopsy is performed. Tubules show loss of brush border, loss of nuclei, and tubular cast formation. There are no other changes. What is the most likely etiology for this patient's "primary nonfunction"?

    A. Acute cellular rejection   B. Hyperacute rejection

    C. Chronic rejection   D. Acute tubular necrosis (ATN)

    E. Recurrent disease

10. A kidney biopsy specimen that shows subendothelial granular electron-dense deposits is characteristic of which disease state?

    A. Rapidly progressive glomerulonephritis

    B. Poststreptococcal glomerulonephritis

    C. Membranous glomerulonephritis

    D. Systemic lupus erythematosus (SLE)

    E. Goodpasture's syndrome

11. Characteristics of Sjögren's syndrome include all of the following EXCEPT

    A. swelling of the lacrimal and salivary glands

    B. formation of epimyoepithelial islands

    C. association with rheumatoid arthritis

    D. metastasis to regional lymph nodes

    E. development of malignant lymphoma

Questions

1. What is an opportunistic infection?
2. What is Kaposi's sarcoma?
3. What are the nature and consequences of infection with the HIV virus?
4. What types of neoplasm are encountered in AIDS?
5. What is the mechanism of the graft versus host (GVH) reaction?
6. What forms of graft rejection affect a transplanted kidney?
7. Describe the histological changes in the donor kidney associated with chronic rejection.
8. What is the cause of Down's syndrome?
9. What are the essential features of cytomegalovirus infection?
10. What is Sjögren's syndrome?

第十一章　泌尿系统疾病

一、大　体　观　察

1. 快速进行性肾小球肾炎(RPGN)

(1) 简要说明

1) 伴有严重肾小球损伤的综合征,没有明确病因。

2) 伴有严重少尿的肾功能衰竭,在数周至数月内死亡。

(2) 大体所见:肾脏体积增大,苍白色,肾脏表面可见皮质下出血。

2. 慢性肾小球肾炎

(1) 简要说明

1) 慢性肾小球肾炎是各型肾小球肾炎的最终阶段。

2) 这些肾炎类型包括:链球菌感染后肾小球肾炎、快速进行性肾小球肾炎、膜性肾小球肾炎、局灶性肾小球硬化、膜增生性肾小球肾炎等。

(2) 大体所见:肾脏体积减小,表面呈细颗粒状,皮质变薄。

3. 硬化性肾小球肾炎(固缩肾)

(1) 简要说明:可发生于各种肾小球疾病的终末阶段。

(2) 大体所见:由于弥漫性肾小球玻璃样变性伴有肾小管萎缩以及间质纤维化,肾脏体积缩小、质地变硬(固缩肾),肾脏表面呈细颗粒状,患者慢性肾功能衰竭。

4. 慢性肾盂肾炎

(1) 简要说明

1) 肾盂肾炎:一种肾脏的感染,主要累及肾小管、肾间质和肾盂。慢性肾盂肾炎的病变更加复杂,细菌感染、膀胱尿道反流以及尿道阻塞都与其发病有关。

2）慢性小管间质性炎症和肾盂、肾盏的瘢痕形成。

（2）大体所见：肾盏外形不规则，可见瘢痕。

5. 肾细胞癌

（1）简要说明

1）肿瘤来源于肾小管上皮细胞，吸烟是最重要的危险因素。好发于老年男性。

2）典型症状：血尿、腰痛和肿块。

3）肾癌分型：透明细胞癌（70%~80%），颗粒细胞型，混合型。

（2）大体所见

1）肾脏皮质的不规则突出的肿块，膨胀性生长压迫周围肾脏实质形成假包膜。

2）切面常见出血、坏死、囊性变，呈灰白色或黄色。

6. 肾鳞状细胞癌

（1）简要说明

1）肿瘤细胞聚集成有显著的巢状浸润灶，周围由成纤维细胞或纤维间质包绕。

2）和肾结石有关。

（2）大体所见：灰白色，体积较大、实性、乳头状、境界不清的肿块。切面可见出血和坏死。

7. 膀胱移行细胞癌

（1）简要说明

1）好发于男性。

2）多见于吸烟和长期暴露于工业致癌物的人群中。

3）临床表现为血尿和腰痛。

（2）大体所见：从单纯乳头状到结节状，扁平状，也可以是混合型。

二、镜　下　观　察

1. 快速进行性肾小球肾炎（RPGN）（新月体性肾小球肾炎）

（1）Bowman 囊内细胞大量的增生（新月体形成），累及多数的肾小球，迅速出现肾功能衰竭。

Bowman 囊内新月体形成，从局灶阶段性壁层上皮细胞增生到弥漫性新月体形成环绕 Bowman 囊。

（2）细胞、纤维细胞或纤维性新月体。一些肾小球硬化。

（3）早期肾小管无明显病变，尔后肾小管萎缩，纤维化或瘢痕形成，肾小管内可见透明管型。

（4）间质水肿伴有单核细胞浸润。也可表现出血和间质的慢性炎症反应。

2. 结节性肾小球硬化

（1）肾小管：Armanni-Ebstein 改变（肾小管上皮细胞之间出现糖原沉积）。

（2）间质的病变取决于是否有感染。

（3）肾小球：血管球的系膜细胞和内皮细胞区出现均质、伊红染色、球状结节。毛细血管分布于周边。

（4）弥漫性毛细血管内肾小球硬化：伊红染的膜基质增多。

（5）球囊小滴：Bowman 囊出现伊红染小滴。

（6）纤维帽：血管球的毛细血管襻的内腔出现嗜伊红染、蜡状的脂质沉积。

3. 固缩肾

（1）广泛的肾小球硬化，一些肾小球的硬化是球性的。

（2）周围肾小球萎缩和间质纤维化。

（3）动脉出现硬化。

4. 慢性肾盂肾炎

（1）在瘢痕区，肾小管上皮细胞萎缩扩张，其中含有均质、嗜伊红染的管型，形似甲状腺组织。炎症反应轻微。

（2）肾小球变化多样：Bowman 囊增厚，囊外纤维化，血管球萎缩、硬化和玻璃样变性，增生性改变和坏死。

（3）间质的慢性炎性浸润和不同程度的纤维化。在非瘢痕区，肾小球和血管显示缺血性改变。

5. 肾细胞癌

（1）透明细胞：由于胞浆富含脂质和糖原而透明。细胞境界清晰，细胞之间结合紧密。

（2）颗粒细胞：由于含有大量线粒体而使胞浆内出现大量粉红色颗粒。

（3）细胞排列成片状、巢状、条索状和腺管状或乳头状，背景含有丰富的毛细血管，被纤维组织所分割。

（4）细胞和核的多形性小，核分裂象少。

（5）坏死、纤维化、胆固醇沉积（可以出现异物反应）、出血、钙化或囊性变。

6. 肾鳞状细胞癌

（1）肿瘤细胞聚集成有突起的巢状浸润灶，周围由成纤维细胞或纤维间质包绕。

（2）肾肿瘤伴有过度角化（层状伊红染的物质），注意鉴别正常肾实质和肾盂移行上皮细胞的鳞状上皮化生（缺乏异型增生）。角化的鳞癌细胞伴有边缘浸润。注意扩张的肾小管其上皮细胞萎缩。

7. 肾脏 Wilm 瘤　　通常包含三种成分：胚基、间质和上皮细胞。

其他特点包括：10%是双侧或多发性。相对孤立，境界清楚的肿块。胚基型最多见。

多数为卵圆形或圆形的深染的癌细胞，胞浆少。一些病例可见梭形细胞伴有嗜酸性间质提示间质的分化。局灶的腺腔形成提示上皮细胞分化。

8. 膀胱移行细胞癌

乳头型或非乳头型

乳头型（外生病灶）：中间为纤维血管轴心，其外分布有多层肿瘤细胞，呈菜花状。

非乳头型：光滑或轻微突起的病灶伴有广泛的浸润。

其他：根据 WHO 分级：

1 级：细胞层次增加，显示一定的异型性。

2 级：细胞层次增加，有可见核分裂象。癌细胞多形、深染，失去极性，但仍可以辨认出移行上皮起源。

3级:很多肿瘤细胞显示间变,浅层上皮细胞显示松散和分离。出现瘤巨细胞。局灶的鳞状上皮或腺上皮化生。

三、思 考 题

（一）选择题

选一个字母代表的最合适答案。

1. 脂性肾病的特点是肾小球中哪种成分超微结构的改变

    A. 内皮层   B. 上皮层   C. 肾小球膜   D. 血管   E. 基底膜

2. 下面哪种准确地描述了膜性肾小球病的特点?

    A. 它是引起儿童肾病综合征的常见原因

    B. 受累病人常可出现急性肾衰

    C. 病理学特点的描述是"弥漫性增生性肾小球肾炎"

    D. 对类固醇激素的治疗效果较好

3. 细菌可通过哪种途径到达肾引起慢性非阻塞性肾盂肾炎

    A. 血流   B. 淋巴液   C. Batson 丛   D. 膀胱输尿管反流   E. 动静脉短路

4. 患有链球菌感染后肾小球肾炎的病人的免疫荧光标记的肾组织可见

    A. 颗粒状 IgG 沉积   B. IgG 线状沉积   C. IgA 颗粒状沉积

    D. 链球菌抗原的线状沉积   E. 链球菌抗原的颗粒状沉积

5. 患有肾细胞癌的病人哪种说法是正确的

    A. 在早期有临床症状

    B. 在大多数的病人出现血尿、侧腹的疼痛、侧腹的肿块

    C. 组织病理学的特点是透明细胞癌

    D. 很少发生转移,当出现转移时也局限在肾周

    E. 肾细胞癌的肉眼形态学经常表现为实体的灰白色的肿瘤;脂质成分很少

6. 一位病人在医生办公室主诉有血尿。外科医生选择用膀胱内镜检查作为诊断病情的一种方法。在检查中发现膀胱的左侧壁有许多 3mm 的病灶,决定取活组织检查,然后将标本送外科病理实验室诊断。关于这种病变的哪种病理描述对病人诊断有提示作用

    A. 肿瘤乳头有七层上皮细胞

    B. 有明显多形性核细胞的乳头浸润达骨骼肌深部

    C. 固有膜层有致密的炎症改变了正常尿道上皮的排列,形成息肉样团块

    D. 伴有中等多行性核的肿瘤乳头局限于黏膜内

    E. 弥漫性膀胱腺炎

7. 下面的哪项不是肾病综合征的临床特点

    A. 蛋白尿   B. 低血清白蛋白血症   C. 红细胞减少

    D. 高血脂   E. 水肿

8. 下面关于感染后弥漫性毛细血管性肾小球肾炎的描述哪项不正确

    A. A 组 β 溶血性链球菌感染后可引起该病

B. 在电子显微镜下可见到大的免疫复合物沉积在上皮下

C. 组织学上表现为弥漫增生性肾小球肾炎

D. 临床表现为急性肾炎

E. 主要累及儿童可进展到慢性肾衰

9. 除了哪项都可引起肾盂积水

A. 慢性肾静脉血栓　　　　B. 大的子宫平滑肌瘤　　　　C. 肾结石

D. 良性前列腺增生　　　　E. 输尿管的乳头状移行细胞癌

（二）问答题

1. 什么是肾小球肾炎？

2. 肾小球肾炎的分类。

3. 肾小球肾炎的临床进展怎样？

4. 肾小球肾炎的病因有哪些？

5. 肾小球肾炎中免疫复合物是如何检测的？它们分布在哪里？

6. 什么是轻微病变性肾炎？

7. 请描述肺出血-肾炎综合征中肾脏的病变。

8. 请对肾脏的原发性肿瘤进行分类。

9. 请描述肾腺癌的大体及镜下特点。

10. 请描述肾母细胞瘤的大体及镜下表现。

11. 什么是肾盂肾炎？

12. 诱发肾盂肾炎的因素有哪些？

13. 请描述急性肾盂肾炎的病理变化。

14. 什么是慢性肾盂肾炎？

15 膀胱肿瘤的大体表现是什么？

16. 请描述膀胱肿瘤的镜下表现。

Chapter 11   Diseases of the Kidney and Its collecting System

Gross Findings

1. Rapidly progressive glomerulonephritis (RPGN)

(1) Brief Descriptions

1) A syndrome associated with severe glomerular injury and does not denote a specific etiologic form of glomerulonephritis.

2) Loss of renal function associated with severe oliguria and death from renal failure within week to months.

(2) Gross Findings: The kidney is enlarged and pale, often with petechial hemorrhages on the cortical surface. s.

2. Chronic glomerulonephritis

(1) Brief Descriptions

1) Chronic glomerulonephritis is best considered an end-stage pool of glomerular disease fed by a number of streams of specific types of glomerulonephritis.

2) Poststreptococcal GN, rapidly progressive GN, membranous GN, focal glomerulosclerosis, membranoproliferative GN, ···etc. chronic GN.

(2) Gross Findings: Small, firm kidney with granular subcapsular surface. and narrowed cortex.

3. Sclerosing glomerulonephritis(Contracted kidney)

(1) Brief Descriptions: It may be caused by many types of glomerular diseases at their end-stage.

(2) Gross Findings: Owing to histologically diffuse glomerular hyalinization with tubular atrophy and interstitial fibrosis, The kidneys are small and contracted (Small-sized kidney), with granular appearance of external surface. The patients present with chronic renal failure.

4. Chronic pyelonephritis

(1) Brief Descriptions

1) Pyelonephritis: an infection of the kidney which affects tubules, interstitium, and renal pelvis.

Chronic pyelonephritis is a more complex disorder: bacterial infection, vesicoureteral reflux, obstruction are involved in its pathogenesis.

2) Chronic tubulointerstitial inflammation and renal scarring are associated with pathologic involved of the calyces and pelvis.

(2) Gross Findings: Scars are seen overlying a blunted or deformed calyx.

5. Renal cell carcinoma

(1) Brief Descriptions

1) Tumors arise from tubular epithelial cells; Tobacco is the most prominent risk factor; often in older; preponderance in men.

2) Classic symptoms: hematuria, loin pain and mass.

3) Classification of RCC: clear cell type (70% to 80%); granular cell type and mixed type.

(2) Gross Findings

1) Protruding from renal cortex, as an irregular, bosselated mass, expansile growth with compressing adjacent renal parenchyma into a pseudocapsule.

2) Cut surface often hemorrhagic, grayish white to yellow, and cystic change or necrosis.

6. Squamous cell carcinoma of kidney

(1) Brief Descriptions

1) Infiltration of tumor cells with a spiky or angular outline which are surrounding by a fibro-blastic or fibrous stroma.

2) Related to renal stone.

(2) Gross Findings: Large, solitary, papillary, ill-circumscribed mass with grey -white color. Necrosis and hemorrhage is in cut surface.

7. Transitional cell carcinoma of bladder

(1) Brief Descriptions

1) Male predominance.

2) Most common in order individuals and tobacco and industrial carcinogen exposure are risk factors.

3) Symptoms and signs including hematuria and flank pain.

(2) Gross Findings: Varied from purely papillary to nodular, or flat pattern, even mixed architecture.

Micro Findings

1. Rapidly progressive glomerulonephritis (RPGN) (crescentic glomerulonephritis)

(1) Massive proliferation of cells (crescent formation) in Bowman's space, affecting a high percentage of glomeruli, and quickly develop renal failure.

Crescent on the inside of Bowman's capsule, from a focal and segmental accumulation of a few cells lining Bowman's capsule to extensively circumferential involvement.

(2) Cellular, fibrocellular or fibrotic crescent. Some glomerulus demonstrates sclerosing change.

(3) Minimal change in tuft and tubules in early stage, then tubular atrophy, fibrosis and scarring in progressive patients. Hyaline casts in renal tubules.

（4）Edematous interstitium with mononuclear cells infiltration. Or hemorrhagic and chronic inflamed stroma.

2. Nodular glomerulosclerosis

（1）Tubules: Armanni-Ebstein change（glycogen deposits within tubular epithelial cells）.

（2）Variable change of interstitium depending on infection or not.

（3）Glomeruli: Acellular, homogeneous, eosinophilic, globular nodules in the mesangial or intercapillary region of a glomerular tuft with capillary displaced to the periphery.

（4）Diffuse intercapillary glomerulosclerosis: increasing eosinophilic mesangial matrix materials.

（5）Capsular drop: eosinophilic small nodules on Bowman's capsule.

（6）Fibrin cap: eosinophilic, waxy, fatty structure within the lumen of one or more capillary loops of glomerular tufts.

3. Contracted kidney

（1）Extensive global sclerosis of glomeruli. Some glomeruli are totally sclerosis.

（2）Surrounding tubular atrophy and interstitial fibrosis.

（3）Vascular change with arteriosclerosis.

4. Chronic pyelonephritis

（1）In scared areas, dilated, atrophic tubules lined by atrophic epithelium and containing homogeneous eosinophilic casts likened to thyroid tissue（thyroidization）, and with scant inflammation in these areas.

（2）The glomeruli show very variable changes: thickening of Bowman's capsule, fibrosis outside the capsule, collapse or solidification of tuft, sclerosis or hyalinosis of tuft, proliferative change and necrosis.

（3）Chronic inflammatory infiltration in interstitium and variable degree of fibrosis.

In non-scarred tissue, the glomeruli and vessels may show ischemic change.

5. Renal cell carcinoma

（1）Clear cell:Clear cytoplasm due to high contain of lipid & glycogen. Prominent cell borders and tightly adherent to neighboring cells.

（2）Granular cell: pink granular cytoplasm due to high content of mitochondria.

（3）Arrange in sheets, nests, cords, tubular or papillary pattern with a fine capillary vascular background, and separated by fibrous septi.

（4）Little cellular or nuclear pleomorphism or mitosis.

（5）Necrosis, fibrosis, cholesterol deposit（may with foreign body reaction）, hemorrhage, calcification or cystic change.

6. Squamous cell carcinoma, kidney

（1）Infiltration of tumor cells with a spiky or angular outline which are surrounding by a fibroblastic or fibrous stroma.

（2）Renal tumor with extensive keratinization（layered eosinophilic materials）;note differentiated between normal renal parenchyma and squamous metaplasia of renal pelvic transitional epithelium（lack of dysplasia）. Keratinized squamous cancer cells with infiltrating borders; note dilated atrophic ducts.

7. Wilms' tumor, Kidney

Classic triphasic components: blastemal.,stromal, epithelial cell type.

Others:10% are bilateral or multiple.

Relatively solitary well-circumscribed mass. The most are Blastemal type.

Most are oval to round hyperchromatic cancer cells with scanty cytoplasm. Some area shows more spindle cells type with eosinophilic stroma indicating stromal differentiation. Focal glandular formation is seen toward epithelial differention.

8. Transitional cell carcinoma of bladder

Papillary and non-papillary type:In papillary type (exophytic lesion): a thin core of fibro-vascular tissue covered by layers of tumor cells, like a molded cauliflower.

In non-papillary type: a smooth or slightly bulging lesion with extensive invasion.

Others:

According to WHO grading system:

Grade 1: increase in number of layers of cells showing some atypia.

Grade 2: The number of layers of cells increased, as in the number of mitosis. Cancer cells show pleomorphism, hyperchromatism, and loss of polarity but are still recognizable as of transitional origin.

Grade 3: Many of the tumor cells show anaplastic change with loosening and fragmentation of the superficial layers of the cells. Giant cancer cells may be present. Focal squamous or glandular metaplasia.

Study Questions

Choose Tests

Directions: Each of the numbered items or incomplete statements in this section is followed by answers or by completions of the statement. Select the one lettered answer or completion that is best in each case.

1. Lipoid nephrosis of the kidney characteristically produces ultrastructural changes in which renal glomerular element?

   A. Endothelium   B. Epithelium   C. Mesangium

   D. Blood vessels   E. Basement membrane

2. Which statement best characterizes membranous glomerulopathy?

   A. It is the most common cause of nephrotic syndrome in children

   B. Affected patients usually present with acute renal failure

   C. The characteristic pathology is best described as "diffuse proliferative glomerulonephritis"

   D. Electron microscopy demonstrates numerous subepithelial immune-type deposits

   E. It usually is responsive to steroid therapy

3. In most cases of nonobstructive chronic pyelonephritis, bacteria reach the kidney via

   A. the bloodstream   B. the lymphatics   C. Batson's plexus

   D. vesicoureteral reflux   E. aberrant arteriovenous shunts

4. An immunofluorescence-stained kidney speci- men from a patient with poststreptococcal glomerulonephritis is likely to show

   A. granular deposits of immunoglobulin G (IgG)

   B. linear deposits of IgG

   C. granular deposits of IgA

D. linear deposits of streptococcal antigen

E. granular deposits of streptococcal antigen

5. Which statement is true of a patient with renal cell carcinoma?

   A. Clinical presentation is usually at an early stage

   B. The combination of hematuria, flank pain, and flank mass is found in the majority of patients

   C. The classic histopathology is that of clear cell carcinoma

   D. Metastases are rare and, when present, are usually confined to the perirenal area

   E. The gross morphology of renal cell carcinoma is usually that of a solid gray-white tumor, indicating its low lipid content

6. A patient presents at the physician's office complaining of intermittent hematuria. As a Board certified urologist, the physician elects to perform a cystoscopic examination as part of this patients evaluation. He sees several 3-mm exophytic lesions in the left lateral wall of the bladder, decides to biopsy them, then sends them to the surgical pathology laboratory for expert evaluation. Which pathologic description of these lesions would be most ominous for the patient's prognosis?

   A. Papillary tumor lined by seven layers of cytologically bland epithelium

   B. Papillary groups with marked nuclear pleomorphism infiltrating through skeletal muscle

   C. Dense inflammation of lamina propria lifting normal-appearing urothelium and forming polypoid mass

   D. Papillary tumor with moderate nuclear pleomorphism confined to the mucosa

   E. Extensive cystitis glandularis

7. All of the following clinical features are likely to be found in nephrotic syndrome EXCEPT

   A. proteinuria   B. hypoalbuminemia   C. red cell casts

   D. hyperlipidemia   E. edema

8. All of the following statements regarding postinfectious glomerulonephritis are true EXCEPT

   A. the disease follows infection with group A β-hemolytic streptococci

   B. large subepithelial immune-type deposits are seen by electron microscopy

   C. the histologic picture is that of diffuse proliferative glomerulonephritis

   D. the clinical picture is characteristic of acute nephritis

   E. most affected children progress to chronic renal failure

9. All of the following are causes of hydronephrosis EXCEPT

   A. chronic renal vein thrombosis   B. large uterine leiomyoma

   C. renal calculi   D. benign prostatic hypertrophy

   E. papillary transitional cell carcinoma of the ureter

Questions

1. What is glomerulonephritis?

2. Classify the glomerulonephritides.

3. How do the glomerulonephritides usually behave?

4. What are the causes of the glomerulonephritides?

5. How are the immune complexes which occur in the glomerulonephritides detected in the kidney and where are they localised?

6. What is minimal change disease?

7. Describe the glomerulonephritis of Goodpasture's syndrome.

8. Classify the primary tumors of the kidney.

9. Describe the macroscopic and microscopic features of a renal adenocarcinoma.

10. Describe the macroscopic and microscopic appearances of a nephroblastoma.

11. What is pyelonephritis?

12. What factors predispose to the development of pyelonephritis?

13. Describe the pathology of acute pyelonephritis.

14. What is chronic pyelonephritis?

15. What is the gross appearance of a vesical tumour?

16. Describe the microscopic appearance of a vesical tumour.

第十二章　生殖系统和乳腺疾病

大体观察

1. 宫颈鳞状上皮原位癌
2. 宫颈鳞状细胞癌
3. 子宫内膜异位
4. 子宫体多发性平滑肌瘤
5. 葡萄胎
6. 侵袭性葡萄胎
7. 绒毛膜癌
8. 输卵管异位妊娠
9. 卵巢子宫内膜异位
10. 卵巢成熟囊性畸胎瘤
11. 卵巢浆液性乳头状囊腺瘤
12. 卵巢黏液性囊腺瘤
13. 前列腺腺癌
14. 乳腺导管内癌(导管原位癌)
15. 浸润性导管癌(乳腺硬癌)
16. 浸润性导管癌(乳腺髓样癌)
17. 乳腺黏液癌(胶样癌)
18. 乳腺湿疹样癌(Paget 病)

镜下观察

1. 宫颈上皮内瘤变Ⅲ级(鳞状上皮原位癌)
2. 宫颈鳞状细胞癌
3. 子宫体鳞状细胞癌
4. 宫内膜癌
5. 子宫内膜葡萄胎
6. 子宫内膜侵袭性葡萄胎
7. 子宫体绒毛膜癌
8. 子宫体腺肌病
9. 卵巢子宫内膜异位
10. 输卵管/卵巢异位妊娠
11. 卵巢成熟性囊性畸胎瘤
12. 前列腺结节状增生
13. 前列腺腺癌
14. 乳腺导管内癌
15. 乳腺浸润性导管癌
16. 乳腺黏液癌
17. 乳腺髓样癌
18. 乳腺 Paget 病

一、大 体 观 察

1. 宫颈鳞状上皮原位癌

(1) 简要说明

1) 人类乳头瘤病毒被认为是宫颈肿瘤形成的重要因素。

2) 角化细胞不典型性:核异形性,核周空泡化→鳞状上皮中上层出现病毒细胞病变效应。

3) 分级

不典型增生:轻、中、重度。宫颈上皮内瘤变(CIN):CINⅠ,Ⅱ,Ⅲ。

鳞状上皮内病变(SIL):低级别和高级别。

(2) 大体所见:黏膜增厚、糜烂或没有明显病变。

2. 宫颈鳞状细胞癌

(1) 简要说明

1）95%鳞状细胞癌(SCC)：角化型(高分化)或非角化型(中等分化)。

2）<5%的SCC：低分化小细胞鳞癌或未分化小细胞癌。

3）子宫体可以被宫颈鳞癌直接侵犯。

（2）大体所见

1）外生型：肿瘤突出于宫颈表面，通常呈息肉状赘生物。

2）内生型：肿瘤浸润周围组织，表面突出不明显，形成溃疡或浸润生长。

3.子宫内膜异位

（1）简要说明

1）定义：子宫肌层出现异位的子宫内膜组织。

2）症状：月经过多或痛经，或无明显临床表现。

（2）大体所见：子宫增大，子宫壁不规则增厚。部分病例子宫肌层中可见红褐色血红蛋白沉着。

4.子宫体多发性平滑肌瘤

（1）简要说明

1）女性最常见的肿瘤，也就是俗称的"纤维瘤"。

2）雌激素依赖性：通常在去势治疗或绝经期后肿瘤消退或钙化，在妊娠期瘤体可迅速增大。

3）原因：未知。

（2）大体所见：单发性或多发性，境界清晰，质地实，灰白色，切面呈漩涡状。

5.葡萄胎

（1）简要说明

1）良性、非侵袭性滋养层细胞疾病(GTD)，以绒毛高度水肿和滋养层细胞增生为特征。

2）多数患者妊娠4到5月时阴道流血。

（2）大体所见

1）子宫较正常月份偏大。

2）子宫腔内充满薄壁、水泡状、葡萄状的结构。

6.侵袭性葡萄胎　绒毛高度水肿，滋养层细胞增生并浸润子宫肌层，伴有出血坏死。

7.绒毛膜癌

（1）滋养层上皮异型性增生形成出血性结节，无绒毛结构。

（2）肿瘤广泛地侵犯血管和纤维间质，造成严重的出血和坏死。

（3）可以转移到肺、肝、脑、骨髓，形成多发性转移性结节，出血性伴坏死。

8.输卵管异位妊娠

（1）简要说明

定义：胚胎植入除子宫正常部位以外的其他组织，输卵管最常见(90%)，少见于卵巢和腹腔。

（2）大体所见：输卵管壶腹部扩张，腔内有陈旧性出血。可见输卵管破裂和出血。

9.卵巢子宫内膜异位

（1）简要说明

定义：子宫内膜腺体和间质出现在子宫以外的其他部位。

部位（按发生率高低）：卵巢，子宫韧带，直肠阴道隔、盆腔腹膜，腹部手术瘢痕，少见于脐、阴道、外阴或阑尾。

症状和体征：不孕、痛经、下腹疼痛等。

（2）大体所见

"巧克力囊肿"：中等大小的薄壁囊肿，内含深紫褐色，半固态的黏稠液体。

10. 卵巢成熟囊性畸胎瘤

（1）简要说明

定义：畸胎瘤是来源于多潜能细胞的真性肿瘤，包含来自一个胚层以上的实质细胞，通常包含三胚层成分。

成熟畸胎瘤是指含有分化成熟的各种组织，囊状，良性肿瘤。

（2）大体所见：单囊或多囊，内含毛发、皮脂等。又称"皮样囊肿"。

11. 卵巢浆液性乳头状囊腺瘤

（1）简要说明

1）这是最常见的卵巢囊性瘤变，占卵巢肿瘤的 30%。

2）有三型：良性、恶性、交界性。

（2）大体所见：较大的囊性病灶，突出于卵巢表面，囊内壁光滑，有乳头状突起，充满清亮浆液。

12. 卵巢黏液性囊腺瘤

（1）简要说明

1）这是一个常见的卵巢肿瘤，占所有卵巢肿瘤的 25%，但是恶性相对不常见。

2）为多灶性肿瘤。

（2）大体所见：肿瘤中形成大小不等的多个囊腔，其中充满黏稠黏液，富含糖蛋白。

13. 前列腺腺癌

（1）简要说明

1）前列腺癌是美国男性最常见的恶性肿瘤。

2）好发于前列腺的外周，但也可发生于移行区。

（2）大体所见

1）灰黄色，境界不清，质硬。

2）肿瘤可以浸润精囊腺和其他盆腔器官。

14. 乳腺导管内癌（导管原位癌）

（1）简要说明

1）定义：导管内癌，未侵犯基底膜。

2）五种组织学类型：粉刺癌、实体癌、筛状癌、乳头状和微乳头状。

（2）大体所见

1）病灶难以确定，硬度轻微增加。

2）点状的坏死物质区（粉刺样）。

15. 浸润性导管癌(乳腺硬癌)

(1)简要说明

1)最常见的乳腺恶性肿瘤。

2)多数起源于乳腺终末导管小叶单位,"导管"或"小叶"并不能说明细胞起源的部位。

(2)大体所见

1)肿瘤组织质地硬如石,收缩,浸润周围的乳腺组织。

2)切面可见肿瘤组织放射状浸润周围实质和脂肪组织(蟹足状)。伴有大量胶原增生。

3)由于导管弹力纤维变性而使切面出现"白粉笔状条纹"。

16. 浸润性导管癌(乳腺髓样癌)

(1)肿瘤组织含有大量肿瘤细胞,因而质地软,境界较清,有时出现周围组织的浸润。

(2)切面显示由肿瘤细胞构成的实质,其中心有坏死。

17. 乳腺黏液癌(胶样癌)

(1)简要说明:浸润性乳腺癌,好发于老年女性,生长较慢。短期预后较好。

(2)大体所见:境界清楚,切面由纤细的间隔分割成胶冻状的肿块。体积较大的肿瘤会发生囊性变。

18. 乳腺湿疹样癌(Paget病) 肿瘤累及乳头和乳晕皮肤,其上开裂溃疡,炎性充血水肿,乳头表现为湿疹样改变。

二、镜 下 观 察

1. 宫颈上皮内瘤变Ⅲ级(鳞状上皮原位癌)

(1)上皮全层出现异形性的细胞,细胞核多形性、染色深。整个鳞状上皮层组织结构显示去分化,表现为极性消失。

(2)基底膜完整,无间质浸润。

2. 宫颈鳞状细胞癌

(1)除了上皮层的病灶以外,癌细胞呈巢状浸润深层间质。

(2)肿瘤细胞多形性,核浆比增大,核分裂象增多,出现病理性核分裂象。细胞核染色深,核仁明显。显示肿瘤细胞的异形性。

(3)出现血管侵犯。间质中有炎症细胞浸润。

3. 子宫体鳞状细胞癌

(1)癌巢中有大的上皮样细胞,浸润子宫肌层。

(2)肿瘤细胞的核呈空泡状,核仁明显,核分裂象增多。

4. 宫内膜癌

大部分子宫内膜癌是腺癌,子宫内膜样的腺癌分为三级:

1级分化良好,腺体结构清晰可见。

2级分化中等,腺体组织结构较好,其中混有实性片状的恶性细胞。

3级分化很差,特征是实性片状的癌细胞中很难有可辨认的腺体结构,核的异型性很大,有丝分裂活跃。

大约20%的内膜癌伴有灶性鳞状上皮的化生,称为腺棘皮癌,鳞化上皮恶变时称为腺鳞癌。如前所述,子宫内膜癌的亚型,类似于卵巢的浆液性癌,这种成分大约占有子宫内膜癌的20%,不论组织结构怎样,乳头样浆液性癌和透明细胞癌都归于Ⅲ级。

5. 子宫内膜葡萄胎

(1) 绒毛高度水肿

(2) 绒毛疏松、黏液样,无或仅有发育不良的绒毛血管。

(3) 滋养层细胞增生成片状或团块状。

(4) 严重的出血。

其他描述:

(1) 完全性葡萄胎:几乎全部的绒毛水肿,弥漫性的滋养层细胞增生。

(2) 部分性葡萄胎:一些绒毛水肿,灶性滋养层细胞增生。

6. 子宫内膜侵袭性葡萄胎　水肿的绒毛间质,滋养层细胞增生呈片状或团块状,浸润子宫肌层,引起出血和坏死。

7. 子宫体绒毛膜癌

(1) 滋养层细胞异形增生,无绒毛。

(2) 侵犯血管和纤维间质。

(3) 严重的出血和坏死。

8. 子宫体腺肌病

(1) 异位的子宫内膜组织呈巢状分布在子宫肌层之间,有梭形细胞组成的间质将其与平滑肌束分隔。

(2) 子宫内膜巢必须在子宫内膜和肌层交界处下一个低倍镜视野以上(2~3mm)。

其他描述:

异位的子宫内膜组织(包括腺体和内膜间质)出现在子宫肌层内:腺肌病。

异位的子宫内膜组织出现在子宫以外:子宫内膜异位。

9. 卵巢子宫内膜异位　具有以下三个特征中的两个:内膜腺体和内膜间质,在卵巢实质中有陈旧性出血,可见吞噬有含铁血黄素的巨噬细胞,可以形成囊状病灶(巧克力囊肿)。

10. 输卵管/卵巢异位妊娠

(1) 在输卵管腔或卵巢间质中出现血凝块和绒毛。

(2) 绒毛和滋养层细胞(淡染的间质轴心,外层被覆合体滋养层细胞,内曾被覆细胞滋养层细胞)。

(3) 输卵管异位妊娠时,管壁增厚,出血。

其他:

输卵管妊娠并发破裂是一种临床急症。

11. 卵巢成熟性囊性畸胎瘤

(1) 外胚层:囊状病灶被覆皮肤,含有皮脂腺和毛囊。

(2) 中胚层:纤维和脂肪组织。

(3) 内胚层:甲状腺组织,含有大小不一的成熟的甲状腺滤泡。

12. 前列腺结节状增生

(1) 结节含有增生的腺体和纤维平滑肌间质。

（2）增生的腺上皮形成不规则乳头,但仍包含两层细胞(高柱状上皮和扁平的基底细胞)。

（3）纤维平滑肌间质,包含梭形间质细胞和结缔组织。

（4）腺腔含有分泌物。

13. 前列腺腺癌

（1）不规则、紧密排列的腺体内含有乳头,疏松的筛状或融合的腺样结构,弥漫性浸润在前列腺组织中。

（2）增大的、不规则的、深染或泡状的细胞核,含有显著的核仁和粗糙的染色质。

其他:根据腺体分化以及肿瘤在间质中的生长方式分级。

14. 乳腺导管内癌

（1）扩张的导管基底膜完整,异形增生的上皮细胞阻塞管腔。

（2）一些导管的中央出现坏死物。

（3）筛状生长方式:粉刺癌表现为导管内增生的肿瘤细胞伴有中央坏死物。

（4）肿瘤细胞:细胞松散,异形,核分裂象增多,肿瘤细胞形态一致,缺乏正常的肌上皮细胞。

（5）肿块不易确定,局灶坏死。

15. 乳腺浸润性导管癌

（1）肿瘤细胞多形,核深染。浸润乳腺组织直达周围脂肪组织。

（2）肿瘤细胞排列成条索、片状、巢状或单个细胞排列成不规则的导管。

（3）致密的纤维性间质或促结缔组织增生性间质。

16. 乳腺黏液癌

（1）细胞外的黏液池形成,延伸至邻近组织间隙。

（2）肿瘤细胞岛或单个的肿瘤细胞在黏液池中漂浮。

（3）淡染的黏液形成"黏液湖",其中漂浮着肿瘤细胞岛。

（4）肿瘤细胞呈巢状、筛状或腺样结构。

（5）肿瘤细胞核深染,有些具有明显的核仁。

17. 乳腺髓样癌

（1）肿瘤边界清楚。

（2）大量淋巴细胞浸润。

（3）巨大的多形性肿瘤呈实性、合体样生长,很少间质。

18. 乳腺 Paget 病

（1）肿瘤起源于大的分泌性导管,可累及乳头和乳晕皮肤。

（2）Paget 细胞体积大,高染色质细胞,多形细胞,核周空晕,位于角化的鳞状上皮中。

三、思 考 题

（一）选择题

选一个字母代表的最合适答案。

1. 哪种生殖细胞性肿瘤是最常见的前纵隔恶性肿瘤?

A. 囊性畸胎瘤   B. 胚胎细胞癌   C. 绒癌

D. 精原细胞瘤   E. 内胚窦瘤

2. 关于前列腺肿瘤正确的说法是

A. 它常发生在尿道周围   B. 它与血清绒毛膜促性腺激素的水平上升有关

C. 好发骨转移   D. 许多的前列腺癌是肉瘤   E. 有男性激素的增多

3. 良性结节样增生主要影响哪个前列腺小叶

A. 前叶   B. 后叶   C. 侧叶   D. 中叶

4. 下列哪项是引起男性尿道复发感染的原因

A. 免疫缺陷性疾病   B. 淋病   C. 慢性前列腺炎

D. 肾结石   E. 梅毒

5. 一位 60 岁男性主诉排尿困难。体格检查发现有光滑的、弥漫增大的前列腺腺体。活检发现良性前列腺的肥大。下列哪项可能是出现病人排尿症状的原因

A. 局部神经的浸润   B. 骶神经丛的受压   C. 前列腺组织浸入膀胱壁

D. 尿道受压   E. 尿道上皮的多发性乳头形瘤病

6. 下列除了哪项,关于前列腺癌的说法是正确的

A. 血清酸性磷酸酯酶水平上升   B. 与暴露在环境中的特定的化合物有关

C. 常可发生骨转移   D. 常起源于前列腺的前叶

7. 下列哪种类型的卵巢肿瘤中可发现砂粒体

A. Brenner 肿瘤   B. 生殖细胞性肿瘤   C. 浆液性囊性癌

D. 黏液性囊腺瘤   E. 黏液性囊性癌

8. 在绝经前的妇女最常见的卵巢良性生殖细胞性肿瘤是

A. Brenner 肿瘤   B. 内膜样肿瘤   C. 良性畸胎瘤

D. 黏液性囊腺瘤   E. 囊腺纤维瘤

9. 一个 30 岁女性,子宫内膜活组织检查发现有子宫内膜的增生伴显著慢性子宫内膜炎。这些改变最可能代表下列哪种情况

A. 子宫内膜的癌前病变   B. 黄体生成不足   C. 雌激素过多

D. 是由于子宫内避孕器的作用   E. 内膜癌

10. 一位 40 岁的妇女有卵巢肿块。在手术时在右侧卵巢发现了 5cm 的囊性肿块。在囊肿的表面呈乳头样。下列哪个特点可在浆液性囊腺瘤中区分出交界性肿瘤?

A. 累及另一侧卵巢   B. 累及腹膜   C. 细胞学上不典型性

D. 浸润卵巢基质   E. 砂粒体

11. 一个 35 的妇女在妇产科检查时发现有临床不典型的上皮细胞覆盖在子宫颈。上皮细胞经 Lugol 碘不能着色。阴道的活组织检查发现有宫颈腺体的恶变。这些发现与下列哪个诊断一致?

A. 慢性宫颈炎   B. 尖锐湿疣   C. 宫颈癌

D. 宫颈上皮内的瘤形成   E. 子宫内膜异位症

12. 下列关于绒毛膜癌的说法都是正确的,除哪个

A. 可发生在正常妊娠以后   B. 可引起葡萄胎的发生

C. 由恶性滋养层细胞组成　　　　　D. 用子宫切除和放射治疗

E. 治疗的效果可用人绒毛膜促性腺激素(hCG)的水平进行监测

13. 下列哪个是浸润性乳腺小叶癌的组织学特点？

A. 排列成假腺体　　　　　B. 间质有个别细胞浸润　　　　　C. 乳头样生长

D. 黏液积聚形成黏液池　　　　E. 高细胞性间质伴有不典型的梭形细胞

14. 乳腺腺体的原始结构单位是

A. 小导管　　　　B. 腺泡　　　　C. 窦　　　　D. 小叶　　　　E. 象限

15. 一位女性的一侧乳头出现血性渗出，她最可能发生了

A. 乳头 Pagets 病　　　　　B. 导管内乳头状瘤　　　　　C. 髓样癌

D. 黏液癌　　　　　　　　E. 导管内癌

16. 下列哪项是乳腺癌常见的类型

A. 导管内癌　　B. 髓样癌　　C. 乳头样癌　　D. 黏液癌　　E. 导管浸润癌

17. 诊断小叶原位癌时哪种说法是正确的

A. 要行腋窝淋巴结清扫

B. 可行切除术和放射治疗

C. 在患有一侧乳腺原位癌的病人中有 20% 的病人经过仔细的体格检查可在对侧的乳房发现肿块

D. 病人有很高的风险发展为浸润性的乳腺癌

E. 在绝经前的女性这种病变不多见

18. 目前，引起 50 岁以上的妇女死亡的最常见原因是

A. 白血病　　　　B. 心肌梗死　　C. 乳腺癌　　　　D. 肺癌　　　　E. 宫颈癌

19. 除了哪项都是影响乳腺癌病人预后的重要因素

A. 病人的年龄　　　　　B. 肿瘤的组织学类型　　　　C. 肿瘤中出现雌激素受体

D. 出现转移　　　　　　E. 局限在乳腺

20. 除了哪项都可能是青少年发生男子乳腺发育的原因

A. 小叶增生　　　　　B. 外源的雌激素　　　　C. 一些睾丸肿瘤

D. 青春期　　　　　　E. 肝硬化

(二) 问答题

1. 什么是子宫内膜异位症和子宫腺肌病？

2. 子宫体癌主要的临床及病理特征是什么？

3. 子宫颈常见的恶性肿瘤有哪些？它们的病因是什么？

4. 请描述对预示子宫颈癌变有意义的组织学表现。

5. 宫颈上皮不典型增生(宫颈上皮内瘤变，CIN)的组织学特点是什么？

6. 发生于卵巢的肿瘤有哪些？

7. 什么是 Meig 征？

8. 哪些肿瘤是胎盘源性的？

9. 什么是葡萄胎？

10. 哪些原因可以引发女性乳房肿块？

11. 最常见的乳房良性肿瘤是什么？请对其进行描述。

12. 乳腺癌的病因有哪些？

13. 请对乳腺癌进行分类。

14. 什么是炎性乳腺癌？

15. 什么是乳头 Paget 病？

16. 什么是雌激素受体以及它们在乳腺癌中的意义是什么？

17. 男性会发生乳腺癌吗？

18. 男性乳房肿大的可能原因有哪些？

19. 男性乳房发育的原因及表现是什么？

Chapter 12   Diseases of the Genital System and Breast

Gross Findings
1. Squamous cell carcinoma in situ of cervix
2. Squamous cell carcinoma of cervix
3. Adenomyosis of uterine corpus
4. Multi leiomyoma, Uterine corpus
5. Hydatidiform mole
6. Invasive mole
7. Choriocarcinoma
8. Ectopic gestation, Fallopian tube
9. Endometriosis, Ovary
10. Mature cystic teratoma, Ovary
11. Serous papillary cystadenoma, ovary
12. Mucinous cystanenoma, ovary
13. Adenocarcinoma of prostate
14. Intraductal carcinoma of breast (Ductal carcinoma in situ.)
15. Infiltrating ductal carcinoma, (Breast scirrhous carcinoma)
16. Infiltrating ductal carcinoma (Breast medullary carcinoma)
17. Mucinous carcinoma, Breast (Colloid carcinoma.)
18. Eczematoid carcinoma of breast (paget's disease)

Micro Findings
1. Intraepithelial neoplasm Grade Ⅲ (Squamous cell carcinoma in situ)
2. Squamous cell carcinoma of cervix
3. Squamous cell carcinoma Uterine Corpus
4. Endometrial carcinomas
5. Hydatidiform mole
6. Invasive hydatidiform mole
7. Choriocarcinoma
8. Adenomyosis
9. Endometriosis
10. Ectopic gestation
11. Mature cystic teratoma
12. Nodular hyperplasia of prostate.
13. Adenocarcinoma
14. Intraductal carcinoma
15. Infiltrating ductal carcinoma
16. Mucinous carcinoma
17. Medullary carcinoma of the breast
18. Paget's disease of the breast

Gross Findings

1. Squamous cell carcinoma in situ of cervix

(1) Brief Descriptions

1) Human papilloma virus (HPV) is currently considered and important factor in cervical oncogenesis.

2) Koilocytic atypia: nuclear atypia and perinuclear vacuolization → viral "cytopathic" effect; in the upper and middle lining squamous epithelium.

3) Classification:

Dysplasia: mild, moderate and severe. Cervical intraepithelial neoplasia (CIN): CIN I, Ⅱ, Ⅲ. Squamous intraepithelial lesion (SIL): low-grade and high-grade.

(2) Gross Findings:The mucosa thicken and erosion or no significant lesion.

2. Squamous cell carcinoma of cervix

(1) Brief Descriptions

1) 95% of squamous cell carcinoma (SCC): keratinizing (well-differentiated) or nonkeratinizing (moderately differentiated) patterns.

2) <5% of SCC: poorly differentiated small cell squamous or small cell undifferentiated carcinomas.

3) The uterine corpus can be directly invaded by SCC of cervix.

(2) Gross Findings

1) Exophytic pattern: the tumor grows out from the surface., often as a polypoid excrescence.

2) Endophytic pattern: the tumor infiltrates into the surrounding structures, without much surface. growth, ulcerating or infiltrative patterns.

3. Adenomyosis of uterine corpus

(1) Brief Descriptions

1) Definition: ectopic islands of endometrial tissue in the myometrium.

2) Symptoms: menorrhagia or dysmenorrhea; general and not diagnostic.

(2) Gross Findings: Uterine enlargement and irregular thickening of the uterine wall, with red-brown blood pigmentation within the myometrium in some cases.

4. Multi leiomyoma, Uterine corpus

(1) Brief Descriptions

1) The most common tumors in women and are referred to in colloquial usage as fibroids

2) Estrogen responsive; they regress or even calcify after castration or menopause and may undergo rapid increase in size during pregnancy

3) Cause: unknown

(2) Gross Findings: Solitary or multiple Circumscribed, firm, grayish-white, whirled appearance in cut surface.

5. Hydatidiform mole

(1) Brief Descriptions

1) Benign, noninvasive trophoblastic disease (GTD), characterized by cystic swelling of the chorionic villi with variable trophoblastic proliferation.

2) Most patients present in the fourth or fifth month of pregnancy with vaginal bleeding.

(2) Gross Findings

1) The uterus usually larger than the stage of pregnancy.

2) The uterine cavity is filled with a delicate friable mass of thin-walled, cystic, grape-like structures.

6. Invasive mole   Hydropic swelling of chorionic villi and masses of trophoblasts infiltrate the myometrium with severe hemorrhageand necrosis.

7. Choriocarcinoma

(1) Atipal proliferation of trophoblasts form hemorrhagic nodular without. chorionic villi

(2) Tumor extensively invated vascular and fibrous stroma with severe hemorrhage and necrosis.

(3) Tumor metastasizes to the lungs, liver, brain, kidney, bone marrow and other organs, that matastatic modular are formation with hemorrhage, necrosis and secondary inflammatory infiltration.

8. Ectopic gestation, Fallopian tube

(1) Brief Descriptions: Implantation of the fetus in any sites other than normal uterine location, most common in the fallopian tubes (90%), rarely in the ovary or abdominal cavity.

(2) Gross Findings: The fallopian tube shows engorgement in ampulla portion with old blood clots in the lumen.

Tubal rupture and Hemorrhage may be seen.

9. Endometriosis, Ovary

(1) Brief Descriptions

Definition: presence of endometrial glands or stroma in abnormal locations outside the uterus.

Sites (in desecnding order of frequency): ovaries, uterine ligaments, rectovaginal septum, pelvic peritoneum, laparotomy scars, rarely in the umbilicus, vagina, vulva, or appendix.

Symptoms and signs: infertility, dysmenorrhea, pelvic pain, and other problems.

(2) Gross Findings

"Chocolate cysts": a moderately thin-walled cyst containing dark purple-brown, semisolid, sticky material.

10. Mature cystic teratoma, Ovary

(1) Brief Descriptions

Definition: Teratoma is true neoplasm derived from totipotential cells and composed of a variety of parenchymal cell types representative of more than one germ layer, usually all three.

Mature teratoma: teratoma composed of mature elements indistinguishable with normal tissue; benign and cystic.

(2) Gross Findings

Uniloculated or multiloculated cystic cavities filled with fatty or sebaceous material and hair → "dermoid cyst"

11. Serous papillary cystadenoma, ovary

(1) Brief Descriptions

1) It is the commonest cystic lesion in ovary, account for 30% of all ovarian tumors.

2) There are benign, borderline, and malignant.

(2) Gross Findings: Larger cystic lesion project from the ovarian surface., cystic wall is smooth with small papillary projections with clear serous.

12. Mucinous cystanenoma, ovary

(1) Brief Descriptions

1) It is common, accounting for about 25% of all ovarian neoplasias, but malignant is relatively uncommon..

2) Multiloculated tumors..

(2) Gross Findings: Tumor are characterized by more cysts of variable size, that filled with sticky mucinous rich in glycoproteins.

13. Adenocarcinoma of prostate

(1) Brief Descriptions

1) Carcinoma of the prostate is the most common form of cancer among men in the US.

2) Tends to occur in peripheral parts of the gland but also may occur in the transition zone.

(2) Gross Findings

1) Gray or yellowish, poorly delineated, firm areas.

2) Carcinoma invades the seminal vesicles and may extend into other pelvic organs.

14. Intraductal carcinoma of breast (Ductal carcinoma in situ.)

(1) Brief Descriptions

Definition: Ductal carcinoma with intact basement membrane.

Five architectural subtypes: comedocarcinoma, solid, cribriform, papillary, and micropapillary.

(2) Gross Findings

1) Poorly defined focus of slightly increased consistency

2) Punctate areas of necrotic material (comedone-like)

15. Infiltrating ductal carcinoma, (Breast scirrhous carcinoma)

(1) Brief Descriptions

1) The largest group of malignant breast tumors.

2) All carcinomas are thought to arise from the terminal ductlobular unit, and "ductal" and "lobular" no longer imply a site or cell type of origin.

(2) Gross Findings

1) The tumor of stony-hard consistency is retracted and infiltrating the surrounding breast substance.

2) In cut surface showing radiating through the surrounding parenchyma into the fat (crab-like configuration). with a large volume collagefibron proliferation

3) "Chalky streaks" on the cut surface due to duct elastosis.

16. Infiltrating ductal carcinoma (Breast medullary carcinoma)

(1) The tumor of soft consist of a large volume carcinoma cells with well circumscribed, sometimes infiltrating the surrounding breast substance.

(2) On cut surface showing carcinoma cells consist of tumor parenchyma with necrosis in the center of tumor.

17. Mucinous carcinoma, Breast (Colloid carcinoma.)

(1) Brief Descriptions: Invasive carcinoma of breast; tends to occur in older women and grows slowly; pure form with an excellent short-term prognosis.

(2) Gross Findings: Well circumscribed and formed by a currant jelly-like mass held together by delicate septa.

Cystic degeneration has been reported in relatively large tumors.

18. Eczematoid carcinoma of breast (paget's disease)   Paget's disease involve the skin of the nipple and areola, that is fissured, ulcerated, and oozing, with an accompanying inflammatory, hyperemia and edama. The nipple shows eczematoid changes.

Micro Findings

1. Intraepithelial neoplasm Grade Ⅲ (Squamous cell carcinoma in situ)

(1) Full-thickness severely dysplasia keratinocytes with hyperchromatic and pleomorphic nuclei. without any differentiation: altered polarity, in the entire thickness of squamous epithelium.

(2) Basement membrane is intact, no stromal invasion.

2. Squamous cell carcinoma of cervix

(1) In addition to the mucosa lesion, the tumor cells are arranged in cell nests infiltrating to deep stomal tissue.

(2) The tumor cells: pleomorphism, increased N/C ratio, increased mitotic figures, atypical mitosis. The nuclei show hyperchromatism and contain prominent nucleoli. Anaplastic tumor cells

(3) Vascular invasion is present. Inflammatory cell in the fibrous stroma.

3. Squamous cell carcinoma Uterine Corpus

(1) Tumor nests composed of large epidermoid cell infiltrate the myometrium.

(2) Tumor cells with vesicular nuclei, conspicuous nucleoli and increased mitotic figures.

4. Endometrial carcinomas

Most endometrial carcinomas (about 85%) are adenocarcinomas with three-step grading system

Well differentiated (grade 1), with easily recognizable glandular patterns;

Moderately differentiated (grade 2), showing well-formed glands mixed with solid sheets of malignant cells;

Poorly differentiated (grade 3), characterized by solid sheets of cells with barely recognizable glands and a greater degree of nuclear atypia and mitotic activity.

Up to 20% of endometrioid carcinomas contain foci of squamous differentiation. Squamous elements may be histologically benign-appearing(adenoacanthoma).

when Squamous elements is maligament (adenosquamous carcinomas).

As mentioned earlier, a subset of endometrial cancers resemble serous carcinomas of the ovary. They comprise approximately 20% of endometrial carcinornas. Papillary serous carcinomas and clear cell carcinomas are managed as grade 3 carcinomas irrespective of histologic pattern.

5. Hydatidiform mole

(1) Hydropic swelling of chorionic villi.

(2) Loose and myxomatous stroma with absence or inadequate development of vascularization of villi.

(3) Proliferation of trophoblasts. Sheets and masses of trophoblasts.

(4) Severe hemorrhage.

Others:

(1) Complete mole: all or most of the villi are edematous and diffuse trophoblastic hyperplasia.

(2) Partial mole: some villi are edematous + focal trophoblastic hyperplasia.

6. Invasive hydatidiform mole　Hydropic swelling of chorionic villi and Sheets and masses of trophoblasts infiltrate the myometrium with severe hemorrhageand necrosis.

7. Choriocarcinoma

(1) Atipal proliferation of trophoblasts without. chorionic villi;

(2) Vascular and fibrous stroma invasion;

(3) Severe hemorrhageand necrosis.

8. Adenomyosis

(1) Ectopic nests of endometrial glands enclosed within a spindle cell stroma between the muscle bundles of the myometrium.

(2) The nests should be one low power field or more (2. to 3. mm) below the endomyometrial junction.

Others:

Ectopic endometrial tissue(includes endometrial glands and endometrial stroma) in the myometrium of uterus: adenomyosis.

Ectopic endometrial tissue in abnormal location outside the uterus: endometrisis.

9. Endometriosis　Two of the three following features: endometrial glands. and endometrial stroma. in the ovarian parenchyma.

Old hemorrhage with hemosiderin-laden macrophage. may form cystic lesion ("chocolate cysts").

10. Ectopic gestation

(1) Blood clot and chorionic villi in the lumen of the tube or in the ovarian stroma

(2) Chorionic villi and trophoblasts (with its pale-staining core of myxoid tissue covered with a thin (outer) layer of syncytiotrophoblasts & (inner) cytotrophoblasts).

(3) Thickening and hemorrhage of the tubal wall in tubal pregnancy.

Others: Rupture of a tubal pregnancy constitutes a medical emergency.

11. Mature cystic teratoma

(1) Ectoderm: The cystic lesion is lined by skin with its sebaceous glands and hair follicles.

(2) Mesoderm: fibrous and fatty tissue.

(3) Endoderm: thyroid tissue with mature thyroid follicles of various sizes.

12. Nodular hyperplasia of prostate.

(1) Nodules are composed of proliferating glands and fibromusculoar stroma.

(2) Hyperplastic glandular epithelium form irregular papillae, but remains two cell layers (tall columnar epithelial cells and flattened basal cells.)

(3) Fibromusculoar stroma. are composed of spindled stromal cells and connective tisses.

(4) Glandular lumina contain secretory material.

13. Adenocarcinoma, Prostate

(1) Irregular, closely packed glands with papillary, loosely cribriform or fused glandular tumor, raggedly infiltrated in prostate tissue.

(2) Enlarged, irregular, hyperchromatic or vesicular nuclei with prominent nucleoli and coarse chromatin

Others:Grading base on the degree of glandular differentiation & the growth pattern of the tumor in relation to the stroma.

14. Intraductal carcinoma

(1) Dilated ducts with intact basement membrane and filled with neoplastic anaplastic epithelial cells that plug lumina.

(2) Presence of central necrosis in some ducts.

(3) Cribriform pattern Comedocarcinoma showing intraductal proliferation of malignant cells with central necrosis.

(4) Tumor cells: loosely cohesive, cytologic atypia, increased mitotic figures. The tumor cells showing monomorphic appearance and lacking normal myoepithelial cells. Cellular atypia.

(5) Poorly defined tumor mass with focal necrosis

15. Infiltrating ductal carcinoma

(1) The tumor cells are pleomorphic and have hyperchromatic nucleus and infiltrate the breast tissue into the adjacent adipose tissue.

(2) The tumor cells are arranged in cords, sheets, nests or as individual cells with focal irregular ductal formation.

(3) Densely fibrotic to desmoplastic stroma.

16. Mucinous carcinoma

(1) Extracellular mucin pooling that dissect and extend into the contiguous tissue spaces and planes of cleavage.

(2) Small islands and isolated neoplastic cells are floating within a sea of mucin.

(3) Lakes of slightly staining mucin with island of neoplastic cells floating.

(4) The neoplastic cells arrange in nests, cribriform or glandular pattern.

(5) Tumor cells have hyperchromatic nuclei and some have distinct nucleoli.

17. Medullary carcinoma of the breast

(1) A well-circumscribed margin.

(2) A number of lymphocyte infiltration.

(3) Large, pleomorphic tumor cells growing in solid, syncytium-like with scant stroma.

18. Paget's disease of the breast

(1) The tumor arises with in the large excretory ducts and extends to involve the skin of the nipple and areola.

(2) Paget's cells appear as large, pale hypercuromatic cell and pleomorphic nuclei surrounded a clear halo, located within the overlying keratinizing squamous epithelium.

Study Questions

Choose Tests

Directions: The numbered item or incomplete statement in this section is followed by answers or by completions of the statement. Select the one lettered answer or completion that is best in this case.

1. Which germ cell tumor is the most common malignant tumor of the anterior mediastinum?

　A. Cystic teratoma　　　　B. Embryonal cell carcinoma　　　C. Choriocarcinoma

　D. Seminoma　　　　　　　E. Endodermal sinus tumor

2. Which statement is true of prostatic cancer?

　A. It most commonly arises in a periurethral location

　B. It is associated with an elevated human chorionic gonadotropin (hCG) serum level

　C. Bone is a common metastatic site

　D. Most prostate cancers are sarcomas

　E. Androgen supplementation is indicated

3. Which prostatic lobe is most often affected by benign nodular hyperplasia?

　A. Anterior lobe　　　B. Posterior lobe　　　C. Lateral lobe　　　D. Middle lobe

4. Which condition probably is the most common cause of recurrent urinary tract infections (UTIs) in men?

　A. Immunodeficiency disorders　B. Neisserial gonorrhoeae　　C. Chronic prostatitis

　D. Kidney stones　　　　　　　E. Syphilis

5. A 60-year-old man complains of difficulty with urination. Physical examination reveals a smooth, diffusely enlarged prostate gland. A biopsy reveals benign prostatic hypertrophy (BPH). Which is the most likely etiology of the patient's urinary symptom?

　A. Perineural invasion of local nerves　　B. Compression of sacral nerve roots

　C. Infiltration of prostatic tissue into the bladder wall

　D. Urethral compression　　　　　　E. Papillomatosis of urethral epithelium

6. All of the following statements concerning prostatic carcinoma are generally accepted as true EXCEPT

　A. serum acid phosphatase levels can be elevated

　B. it is linked to environmental exposure to certain compounds

　C. metastatic bone disease is a common outcome

　D. it most often originates in the anterior lobe of the gland

7. Psammoma bodies are most often found in which type of ovarian cancer?
   A. Brenner tumor　　　　B. Germ cell tumor　　　　C. Serous cystadenocarcinoma
   D. Mucinous cystadenoma　E. Mucinous cystadenocarcinoma

8. The most common benign germ cell tumor of the ovaries in premenopausal women is
   A. Brenner tumor　　　　B. Endometrioid tumor　　　C. benign teratoma
   D. mucinous cystadenoma　　E. cystadenofibroma

9. The endometrial biopsy specimen obtained from a 30-year-old woman shows a proliferative-phase endometrium with evidence of chronic endometritis. This finding most likely represents
   A. a premalignant endometrial lesion　　B. an inadequate luteal phase
   C. a hyperestrogenic state　　　　　　　D. the effects of an intrauterine device (IUD)
   E. Endmetrial carcinoma

10. A 40-year-old woman presents with an ovarian mass. At surgery, a 5-cm cystic mass is found attached to the right ovary. The surface of the cyst is grossly papillary. Which feature distinguishes a borderline serous tumor from a serous cystadenocarcinoma?
    A. Involvement of the other ovary　　B. Involvement of the peritoneum
    C. Cellular atypia　　　　　　　　　D. Invasion of ovarian stroma
    E. Psammoma bodies

11. During a gynecologic examination, a 35-year old woman is found to have clinically atypical epithelium covering the majority of the cervix and the proximal vagina. The epithelium does not stain with Lugol's iodine. A biopsy of the vagina reveals benign endocervical glands. These findings are consistent with a diagnosis of
    A. chronic cervicitis　　B. condyloma acuminatum　　C. cervical carcinoma
    D. cervical intraepithelial neoplasia　　　　　　　E. endometriosis

12. All of the following statements about choriocarcinoma are true EXCEPT
    A. it may occur after a normal pregnancy　　B. it can arise in a hydatidiform mole
    C. it consists of malignant trophoblasts
    D. it is treated with hysterectomy and radiation therapy
    E. response to therapy is monitored by human chorionic gonadotropin (hCG) levels

13. Which histologic feature is the hallmark of invasive lobular carcinoma of the breast?
    A. Its arrangement in pseudoglands
    B. Individual cell infiltration of the stroma
    C. Papillary outgrowths
    D. Pools of mucinous material
    E. Highly cellular stroma with atypical spindle cells

14. The primary structural unit of the mammary gland is known as the
    A. ductule　　B. acinus　　C. sinus　　D. lobule　　E. quadrant

15. A woman who presents with a bloody discharge from one nipple is most likely to have
    A. Paget's disease of the nipple　　　B. intraductal papilloma
    C. medullary carcinoma　　　　　　　D. mucinous carcinoma
    E. intraductal carcinoma

16. Which of the following is the most common type of breast carcinoma?
    A. Intraductal　　B. Medullary　　C. Papillary　　D. Mucinous　　E. Infiltrating ductal

17. Which statement would be true for the diagnosis of lobular carcinoma in situ?

A. Axillary lymph node dissection is indicated

B. Excision and radiation therapy are indicated

C. Careful physical examination will reveal masses in the contralateral breast in 20% of patients with lobular carcinoma in situ in one breast

D. The patient is at increased risk of invasive breast cancer

E. This finding is unusual in premenopausal women

18. Presently, in the United States, the most common cause of death in women beyond the fifth decade is

A. leukemia　　　　　B. myocardial infarction　　　C. breast carcinoma

D. lung carcinoma　　　E. cervical carcinoma

19. Important prognostic factors for patients with breast carcinoma include all of the following EXCEPT

A. age of the patient　　　　　　　　　　B. histologic tumor type

C. presence of estrogen receptors in the tumor　D. presence of metastases

E. location within the breast

20. All of the following are possible etiologies of a teenager's gynecomastia EXCEPT

A. lobular hypertrophy　　　　B. exogenous estrogen

C. some testicular tumors　　　D. puberty

E. cirrhosis of the liver

Questions

1. What is endometriosis and adenomyosis?

2. What are the salient clinical and pathological features of carcinoma of the body of the uterus?

3. What are the common malignant tumors of the cervix and what is their aetiology?

4. Describe the significance of the histological appearances occurring in the cervix uteri which are considered to herald malignant changes.

5. What are the histological features of cervical epithelial dysplasia (Cervial Intraepithelial Neoplasia; CIN)?

6. What tumors may arise in the ovaries?

7. What is Meig's syndrome?

8. What tumors of placental origin occur?

9. What is a hydatidiform mole?

10. What may cause a lump in the female breast?

11. What is the commonest benign breast tumour? Describe it.

12. What are the aetiological factors involved in the development of breast cancer?

13. Classify breast cancers.

14. What is an inflammatory carcinoma of breast?

15. What is Paget's disease of the nipple?

16. What are oestrogen receptors and what is their significance in breast cancer?

17. Can a man develop carcinoma of the breast?

18. What are the likely reasons for swellings in the male breast?

19. What are the causes and appearances of gynaecomastia?

第十三章 内分泌系统疾病

大体观察

1. 结节性甲状腺肿
2. 亚急性甲状腺炎
3. 桥本甲状腺炎
4. 甲状腺滤泡状腺瘤
5. 甲状腺乳头状癌
6. 甲状腺髓样癌
7. 肾上腺嗜铬细胞瘤

镜下观察

1. 结节性甲状腺肿
2. 亚急性甲状腺炎
3. 桥本甲状腺炎(慢性淋巴细胞性甲状腺炎)
4. 甲状腺滤泡状腺瘤
5. 甲状腺乳头状癌
6. 甲状腺髓样癌
7. 肾上腺皮质腺瘤
8. 肾上腺嗜铬细胞瘤

一、大 体 观 察

1. 结节性甲状腺肿

(1) 简要说明

1) 复合性增生合并退化造成甲状腺的不规则增大。

2) 甲状腺增生的原因包括:①促甲状腺素 TSH;②TSH 受体的抗体;③缺碘;④食物中有甲状腺肿原;⑤药物。

3) 非毒性甲状腺肿呈地方分布,也可以散发。

(2) 大体所见

1) 多叶状、不对称的腺体增大。

2) 切面可见不规则的结节,含有数量不等的棕色的胶胨状物质。

2. 亚急性甲状腺炎

(1) 简要说明

1) 肉芽肿性甲状腺炎或 Dequervain 甲状腺炎。

2) 好发于 30~50 岁的妇女。

3) 由病毒感染或病毒感染后的炎症引起。

4) 突发的甲状腺肿大、疼痛。病程分三个阶段(甲状腺功能亢进、甲状腺功能减退、痊愈)

(2) 大体所见

1) 腺体的病变部位不对称或不均匀。

2) 切面可见坚实的,不规则的黄白色病灶,或一些分界不清的结节(数毫米至数厘米)。

3. 桥本甲状腺炎

(1) 简要说明

1）这种疾病多发于 45~65 岁的女性,性别比女 :男为 10 ∶1~20 ∶1。

2）自身免疫性甲状腺炎或淋巴瘤样甲状腺肿。

3）症状和体征:甲状腺功能正常或减退。

（2）大体所见

1）甲状腺对称性肿大,切面黄白色。

2）包膜完整。

4. 甲状腺滤泡状腺瘤

（1）病变要点

1）起源于甲状腺滤泡上皮。

2）多数病例并非癌前病变。

（2）大体所见:界限清晰的结节,有完整的结缔组织包膜,切面柔软,灰黄色或棕黄色。

5. 甲状腺乳头状癌

（1）简要说明

1）最常见的甲状腺癌类型。

2）好发于 20~40 岁,与以往的放射性碘接触有关。

（2）大体所见:实性、坚硬、灰白色、分叶状病灶,中心有硬化。

6. 甲状腺髓样癌

（1）简要说明

1）起源于滤泡旁细胞,C 细胞,分泌降钙素。

2）散发性(80%),多发性内分泌腺瘤综合征 IIA 或 IIB。

3）单侧(散发病例),两侧或多中心(家族病例)。

（2）大体所见

1）分界清楚,灰白色病灶。

2）大小变化大,小的仅肉眼可见,大者取代整个甲状腺组织。大的病灶境界清楚,但没有包膜。

7. 肾上腺嗜铬细胞瘤

（1）简要说明

1）由嗜铬细胞组成的少见的肿瘤,具有合成和分泌儿茶酚胺类物质的功能。

2）属于肾上腺髓质的神经节肿瘤。

3）10% 肿瘤是恶性,10% 双侧,10% 在肾上腺以外。

（2）大体所见

1）局限于肾上腺内小的,境界清楚的病灶,可以大到重达数公斤的出血性肿块。

2）将新鲜组织置于重铬酸钾溶液中:深棕色。

二、镜下观察

1. 结节性甲状腺肿

（1）由扁平的、静止的上皮细胞形成的富含胶质的滤泡,部分滤泡上皮增生和肥大。

（2）变质性改变:出血、纤维化、钙化和囊性变。

2. 亚急性甲状腺炎

（1）不同分期表现各异。

（2）起初，滤泡上皮脱落，变性，胶质耗竭，然后出现以单个核细胞浸润和微脓肿形成为主要特征的急性炎症反应。

（3）滤泡上皮细胞消失，被组织细胞和巨细胞取代（滤泡完全变性后在胶质周围出现的异物巨细胞）。

（4）间质纤维化，并有淋巴细胞、浆细胞和组织细胞的浸润。

3. 桥本甲状腺炎（慢性淋巴细胞性甲状腺炎）

（1）滤泡上皮细胞嗜酸性变，形成体积小而萎缩的甲状腺滤泡伴滤泡细胞的嗜酸性化生，从淡粉红色细胞到胞浆丰富含粉红色颗粒状的嗜酸性细胞。

（2）间质中有淋巴浆细胞浸润，并出现显著的生发中心。

（3）缺乏结缔组织，轻微增厚的小叶间间隔。

4. 甲状腺滤泡腺瘤

（1）分化良好血管化的肿瘤压迫周围的腺体。

（2）各种继发性变化：可以有出血、纤维化、水肿、钙化、骨形成和囊性变。

（3）完整的纤维性包膜，未见肿瘤包膜和血管浸润。

（4）肿瘤的生长方式：

1）实性/小梁状：少或无滤泡形成。

2）微滤泡：小的滤泡形成，有少量胶质。

3）正常滤泡（单纯型）：滤泡大小接近非肿瘤性腺体。

4）巨滤泡（胶样型）：大滤泡，含有大量胶质。

（5）肿瘤细胞多角形，核染色正常，圆形或卵圆形的核仁。细胞境界清晰，具有中等量的嗜酸性或嗜双色性胞浆。

5. 甲状腺乳头状癌

（1）基于组织学和细胞学特征命名。

（2）中央是纤维血管轴心，周围被覆肿瘤性上皮细胞，形成乳头。

（3）在乳头轴心、纤维间质或肿瘤细胞之间出现砂粒体。

（4）肿瘤细胞核特征：圆形或稍呈卵圆形。

淡染、透明、空亮或毛玻璃样外观：核空淡伴有不规则增厚的核膜。

假包涵体：胞膜内陷，深染，形成嗜酸性，包涵体样的结构。边缘清晰，偏于一侧，压迫细胞核，使之偏于一侧形成新月体样外观。

核沟形成：咖啡豆样核。

6. 甲状腺髓样癌

（1）由富含毛细血管的间质分割肿瘤细胞巢。

（2）圆形、卵圆形、多角形或梭形的细胞，具有一致圆形或卵圆形核，细胞境界不清的嗜酸性或嗜双色性，均匀的胞浆。

（3）淀粉样沉积，用刚果红染色后在偏振光显微镜观察显示绿光的双折射。

7. 肾上腺皮质腺瘤

（1）肿瘤由一致的大细胞组成,排列成巢状或小梁状。

（2）细胞胞浆富含脂质,细胞核小而一致。

（3）细胞核增大和多形性常见,但核分裂象少见。

（4）境界清楚的结节状肿块,肾上腺腺体受压在周围。

8. 肾上腺嗜铬细胞瘤

（1）境界清楚的肿瘤细胞巢被纤细的血管纤维间质所分割,其中含有淀粉样沉积物。

（2）细胞大小形状不一,胞浆呈细颗粒状,嗜碱性或嗜酸性,或含有脂质。

（3）圆形或卵圆形核,核仁明显,由于胞浆内陷有时形成包涵体样结构。

（4）出现巨大的核或高染色质性并不代表恶性的表现。

三、思 考 题

（一）选择题

选一个字母代表的最合适答案。

1. 对糖尿病性肾病的描述正确的是

    A. 它的特点是肾小球基底膜的弥漫性变薄

    B. 常有其他器官在显微镜下的改变

    C. 病人常有肾病

    D. 在几年以后病变可缓解

    E. 在荧光免疫检验法中可见肾小球有 IgG 的沉积

2. 原发性甲状腺癌在甲状腺内出现的多发性病灶是

    A. 乳头样癌和髓样癌   B. 滤泡性癌和乳头样癌

    C. 髓样癌和滤泡性癌   D. 间变性癌和乳头样癌

3. 下列除了哪个都是间变性甲状腺癌的特点

    A. 占了甲状腺癌的 5%   B. 原来肿瘤的恶性变

    C. 年轻人易受累及   D. 在诊断时肿瘤常超出甲状腺被膜

    E. 病人预后差

（二）问答题

1. 甲状腺肿的类型有哪些?

2. "结节性甲状腺肿"的含义是什么?

3. "胶体甲状腺肿"的含义是什么?

4. 引起单纯性甲状腺肿的原因有哪些?

5. 毒性甲状腺肿的组织学表现是什么?

6. 请描述慢性淋巴结样甲状腺炎(桥本甲状腺炎)的大体及镜下表现。

7. 请对甲状腺肿瘤进行分类。

8. 甲状腺滤泡性癌的主要病理学特征是什么?

9. 甲状腺乳头状癌的主要病理学特征是什么?

10. 请描述甲状腺髓样癌的主要特点。

11. 与糖尿病有关的肾脏改变有哪些?

12. 哪些原因引起肾上腺的损伤？

13. 什么是艾迪生病？

14. 哪些综合征与肾上腺皮质激素过量分泌有关？

15. Cushing 综合征与库欣病有何区别？

16. 什么是原发性醛固酮增多症(Conn 综合征)？

17. 什么是多发性内分泌腺瘤(MEN)综合征？

Chapter 13   Disorders of the Endocrine System

Gross Findings
1. Nodular goiter of thyroid
2. Subacute thyroiditis
3. Hashimoto's thyroiditis, Thyroid
4. Follicular adenoma,of thyroid
5. Papillary carcinoma of thyroid
6. Medullary carcinoma of thyroid
7. Pheochromocytoma of adrenal gland

Micro Findings
1. Nodular goiter
2. Subacute thyroiditis
3. Hashimoto's thyroiditis (chronic lymphocytic thyroiditis)
4. Follicular adenoma
5. Papillary carcinoma
6. Medullary carcinoma
7. Adrenocortical adenoma
8. Adrenal gland Pheochromocytoma

Gross Findings

1. Nodular goiter of thyroid

(1) Brief Descriptions

1) Recurrent episodes of hyperplasia and involution combine to produce irregular enlargemen of the thyroid.

2) Hyperplasia of the thyroid gland may result from hyperstimulation by: ①TSH, ②Ab to TSH receptor, ③iodine deficiency, ④goitrogens in food, or ⑤drugs.

3) Nontoxic goiter. Sporadic and endemic forms.

(2) Gross Findings

1) Multilobulated, asymmetrically enlarged glands.

2) Cut section: irregular nodules with variable amounts of brown and gelatinous colloid.

2. Subacute thyroiditis

(1) Brief Descriptions

1) Granulomatous thyroiditis or Dequervain thyroiditis.

2) Frequent in women between the ages of 30 and 50.

3) Caused by a viral infection or a postviral inflammatory process.

4) Sudden onset of painful enlargement of thyroid with 3 phases of course. (hyperthyroid, hypothryoid & recovery).

(2) Gross Findings

1) Asymmetrical or uneven involvement of the gland.

2) Firm & irregular white-tan lesion or several small poorly demarcated nodules (from several mm to a few cm) on cut surface.

3. Hashimoto's thyroiditis, Thyroid

(1) Brief Descriptions

1) This disorder is most prevalent between 45 and 65 years of age and is more common in women than in man, with a female predominance of 10 :1 to 20 :1.

2) Autoimmune thyroiditis & struma lymphomatosa.

3) Symptoms and signs: euthyroidism or hypothyroidism.

(2) Gross Findings

1) Symmetric enlargement with tan yellow cut surface..

2) Intact capsule.

4. Follicular adenoma of thyroid

(1) Brief Descriptions

1) Derived from follicular epithelium.

2) Not forerunners of cancer except in the exceptional instance.

(2) Gross Findings: Well demarcated nodule with a intact fibrous capsule bulging cut surface with a soft, grayish, tan, or brown appearance.

5. Papillary carcinoma of thyroid

(1) Brief Descriptions

1) Most common form of thyroid cancer.

2) Twenties to forties, associated with previous exposure to ionizing radiation.

(2) Gross Findings: Solid, firm, grayish white lobulated lesion with sclerotic center.

6. Medullary carcinoma of thyroid

(1) Brief Descriptions

1) Derived from the parafolliular cells, C cell, secrete calcitonin.

2) Sporadically (80%), MEN syndrome IIA or IIB.

3) One lobe (sporadic), bilaterality and muticentricity(familial).

(2) Gross Findings

1) Well circumscribed, gray-white lesion.

2) Range in size, they may be barely visible or may replace the entire thyroid, the larger lesions are sharply circumscribed but not encapsulated.

7. Pheochromocytoma of adrenal gland

(1) Brief Descriptions

1) Uncommon neoplasm composed of chromaffin cells: synthesize and release catecholamine.

2) Paraganglioma of adrenal medulla.

3) 10% tumor: 10% malignant, 10% bilateral, 10% extra-adrenal.

(2) Gross Findings

1) Small, circumscribed lesions confined to the adrenal to large hemorrhagic masses weighing kilogram.

2) Incubation of fresh tissue with potassium dichromate solution: dark brown color.

Micro Findings

1. Nodular goiter

(1) Colloid rich follicles lined by flatten, inactive epithelium and areas of follicular epithelial hypertrophy and hyperplasia.

(2) Degenerative changes: hemorrhage, fibrosis, calcification, and cystic.

2. Subacute thyroiditis

(1) Vary with the phase.

(2) Initially, desquamation or degeneration of follicular epithelium with colloid depletion, then acute inflammatory response with PMNs & microabscesses.

(3) Then follicular epithelium disappear & replaced by a rim of histiocytes & giant cells (foreign body giant cells form around remnants of colloid after follicle degenerate completely).

(4) Interstitial fibrosis & infiltration of lymphocytes, plasma cells, & histiocytes.

3. Hashimoto's thyroiditis(chronic lymphocytic thyroiditis)

(1) Oxyphilic change of follicular epithelium: small & atrophic thyroid follicles with oxyphilic metaplasia of follicular cells ranging from pale pink staining cells with abundant cytoplasm to oxyphilic cells with pink granular cytoplasm.

(2) Lymphoplasmcytic infiltration with prominent germinal centers in the stroma.

(3) Scanty connective tissue with slightly thickening of inter-lobular septi.

4. Follicular adenoma

(1) Well-vascularized tumor compression the surrounding gland.

(2) Variable secondary degenerative changes: hemorrhage, fibrosis, edema, calcification, bone formation or cystic change.

(3) Intact fibrous capsule without capsular or vascular invasion.

(4) Growth pattern of tumor:

1) Solid/trabecular: cellular areas with few or no follicles formed.

2) Microfollicular: small follicles with minimal amount of colloid.

3) Normofollicular (simple): the size of the follicles approaches that of non-neoplastic glands.

4) Macrofollicular (colloid): larger follicles with full colloid.

(5) Tumor cells are polygonal with normochromatic, round to oval nucleoli; well defined cell border with moderate amount acidophilic to amphophilic cytoplasm.

5. Papillary carcinoma

(1) Based on characteristic architecture & cytological feature.

(2) Papillae formed by a central fibrovascular stalk & covered by neoplastic epithelial cells.

(3) Psammoma bodies in the papillary stalk, fibrous stroma or between tumor cells.

(4) Nuclear features: Round to slight oval shape.

Pale, clear, empty or ground glass appearance: empty of nucleus with irregular thickened inner aspect of nuclear membrane.

Pseudo-inclusion: deep cytoplasmic invagination and result in nuclear acidophilic, inclusion-like round structures, sharply outlined and eccentric, with a crescent-shaped rim of compressed chromatin on the side.

Grooves: coffee-bean like.

6. Medullary carcinoma

(1) Nests of cells separated by stroma with prominent small capillary vasculature.

(2) Round or oval or angulated or spindle cells with uniform, round to oval nuclei & ill-defined eosinophilic or amphophilic and finely cytoplasm.

(3) Amyloid deposition which show green birefringence in polarized light after Congo red stain.

7. Adrenocortical adenoma

(1) Adenomas are composed of uniform large cells arranged in nests and trabeculae.

(2) The cells have abundant lipid-filled cytoplasm and small uniform nuclei.

(3) Nuclear enlargement and pleomorphism are common, but mitotic figures are rare.

(4) Well-circumscribed nodular masses with adrenal gland compressed to the periphery

8. Adrenal gland Pheochromocytoma

(1) Arranged in well-defined nests (zellballen) bounded by delicate fibrovascular stroma, which may contain amyloid.

(2) Cells vary in size & shape & have a finely granular & basophilic or eosinophilic or lipid-containing cytoplasm.

(3) Round or oval vesicular nuclei with prominent nucleoli & sometimes. Inclusion-like structure due to deep cytoplasmic invagination.

(4) Nuclear gigantism & hyperchromasia are not an expression of malignancy.

Study Questions

Choose Tests

Directions: Each of the numbered items or incomplete statements in this section is followed by answers or by completions of the statement. Select the one lettered answer or completion that is best in each case.

1. Which statement about diabetic nephropathy is true?

   A. It is characterized by diffuse thinning of the glomerular basement membrane (GBM)

   B. It usually is accompanied by microangio pathic changes in other organs

   C. Affected patients most often present with nephritis

   D. The disease usually remits after a few years

   E. A granular pattern of glomerular IgG deposits characteristically is seen on immunofluorescent studies

2. The primary thyroid carcinomas that show multiple intrathyroidal foci are

   A. papillary carcinoma and medullary carcinoma

   B. follicular carcinoma and papillary carcinoma

   C. medullary carcinoma and follicular carcinoma

   D. anaplastic carcinoma and papillary carcinoma

3. All of the following features characterize anaplastic thyroid carcinoma EXCEPT that

   A. it accounts for about 5% of thyroid cancer.

   B. the malignancy typically arises in a preexisting tumor.

   C. young adults primarily are affected.

   D. the tumor typically extends beyond the thyroid capsule at diagnosis.

   E. affected patients have a very poor prognosis.

Questions

1. What types ot goitre are recognized?

2. What is meant by the term 'nodular goitre'?

3. What is meant by the term 'colloid goitre'?

4. What are the causes of a simple goitre?

5. What are the histological appearances of a toxic goitre?

6. Describe the gross and microscopic appearances in chronic lymphocytic thyroiditis (Hashimoto's thyroiditis).

7. Classify tumors of the thyroid.

8. What are the chief pathological features of follicular carcinoma of the thyroid?

9. What are the chief pathological features of a papillary carcinoma of the thyroid?

10. Describe the chief features of medullary carcinoma of the thyroid.

11. What renal changes are associated with diabetes?

12. What causes destruction of the adrenal gland?

13. What is Addison's disease?

14. What syndromes are associated with the excessive secretion of cortical adrenal hormones?

15. What is the difference between Cushing's syndrome and Cushing's disease?

16. What is primary hyperaldosteronism (conn's syndrome)?

17. What are the multiple endocrine neoplasia (MEN) syndromes?

第十四章 神经系统疾病

一、大 体 观 察

1. 流行性脑脊髓膜炎　脑表面化脓性渗出,血管扩张充血、淤血。

2. 流行性乙型脑炎

(1) 简要说明:经虫媒病毒,动物宿主和蚊虫叮咬传播。

(2) 大体所见

1) 急性病例:脑的充血和肿胀。

2) 慢性病例:脑软化灶和钙盐沉积。

3. 脑梗死　脑梗死的形态学改变发生在血管阻塞后 6~12 小时,梗死灶表现为软化灶形成和周围组织水肿。

4. 颅内出血破入侧脑室　颅内大量出血,破入侧脑室。

5. 脑多形性胶质母细胞瘤

(1) 简要说明

1) 星形细胞肿瘤:主要由肿瘤性星形细胞组成。

2) WHO 分级:弥漫性星形细胞瘤(WHO Ⅱ级),间变性星形细胞瘤(WHO Ⅲ级),胶质母细胞(WHO Ⅳ级)。

3) 多形性胶质母细胞瘤:高侵袭性,预后差(平均生存期 1 年),不规则浸润灶。

(2) 大体所见:坚硬的白色病灶,有黄色的坏死软化灶,同时可见囊性变和出血。

6. 小脑髓母细胞瘤

(1) 简要说明

1) 定义:小脑肿瘤。

2) 好发于儿童,预后较差由大量未分化小细胞组成。

（2）大体所见

1）儿童好发于小脑正中线,成人更多见于小脑侧叶。

2）境界清楚,灰色,易碎。

3）由于肿瘤生长迅速导致脑积水。

4）可以通过脑脊液扩散。

7. 脑膜瘤

（1）简要说明

1）起源于蛛网膜的脑膜细胞。

2）组织学类型:合体型、纤维型、过渡型、砂粒体型、血管瘤型等。

（2）大体所见

1）有包膜,与正常脑膜分界清楚的圆形肿块,容易分离。

2）由于含有大量纤维,而且出血和坏死较少,所以质地坚硬。

3）肿瘤上的骨组织发生增生反应性骨增厚。

8. 恶性脑膜瘤

（1）复发和局部侵袭的生物学行为。有时出现坏死和出血。

（2）通常是致命的,平均生存期少于两年。

二、镜 下 观 察

1. 流行性脑脊髓膜炎

（1）蛛网膜下腔出现大量中性粒细胞(脓性渗出物)。

（2）其下的脑组织或脊髓组织出现轻微水肿和充血。

2. 流行性乙型脑炎(日本 B 型脑炎)

（1）血管周围淋巴细胞套和脑实质的炎性浸润。

（2）脑水肿和胶质小结形成(胶质细胞增生)。

（3）神经元变性和神经元被噬现象(小胶质细胞或巨噬细胞浸润并吞噬变性的神经元)。

（4）神经元卫星现象:至少 5 个增生的少突胶质细胞围绕在变性的神经元周围。

3. 多形性胶质母细胞瘤

（1）坏死并在坏死周围有假栅栏样结构。

（2）内皮细胞增生以及间变性星形细胞。高细胞性:奇异形核,多核细胞,印戒细胞,瘤巨细胞,核分裂象(变异程度大)。

（3）血管增殖伴有内皮细胞增生。

4. 小脑髓母细胞瘤

（1）Homer Wright 菊心团(假菊心团):细胞卫星状围绕在纤维化区域,其中央没有管腔或血管。

（2）结节状(促结缔组织增生型):暗细胞鞘包围淡染区。

（3）紧密排列的细胞,胡萝卜样的核,核内染色质粗糙。

5. 脑膜瘤

（1）多角形细胞排列成片状或漩涡状。核大,淡染,居中。胞浆丰富,细胞周围有大量胶原纤维。

（2）可见砂粒体。

6. 恶性脑膜瘤

（1）明显的细胞学恶性(核的间变类似于肉类、癌或黑色素瘤)。高细胞性。

（2）核分裂象多见,高核分裂指数>20 /10HPF。

（3）多灶性坏死和失去正常生长方式。

（4）可以侵犯骨组织。

7. 神经鞘瘤(雪旺细胞瘤)

两个不同表现的区域

A 区显示密集排列的梭形细胞,细胞核形成规则排列的栅栏状(Verocay 小体),缺乏分裂象。

B 区显示疏松的黏液样变性区。

变性改变包括血管透明变性和吞噬脂质的巨噬细胞。

三、思 考 题

（一）选择题

选一个字母代表的最合适答案。

1. 小脑的星形细胞瘤的特点是

    A. 多发性的复发灶　　　　　　　　　　B. 生存率低

    C. 在治疗后有长时间的持续性神经功能缺陷

    D. 发生在儿童和青春期的少年

    E. 转化为胶质母细胞瘤

2. 一位 39 岁的男性主诉在 2 年中他感觉到听力进行性下降。除了偶尔有头痛外无其他症状。检查时发现在左侧有严重的感觉神经的听力丧失。X 线在左侧小脑脑桥有 1.5cm 的肿块。这个肿块可能是

    A. 脑膜瘤　　B. 结核脓肿　　C. 胶质母细胞瘤　　D. 神经鞘膜瘤　　E. 肺癌的转移

3. 一位 31 岁的男性出现了运动困难和红细胞记数增加(红细胞增多)。其家族史中有多个成员有肾肿瘤和脑肿瘤。脑的 CT 检查发现在病人的小脑有血管性病灶。可能的诊断是

    A. 星形细胞瘤　　　　　　B. 髓母细胞瘤　　　　　　C. 血管母细胞瘤

    D. 室管膜瘤　　　　　　　E. 多形性胶质母细胞瘤

4. 下列与 Alzheimer 病有关的说法都是正确的除了哪个

    A. 可见脑回萎缩和脑沟变深　　　　　　B. 有明显的小脑的萎缩

    C. 神经纤维缠结是其特点　　　　　　　D. 疾病是长期的、进行性的

    E. 发生在 50~60 岁

（二）问答题

1. 流行性脑脊髓膜炎和乙型脑炎如何鉴别？

2. 什么是 Wallerian 变性？

3. 脑出血的常见部位及其诱因是什么？

4. 动脉瘤形成的原因是什么？

5. 请对神经系统的肿瘤进行分类。

6. 什么是神经鞘瘤？

7. 什么是脑（脊）膜瘤？

Chapter 14　Diseases of the Nervous System

Gross Findings
1. Epidemic cerebrospinal meningitis
2. Epidemic B encephalitis
3. Cerebral infarction
4. Intracranial ventricle hemorrhages
5. Glioblastoma multiforme, Cerebrum
6. Medulloblastoma, Cerebellum
7. Meningioma
8. Malignant meningioma

Micro Findings
1. Epidemic cerebrospinal meningitis
2. Epidemic encephalitis B (Japanese B encephalitis)
3. Glioblastoma multiforme
4. Cerebellum Medulloblastoma
5. Meningioma
6. Malignant meningioma
7. Neurilemma (Schwannomas)

Gross Findings

1. Epidemic cerebrospinal meningitis　Suppurative exudates in surface of brain with blood vessels dilatation and congestion.

2. Epidemic B encephalitis

(1) Brief Descriptions: Arbovirus, animal host and mosquito vectors.

(2) Gross Findings

1) Acute cases: only congestion and swelling of the brain.

2) Chronic cases: areas of cerebral softening and deposition of mineral within brain.

3. Cerebral infarction　The morphology of cerebral infarction happen in 6 to 12 hours after vessels obstruction, Infarction foci show softer and edematous.

4. Intracranial ventricle hemorrhages　Intracranial a large volume bleeding rupture into a ventricle.

5. Glioblastoma multiforme, Cerebrum

(1) Brief Descriptions

1) Astrocytic tumors: tumors composed predominantly of neoplastic astrocytes.

2) WHO grading: diffuse astrocytoma (WHO grade Ⅱ), anaplastic astrocytoma (WHO grade Ⅲ), glioblastoma (WHO grade Ⅳ).

3) Glioblastoma multiforme: high agressive, poor prognosis (mean survival 1 year), and irregular infiltrative lesion.

(2) Gross Findings: There are firm white areas and yellow softer necrotic areas, same time that show cystic change and hemorrhage.

6. Medulloblastoma, Cerebellum

(1) Brief Descriptions

1) Definition: cerebellar neoplasm composed largedly of small undifferentiated cells.

2) Occurs predominantly in children and poor prognosis.

(2) Gross Findings

1) Midline of cerebellum of children and lateral locations more common in adults.

2) Well-circumscribed, gray, friable.

3) Hydrocephalus due to rapid growth of the tumor.

4) May disseminate through CSF.

7. Meningioma,

(1) Brief Descriptions

1) Arising from the meningothelial cell of the arachnoid.

2) Histologic pattern: syncytial, fibroblastic, transitional, psammomatous, angiomatous, etc.

(2) Gross Findings

1) Encapsulated, round masses with a well-defined dura base and easily seperated.

2) Firm to fibrous and lack of hemorrhage and necrosis.

3) Hyperostotic reaction in the overlying bone.

8. Malignant meningioma

(1) Increased tendency of recurrence and locally aggressive behavior. Sometimes with necrosis and hemorrhage.

(2) Usually fatal, with median survivals of less than 2 years.

Micro Findings

1. Epidemic cerebrospinal meningitis

(1) A number of neutrophils in the subarachnoid space (suppurative exudates).

(2) The underlying brain and cord are edematous and moderatelu congested.

2. Epidemic encephalitis B (Japanese B encephalitis)

(1) Perivascular lymphoid cuffing and parenchymal inflammatory infiltrates.

(2) Edematous cerebrum with gliosis (glial cells proliferation).

(3) Neuron degeneration and neurophagia (small glial cells or macrophages infiltrate in degenerated neuron).

(4) Satellitosis: At least 5 proliferative oligodendroglial cells around the degenerated neuron

3. Glioblastoma multiforme

(1) Necrosis and pseudopalisading with necrosis.

(2) Endothelial proliferation & anaplastic astrocytes. Hypercellularity, bazarre nuclei, multinucleated cells, ring-shaped cells, tumor giant cells, mitoses (vary considerably).

(3) The vascular proliferation with endothelial cell hyperplasia

4. Cerebellum Medulloblastoma

(1) Homer Wright rosettes (pseudorosette): cells surround small stellate areas of fibrillarity without a central lumen or blood vessel.

(2) Nodular pattern (desmoplastic variant): mantles of dark cells surround pale island.

(3) Closely packed cells with carrot-shaped nuclei with coarse chromatin.

5. Meningioma

(1) Sheets and whorls of polygonal cells, with large, pale spheroid, central nuclei and abundant cytoplasm supported by collagen stroma.

(2) Psammoma bodies can also be found.

6. Malignant meningioma

（1）Obvious cytological malignancy（Nuclear anaplasia similar to sarcoma, carcinoma or melanoma）and Marked cellullarity

（2）Numerous mitotic figures High mitotic index: >20 mitoses / 10HPF.

（3）Multifocal necrosis and loss of usual growth patterns.

（4）May invade bone.

7. Neurilemma（Schwannomas）

（1）Two different areas intermixed:

Antoni A show densely packed spindlecells, cell nuclei form orderly palisades（Verocay bodies）, absence of mitotic activity.

Antoni B show looser myxoid regions

（2）Degenerative changes include vascular hyalinization and lipidlader macrophages.

Study Questions

Choose Tests

Directions: Each of the numbered items or incomplete statements in this section is followed by answers or by completions of the statement. Select the one lettered answer or completion that is best in each case.

1. Astrocytomas of the cerebellum are characterized by
　　A. multiple recurrences　　　　　　B. poor survival rate
　　C. long-term continued neurologic deficit following therapy
　　D. occurrence in childhood and adolescence
　　E. transformation of glioblastoma

2. A 39-year-old man complains that he has noticed a progressive hearing loss over a 2-year period. Except for occasional headaches, he has no other complaints. Evaluation discloses severe sensorineural hearing loss on the left side. X-rays show a 1. 5 cm mass at the left cerebellopontine angle. The mass is most likely to be a
　　A. meningioma　　　　　　B. tuberculous abscess　　　　　C. glioblastoma
　　D. schwannoma　　　　　　E. metastatic tumor from the lung

3. A 31-year-old man presents with difficulty in locomotion and an elevated red blood cell count（polycythemia）. Family history reveals the presence of kidney and brain tumors in several family members. Computed tomography（CT）of the brain shows a vascular lesion in the cerebellum of this patient. The most likely diagnosis is
　　A. astrocytoma　　　　　　B. medulloblastoma　　　　　　C. hemangioblastoma
　　D. ependymoma　　　　　　E. glioblastoma multiforme

4. All of the following statements concerning Alzheimer's disease are true EXCEPT
　　A. atrophic gyri and enlarged sulci are seen.
　　B. cerebellar atrophy is prominent.
　　C. neurofibrillary tangles are characteristic.
　　D. the disease course is prolonged and progressive.
　　E. it occurs in the fifth and sixth decades of life.

Questions

1. How to distinguish between the epidemic cerebrospinal meningitis and epidemic encepha-

litis B?

2. What is Wallerian degeneration?

3. Where are the common sites in the brain for haemorrhage to occur and what are the predisposing causes?

4. What are the causes of aneurysms of arteries?

5. Classify the tumors of the nervous system.

6. What is a Schwannoma?

7. What is a meningioma?

第十五章 传染病和寄生虫病

大体观察

1. 肺原发综合征
2. 粟粒性结核
3. 局灶性肺结核
4. 浸润性肺结核
5. 慢性纤维空洞性肺结核
6. 肺结核瘤
7. 干酪性肺炎
8. 结核性胸膜炎
9. 肠结核
10. 肠原发综合征
11. 肾结核
12. 结核性脑膜炎
13. 瘤型麻风
14. 肠伤寒
15. 细菌性痢疾(假膜性炎)
16. 宫颈上皮异常增生(尖锐湿疣)
17. 肠阿米巴病
18. 阿米巴肝脓肿
19. 肠血吸虫病
20 血吸虫病性肝硬化
21. 丝虫象皮肿

镜下观察

1. 肺结核结节
2. 结核病慢性纤维空洞
3. 干酪性肺炎
4. 肠结核
5. 淋巴结结核
6. 结核性脑膜炎
7. 皮肤瘤型麻风
8. 肠伤寒
9. 结肠假膜性炎
10. 尖锐湿疣
11. 结肠阿米巴病
12. 肠血吸虫病
13. 血吸虫病性肝硬化

一、大 体 观 察

1. 肺原发综合征　可见肺结核的原发病灶、肺门淋巴结结核和淋巴管炎,三者合称原发综合征,影像学诊断显示哑铃状阴影。

2. 粟粒性结核　结核杆菌通过血流播散,引起肺内和肺外器官(包括肾、脾、肝等)的感染,表现为粟粒样的结核结节播散病灶。

3. 局灶性肺结核　病灶局限于肺尖部。周围有纤维包裹,中央为干酪样坏死灶。

4. 浸润性肺结核　干酪样坏死物通过支气管引流,或经痰液排出,留下急性空洞,空洞壁薄(肉芽组织和干酪样坏死物),含有大量结核杆菌。这些病灶境界不清,灰白色。

5. 慢性纤维空洞性肺结核　空洞壁厚(超过1cm),形态不规则。周围有纤维结缔组织增生。有时有增粗的血管条索通过空洞。可以导致继发性出血。

6. 肺结核瘤 一个直径 2~5cm 的纤维包裹的干酪样坏死灶,位于肺上叶。干酪样坏死灶可发生钙化。

7. 干酪性肺炎 肺内有大量渗出物和大量干酪样坏死物,使肺组织实变,呈灰白色或灰黄色。

8. 结核性胸膜炎 结核性胸膜炎表现为胸膜腔内大量渗出液,没有被完全吸收时,出现纤维组织增生,导致部分胸膜粘连或整个胸膜腔完全闭塞。

9. 肠结核

(1) 病变好发于回盲部。

(2) 椭圆形溃疡环绕肠管分布,有时会出现肠腔狭窄(溃疡型)。

(3) 局部淋巴结增大,伴有干酪性肉芽组织增生,或增生导致结核之肠管增厚(增生型)。

(4) 切面灰白,易碎。

10. 肠原发综合征 包括肠结核的肠壁原发病灶,肠系膜引流区淋巴结炎和肠系膜淋巴管扩张。

11. 肾结核 干酪样坏死灶形成溃疡,切面白色、易碎。

12. 结核性脑膜炎

(1) 软脑膜上散在的白色结节。

(2) 脑底部蛛网膜下腔充满黏稠或纤维性渗出物。使动脉闭塞,并包围颅神经。

13. 瘤型麻风 麻风病灶浸润面部、手和足,导致皮肤增厚,粗糙,成为"狮容"。

麻风侵犯周围神经,如耳大神经导致神经增粗,瘫痪和变形。例如,爪形手、足下垂,鹰状趾和麻痹。

14. 肠伤寒

肠伤寒病变分为四期:

(1) 髓样肿胀期:黏膜上皮糜烂,黏膜下层炎症,淋巴滤泡和伤寒细胞的增生,使肠黏膜表面突出。

(2) 坏死期:肿胀的淋巴组织上方的黏膜坏死。

(3) 溃疡期:坏死物排出,流下卵圆形溃疡,其溃疡长轴与肠管长轴平行。溃疡形成可以导致出血。

(4) 愈合期:表面上皮细胞覆盖溃疡区,没有瘢痕形成及肠腔狭窄。

15. 细菌性痢疾(假膜性炎) 结肠黏膜充血、水肿。纤维性渗出物片状或弥漫性分布于肠黏膜表面,形成灰黄色假膜。

16. 宫颈上皮异常增生(尖锐湿疣)

(1) 简要说明:各型人类乳头瘤病毒(HPV)感染引起的良性病变。

(2) 大体所见:单个或多发性,直径 1 至数毫米,有或无蒂的乳头状赘生物,偶尔融合成菜花状肿块。

17. 肠阿米巴病

(1) 以潜行性病灶和口小底大的烧瓶状溃疡为特征。溃疡边缘呈破絮状,棕褐色,深达黏膜下层或肌层。

（2）溃疡中有广泛的液化性坏死。

（3）溃疡之间的黏膜通常正常或有轻微炎症。

18. 阿米巴肝脓肿　肝右叶的厚壁囊肿,直径可超过 10cm,含有巧克力色,无臭、黏稠的液体。

19. 肠血吸虫病　虫卵在肠壁组织中引起慢性炎症反应,肠壁纤维性增厚或形成溃疡。患者表现为痢疾样症状。

20. 血吸虫病性肝硬化

（1）简要说明:肝脾的血吸虫病主要表现为门静脉周围的纤维化和门静脉高压。

（2）大体所见

1）由于血吸虫色素的沉着使得肝脏颜色变深。

2）血吸虫病性肝硬化主要表现为门管区的纤维化,最终导致干线性的纤维化和窦前性门静脉高压,表现为严重的胃肠道淤血、脾肿大、食管胃底静脉曲张和腹水。

21. 丝虫象皮肿　丝虫引起的慢性淋巴管炎,主要表现为下肢和阴囊的皮肤水肿和纤维化。

二、镜 下 观 察

1. 肺结核结节

（1）主要成分是上皮样细胞和朗汉斯巨细胞,外围是成纤维细胞和淋巴细胞。朗汉斯巨细胞的核呈花环状在嗜酸性胞浆周围排列。

（2）结节中央通常会出现坏死(干酪样坏死)。

其他描述:

结核分支杆菌,$2 \sim 5 \mu m$,直或弯曲的杆状。

通过培养、抗酸染色和杂交技术可以证实。

2. 结核病慢性纤维空洞

（1）空洞壁有三层结构

1）干酪样坏死组织。

2）肉芽组织。

3）纤维结缔组织构成的厚壁。

（2）继发感染时引起炎性浸润。

3. 干酪性肺炎　肺泡腔内充满渗出物和干酪样坏死,引起实变。

4. 肠结核

（1）大的,紧密排列的肉芽肿出现在黏膜层、黏膜下层、肌层甚至浆膜。

（2）干酪样病灶,周围是上皮样细胞,朗汉斯巨细胞,淋巴细胞和外周纤维组织。

5. 淋巴结结核　淋巴结中有干酪样坏死灶和结核性肉芽肿形成。

6. 结核性脑膜炎

（1）慢性炎症反应:淋巴细胞、浆细胞和巨噬细胞浸润。

（2）典型的肉芽肿形成,中央有干酪样坏死,周围有上皮样细胞和朗汉斯巨细胞。

（3）胶质细胞增生。

（4）非炎症区有钙化。

7.**皮肤瘤型麻风**

（1）泡沫细胞:巨噬细胞吞噬了麻风杆菌,胞浆淡染,含有脂质空泡而呈泡沫状。

（2）表皮萎缩,在结节状病灶上方皮肤萎缩变平。

（3）表皮基底细胞以下出现无细胞的透亮区。

（4）出现少量淋巴细胞和血管。

其他描述:

抗酸染色阳性。巨噬细胞内的麻风杆菌平行排列或形成球形团块,也可出现在细胞外,形成麻风球。

8.**肠伤寒**

（1）黏膜表面糜烂。黏膜下淋巴滤泡的炎性增生。

（2）伤寒细胞增生:大的单核细胞吞噬活性增强,其胞浆内含有被吞噬的淋巴细胞、浆细胞、伤寒杆菌、红细胞的碎片,伤寒细胞聚集形成伤寒小结。

9.**结肠假膜性炎**

（1）结肠黏膜损伤糜烂,表面覆盖着斑块状的"假膜",假膜主要由纤维素、中性粒细胞等炎症细胞和坏死组织碎屑组成。

（2）肠隐窝扩张、损伤处被炎性浸润。

10.**尖锐湿疣**

（1）分支状、绒毛状或乳头状的结缔组织间质,被覆增生的上皮细胞。

（2）上皮表层出现过度角化、角化不全和上皮层的增厚(棘皮病)以及表皮突的增厚和延长。

（3）出现典型的核周空泡状的棘细胞(凹空细胞),是 HPV 感染的特征。

（4）这些凹空细胞体积较大,核圆,染色深。

（5）基底膜完整,无间质的侵犯。

（6）间质(真皮)水肿,毛细血管扩张和中等的慢性炎症细胞浸润。

11.**结肠阿米巴病**

（1）肠黏膜形成溃疡,坏死区内水肿、淤血,有显著的嗜酸粒细胞浸润。

（2）阿米巴滋养体圆形,直径 $20 \sim 40 \mu m$,其核为嗜碱性,和红细胞大小相似。一些被吞噬的红细胞碎片见于表层疏松的坏死组织中。

（3）通过过碘酸-雪夫(PAS)染色证实。

其他:最佳诊断方法是通过新鲜粪便中找到吞噬有红细胞的滋养体。

12.**肠血吸虫病**

（1）肠壁组织中有血吸虫卵沉积,引起慢性炎症反应和溃疡部位的纤维组织增生。

（2）肉芽肿形成:肉芽肿的中心是虫卵,虫卵中含有变性或已钙化的毛蚴。有数量不等的散在的巨噬细胞、淋巴细胞、中性粒细胞和嗜酸粒细胞围绕在虫卵周围。这样的结构被称为急性虫卵结节或嗜酸性脓肿。

假结核结节的形成,在钙化的虫卵周围有上皮样细胞、异物巨细胞、淋巴细胞,最终导致结节纤维化。

13. 血吸虫病性肝硬化

（1）虫卵位于门静脉周围，直径 $50\mu m$，早期是嗜酸性脓肿，虫卵周围包围着纤维素样的物质（Hoeppli 现象），随后皮样肉芽肿中央发生坏死，残余虫卵发生钙化。

（2）门静脉系统内的成虫性色素引起的轻微病变，肝脏呈干线性肝硬化。

三、思 考 题

（一）选择题

选一个字母代表的最合适答案。

1. 末端肢体的淋巴水肿可由以下哪个寄生虫感染引起

    A. 结核杆菌   B. 溶组织型阿米巴   C. 伤寒杆菌   D. 血吸虫   E. 班氏丝虫

2. 除了下列哪项，寄生虫感染可累及肝或胆道

    A. 丝虫病   B. 包虫病   C. 阿米巴病

    D. 血吸虫病   E. 华支睾吸虫病

3. 尖锐湿疣性宫颈炎最可能发生在下列哪种病人中

    A. 一个 18 岁有多个性伴侣的女性   B. 一个 38 岁患有卵巢癌的妇女

    C. 一个 20 岁的处女   D. 一个 28 岁患有衣原体感染的母亲

    E. 一个 35 岁患有疱疹性外阴炎的经产妇

4. 一个 35 岁的妇女感觉疲惫。有低热、腹股沟的淋巴结肿大、脓毒性关节炎和出血性丘疹、脓疱疹。皮肤活组织检查发现有严重的中性粒细胞浸润和脓细胞伴显著出血。哪种微生物可能使病人出现这些症状。

    A. 单纯疱疹   B. 人类乳头状瘤病毒   C. 奈瑟氏淋球菌

    D. 结核杆菌   E. 梅毒螺旋体

（二）问答题

1. 淋球菌感染的部位有哪些？

2. 概括结核病的基本病理变化。

3. 比较原发性和继发性结核的特点。

4. 由原发灶播散而来的结核杆菌最常影响身体哪个部位？

5. 肾结核是如何发生的？

6. 概括梅毒瘤的病因和病理变化。

7. 为什么三期梅毒常侵犯主动脉弓？

8. 直肠壁血吸虫病的组织学表现是什么？

9. 请描述阴茎硬下疳。

10. 什么原因引起的淋巴性水肿？

Chapter 15　Infectious Diseases and Parasitosis Diseases

Gross Findings

1. Primary complex of lung
2. Miliary tuberculosis
3. Focal tuberculosis
4. Infiltrating pulmonary tuberculosis
5. Chronic fibrous cavern pulmonary tuberculosis
6. Tuberculoma of lung
7. Caseous pneumonia
8. Tubercule pleurisies
9. Intestinal tuberculosis, Intestine
10. Intestinal primary complex
11. Renal tuberculosis
12. Tuberculous meningitis
13. Lepromatous leprosy
14. Typhoid fever of intestine
15. Bacillary dysentery(Pseudomembranous colitis)
16. Cervical epithelial dysplasia (Condyloma acumi-
    na-
    tum)
17. Enteric amebiasis
18. Amebiic abscess of liver
19. Intestinal schistosomiasis
20. Schistosomiasis cirrhosis of liver
21. Elephantiasis

Micro Findings

1. Tuberculosis, granuloma, Lung
2. Chronic fibrous cavity tuberculosis
3. Caseous pneumonia
4. Intestinal tuberculosis,
5. Tuberculosis of lymph node
6. Tuberculous meningitis, Meninges
7. Lepromatous leprosy skin
8. Interstinal typhoid
9. Pseudomembranous colitis
10. Condyloma acuminatum
11. Colon Amebiasis
12. Intestinal schistosomiasis
13. Schistosomiasis cirrhosis of liver

Gross Findings

1. **Primary complex of lung**　There are tuberculosis foci of Pulmonary lung, hilar lymph nodes lesions and draining lymphangitis,witch total combination called the primary complex this lesions are seen radiographically as "dumb bell" spot.

2. **Miliary tuberculosis**　Owing to tubercle bacilli via the blood stream spread that cause intralung or extralung (including lung kedney, spleen liver etc.) infections and express military disseminated tuberculosis nodules.

3. **Focal tuberculosis**　The lesion mainly localized in the apices of the lungs. Fibrous encapsulation and central caseation.

4. **Infiltrating pulmonary tuberculosis**　The caseous materials in lesions are drained along the air passage or coughed up as sputum.,leaving an acute cavity with thin wall (granulation and caseation) contain amount of bacilli. The lesion express poor circumscribed, with gray-white color.

5. Chronic fibrous cavern pulmonary tuberculosis　The cavity wall is thicker（more than 1cm）with rough irregular lining. Surrounding fibrous connective tissue proliferation, sometimes the thickened vessels are firm cords traversing the cavity,that may cause secondary bleeding.

6. Tuberculoma of lung　2～5cm diameter with fibrous encapsulation caseation lesion localized upper lobe. Caseous lesion may happen. calcification.

7. Caseous pneumonia　In the lung there are amount of exudates and a massive caseation nedrosis express grayish white or yellowish white, that result in the consolidation of lung.

8. Tubercule pleurisies　Tubercule pleurisies express effusive fluid exudates in the pleural space when healing with no complete absorb forming the proliferation of fibrisos tissue, resulting in adhesion of pleura with partial or complete obliteration of the pleural cavity.

9. Intestinal tuberculosis, Intestine

（1）Usually located in the ileocecal area.

（2）Elliptical shape ulcers lying transversely encircling the bowls, sometimes with stenosis of the bowel（ulcer type）.

（3）Local lymph nodes enlarged with caseating granuloma or hyperplastic form of tuberculosis with thickining of the bowed wall（hyperplastic type）.

（4）Cut surface: white & friable.

10. Intestinal primary complex　It compose primary tuberculosis lesion in the wall of intestinal, mesenteric lymphangitis and enlargement of draining mesenteric lymphnodes

11. Renal tuberculosis　The foci of caseation necrosis form ulcer. Cut surface: white & friable

12. Tuberculous meningitis

（1）Discrete,white granules scattered over the leptomeninges.

（2）Gelatinous or fibrinous exudates in subarachnoid spaces often at the base of the brain, obliterating the arteries and encasing cranial nerves.

13. Lepromatous leprosy

（1）leprosy lesions infiltrating the face, hand and feet,result in thickening and wrinkling of the skin produces a characteristic lionine faces.

（2）leprosy lesions involving peripheral great auricular nerves result in nerves enlarged,paralyses and deformities e.g.,claw hands foor drop, claw toes and anaesthesia.

14. Typhoid fever of intestine　Interstinal lesions divides into four stages

（1）Medulloid swelling stages: Including the erosion of the epithelium and mixed inflammation in the lamina proprial lymphoid follicles and typhoid cells proliferation regions standout as projecting areas on the mucosal surface.

（2）Necrosis stages: The mucosa over the swollen lymphoid tissue occur necrosis.

（3）Ulceration stages The necrosis materials shed leaving oval ulcers with their long axes in the direction of bowel flow. Ulcer formation may leading to hemorrhage.

（4）Healing stages The surface. epithelium grows over the ulcerated area,there are no scar formation or contraction of the bowel.

15. Bacillary dysentery（Pseudomembranous colitis）　The colonic mucosa becomes hyperemic and edematous. A fibrinosuppurative exudates patchily or diffusely covers the mucosa and produces a dirty gray to yellow pseudomembrane.

16. Cervical epithelial dysplasia (Condyloma acuminatum)

(1) Brief Descriptions: Benign lesions caused by several types of human papillomavrus (HPV).

(2) Gross Findings: Single or multiple sessile or pedunculated, red papillary excrescences that vary from 1 to several millimeters in diameter, occasionally coalesce into cauliflower like masses.

17. Enteric amebiasis

(1) There are characteristically undermined and a flask shaped ulcer with a narrow neck and broad base. The ulcers have shaggy, yellowish brown edges and a floor foumed by submucous or muscular coats.

(2) In ulcer there are extensive liquefactive necrosis.

(3) The mucosa between ulcers is often normal or mildly inflamed.

18. Amebiic abscess of liver

Amebiic liver abscess: localized in right lobar of liver with thick capsule, it may be exceeding 10cm in diameter. and contain a chocolate-colored, odorless, pasty material likened to anchovy paste.

19. Intestinal schistosomiasis

In the wall of the bowel, the eggs cause chronic inflammations and fibrous thickining or ulceration the patiens express irritation dysenteric symptoms.

20. Schistosomiasis cirrhosis of liver

(1) Brief Descriptions: Mature in the portal venous system causing hepatosplenic schistosomiasis with periportal fibrosis and portal hypertension.

(2) Gross Findings

1) The liver is darkened by schistosoma pigmints deposition.

2) Schistosomiasis cirrhosis of liver predominately express liver fibrosis around portal spaces., eventually leading to a progressive pipestem fibrosis, with presinusoidal portal hypertension and severe congestive, splenomegaly, esophageal varices and ascites.

21. Elephantiasis

Filaria causes chronic lymphadenitis with skin swelling and fibrous of the dependent limb or scrotum.

Micro Findings

1. Tuberculosis, granuloma, Lung

(1) Composed of epithelioid cells and Langhans' giant cells surrounded by a zone of fibroblasts and lymphocytes. Langhans' giant cells: nuclei ring surrounding in eosinophilic cytoplasm.

(2) Some necrosis (caseation) is usually present in the centers of these tubercles.

Others:

(1) Mycobacterium tuberculum(0. 2~0. 5)by(2~5)um, straight or curved rod.

(2) Proved by culture, acid fast stain, or hybridization.

2. Chronic fibrous cavity tuberculosis

(1) There are three layer structures forming cavity wall

1) Caseation necrotic tissue

2) granulation

3）Fibrous connective tissues with thickening vessels

（2）Seecondary infection accompening inflammation infiltrating.

3. Caseous pneumonia   Amount of exudates and a massive caseation necrosis in alveolar spaces with consolidations.

4. Intestinal tuberculosis

（1）Large, closely packed granuloma, in mucosa, submucosa muscularis or extension to serosa

（2）Caseating foci, surrounded by epithelioid cells, Langhans' giant cells, lymphocytes & peripheral fibrosis.

5. Tuberculosis of lymph node   In lymph node there are caseating foci and tuberculositic granuloma formation.

6. Tuberculous meningitis, Meninges

（1）Chronic inflammatory reaction: lymphocytes,plasma cells and macrophages.

（2）Well-formed granuloma with central caseous necrosis surrounded by epithelioid cells and Langhans' giant cells.

（3）Gliosis.

（4）Calcification in inactive area.

7. Lepromatous leprosy skin

（1）foamy lipra cell: macrophages contain many bacilli and exhibit pale lipid vacuolization, foamy cytoplasm.

（2）The epidermic become atrophy and flattening over nodular lesions.

（3）Clear zone show no cells under the basal cells of the epidermis.

（4）A few lymphocytes and blood vessels present.

Others:

Acid-fast stain positive. The bacilli within the macrophages arranged in parallel or globular masses within or outside cells form leprosy globi.

8. Interstinal typhoid

（1）The mucosal surface erosion with inflammation in the lamina proprial lymphoid follicles.

（2）Typhoid cells proliferation: The large mononuclear cells are actively phagocytic and in their cytoplasm remnants of ingested lymphocytes, plasma cells, typhoid bacilli red blood cells, which aggregate form typhoid nodule.

9. Pseudomembranous colitis

（1）The plaquelike adhesion of fibrinopurulent-necrotic debris and mucus to damaged colonic mucosA. Superficial erosion of the mucosa and an adherent "pseudomembrane" "Pseudomembrane" contains amorphous, eosinophilic, fibrin exudate with cellular debris and inflammatory infiltrates.

（2）Supuficial crypts are distended and damaged with inflammatory infiltration.

10. Condyloma acuminatum

（1）A branching, villous or papillary connective tissue stroma covered by a thickened hyperplastic epithelium.

（2）The epithelium shows considerable superficial hyperkeratosis, parakeratosis and thickening of the underlying epidermis（acanthosis）with thickening and elongation of the rete ridges.

（3）Distinct perinuclear clear vacuolization of the prickle cells（koilocytosis）as characteristic of HPV infection.

(4) These vacuolated epithelial cells are relatively large and possess a hyperchromatic, round nucleus.

(5) The basement membrane is intact without invasion of the underlying stroma.

The stroma (dermis) appears edematous with dilated capillaries and a moderately dense, chronic inflammatory infiltrate.

11. Colon Amebiasis

(1) Ulcerated mucosa, edema, congestion and a prominent infiltrate of eosinophils. within necrotic area.

(2) Round organisms of 20~40 um diameter, Trophozoites has one basophilic nuclei about the size of RBC's. some ingested RBCs (erythrophagocytosis), are found in loose surface. debris.

(3) Enhanced recognition by periodic acid-Schiff(PAS)stain.

Others: Diagnosis is best made by identified hematophagous trophozoites in fresh stools.

12. Intestinal schistosomiasis

(1) The schistosoma egg deposit in the wall of bowell and cause a chronic inflammatory re-action and fibrous thicking with ulcerations.

(2) Granulomas formation, the center of granuloma is the schistosoma egg, which contains a miracidium with degeneration or calcifies, there are numerous scattered macrophages,lympho-cytes, neutrophils,and eosinophils around egg, that names an acute egg's guanulomas or eosino-philic abscesses.

Pseudotubercles formation, it is composed of epitheliod cells,forienge giant cells lymphocytes around calcifies egg and eventually fibrous nodules formation.

13. Schistosomiasis cirrhosis of liver

(1) Ova entrapped in portal veins of about 50 um diameter, early with eosinophilic abscess, while the eggs are coated with a rim of fibrinoid material (Hoeppli-Splendore reaction), then an epithelioid granuloma with central necrosis, remaining ova then calcified.

(2) Worm pairs in portal venous system resulting hemozoin pigments & Symmer's clay pip-estem fibrosis.

Study Questions

Choose Tests
Directions: Each of the numbered items or incomplete statements in this section is fol-lowed by answers or by completions of the statement. Select the one lettered answer or completion that is best in each case.

1. Lymphedema of an extremity can be the result of infestation by which parasite?
    A. tubercle bacilli   B. Entamoeba histolytica   C. typhoid bacilli
    D. Schistosoma mansoni   E. Filaria bancrofti

2. Parasitic infections that are likely to involve the liver or bile ducts include all of the fol-low-ing EXCEPT
    A. filariasis   B. echinococcosis   C. amebiasis
    D. schistosomiasis   E. clonorchiasis

3. Condylomatous cervicitis is most likely to be found in which of the following patients?

A. An 18-year-old woman with multiple sex partners

B. A 38-year-old woman with ovarian carcinoma

C. A 20-year-old woman who is a virgin

D. A 28-year-old mother of two with chlamydial infection

E. A 35-year-old multigravida with herpetic vulvitis

4. A 35-year-old woman presents with vague complaints of feeling tired. A low-grade fever, inguinal lymphadenopathy, and a septic accompanied by a ash of hemorrhagic papules are noted. A skin biopsy reveals an intense neutrophic and pus cell infiltrate composed predominantly of hemorrhage. Which microorganism is the most likely etiologic agent of the patient's symptoms?

A. Herpes simplex   B. Human papillomavirus   C. Spirochetes

D. Tubercle bacilli   E. Neisseria gonorrhoeae

Questions

1. What structures are infected by N. gonorrhoeae?

2. Describe the basic pathological lesion in tuberculosis.

3. Compare the primary with the post-primary(secondary) tuberculous lesion.

4. What parts of the body are commonly affected by M. tuberculosis following dissemination from the primary site?

5. How does tuberculosis of the kidney arise?

6. Describe the cause and pathology of a gumma.

7. Why is the aortic arch so commonly affected in tertiary syphilis?

8. what is the histological appearance of schistosomiasis of the rectal wall?

9. Describe a hard chancre of the penis.

10. What are the causes of lymphatic oedema?

各章思考题答案与解释

第一章 细胞、组织的适应和损伤

（一）选择题答案

1- C   2- E

（二）问答题答案

1. 萎缩通常被认为是病理性的,尽管老年性萎缩是否为病理性仍存在争论。退化是生理性,例如胚胎形成期间鳃裂的消失和分娩后子宫恢复到正常大小。

2. 肾盂积水是指肾盂和肾盏的扩张。肾盂扩张时,由于局部肾血流下降,肾单位缺血,肾组织萎缩。首先萎缩的是肾小管,然后是肾小球。肾外肾盂扩张时,肾实质可保持相当长时间的完整性。肾盂积水是慢性尿路阻塞的结果,尿路阻塞可以发生在从肾盂-输尿管接合处到尿道外口的任何部位。

3. 瘘管是在两个空腔脏器或一个空腔脏器和外界之间的异常通道。例如,膀胱结肠瘘并发结肠憩室炎和肛瘘。

4. 溃疡就是上皮或内皮表面连续性的中断。

5. 在两种情况下,器官或组织都增大。其中肥大是由于实质细胞体积增大,增生是由于细胞数量增多。

6. 淀粉样蛋白刚果红染色呈红色,偏振光观察呈果绿色,或通过免疫组织化学检测特殊的淀粉样蛋白。

7. 淀粉样变性是异常糖蛋白在组织的沉积。它通常是原发性的,但也可以继发于:①类风湿性关节炎;②骨髓瘤;③慢性败血症,如慢性骨髓炎或支气管扩张时。淀粉样变性所致死亡常常由于其在肾脏或心脏的沉积导致这些器官衰竭而引起。

8. 肝细胞、心肌细胞和肾小管上皮细胞。

9. ① 核固缩 ② 核碎裂 ③ 核溶解。

10. 坏疽是大块组织坏死继发腐败菌感染,伴颜色发黑。坏疽有三种类型。

(1) 干性坏疽,由于感染较轻,器官或肢体出现干尸化。

(2) 湿性坏疽,由于感染较重,出现严重的坏死和腐败性变化。

(3) 气性坏疽,由于产气杆菌感染,坏死组织中有大量气体。

11. 病理性钙化是指钙盐沉积在骨或牙齿以外的组织。有两种类型:

(1) 营养不良性钙化发生在死亡的或即将死亡的组织内。

(2) 转移性钙化是由于各种原因引起的高钙血症所致正常组织的钙化。

12. 化生是一种分化成熟的组织转变为另一种分化成熟的组织。例如:

(1) 正常情况下由假复层纤毛柱状上皮覆盖的支气管上皮由于吸烟或粉尘的吸入,可转化为鳞状上皮,或在慢性支气管炎的情况下,转化为主要由杯状细胞组成的上皮。

(2) 在尿路结石存在的情况下,尿路的移行上皮可转化为鳞状上皮。

(3) 当胆囊出现结石时,胆囊的腺上皮可转化为鳞状上皮。

(4) 化生可发生在结缔组织,如纤维组织的骨或软骨化生。

13. 凝固性坏死和凋亡的鉴别见下表。

	凝固性坏死	凋亡
刺激	缺氧,中毒	生理性或病理性因素
组织学表现	细胞肿胀,凝固性坏死	单个细胞染色质浓缩
	细胞器破坏	凋亡小体
DNA 破坏	随机,弥漫的	核小体之间
机制	ATP 减少,膜损伤,自由基损伤	基因激活内切酶,蛋白酶
组织反应	周围组织炎症	无炎症,吞噬凋亡小体

14. 老化细胞形态学改变包括:不规则或异常球状核,多形性空泡状的线粒体,内质网的减少,和高尔基体的变形,持续的使脂褐色素的稳定的积聚。

第二章　损伤的修复

(一) 选择题答案

1- D

(二) 问答题答案

1. 并不像以前认为的是由于纤维母细胞产生的胶原的收缩,而是由于水肿的消除和在形成瘢痕之前的肉芽组织的收缩。肉芽组织中的纤维母细胞或肌纤维母细胞是肉芽组织收缩的主要原因。

2. (1) 在骨折断端形成血肿;

(2) 急性炎症的发生;

(3) 粒细胞和组织细胞清除了坏死组织碎屑,例如血肿和死骨片等坏死组织;

(4) 在清除碎屑之后,在骨折断端之间和周围形成肉芽组织;

(5) 肉芽组织的软骨化和骨化使其变得坚硬,因此被称为骨痂。软骨的骨化和骨质的沉积由于缺乏正常的板层结构而被称为编织骨。编织骨既占据原来的骨髓腔也连接密质骨的断端;

(6) 编织骨被重吸收并且被板层骨取代;

(7) 在上一阶段中,同时发生再塑,去除不必要的结构,恢复骨的生理状态。

3. 纤维细胞是一种间质细胞,具有细长的核,处于静止状态。纤维母细胞是纤维细胞的活化形式,比纤维细胞大,能产生胶原。

4. 肉芽组织是由大量毛细血管和增生纤维母细胞,疏松的细胞外基质中含有的炎细胞组成。主要作用:①抗感染,保护创面;②修复创口;③机化包裹坏死组织、炎性渗出物、血栓和其他异物。

第三章 局部循环和血流动力学障碍

（一）选择题答案

1-D 2-D

（二）问答题答案

1. 水肿是过多液体在组织间隙的积聚,肺水肿时液体积聚在肺泡腔。全身性水肿常常伴有胸腔、心包腔和腹腔积液。

2. 循环血流中形成的固体质块。主要由血液成分组成,包括纤维蛋白和血小板,以及红细胞和白细胞的混合物。

3. (1) 内皮或心内膜的损伤;

(2) 血流异常:①血流缓慢;②形成涡流;③血液黏度增高;

(3) 血液成分的改变:①血小板增多;②凝血因子增加;③高脂血症。

4. (1) 血栓,来源于骨盆或髂静脉,或下肢深静脉;

(2) 肿瘤细胞,来源于身体任何部位的原发性肿瘤;

(3) 脂肪,骨折或外伤时;

(4) 羊水,分娩时。

5. 栓子可以是固体、液体、气体,包括血栓栓子、脂肪栓子、空气栓子、氮气栓子、羊水栓子、肿瘤栓子、寄生虫栓子等。

栓子的运行途径主要有5条:

(1) 静脉系栓子可引起肺栓塞或梗死;

(2) 动脉系栓子栓塞于人体的重要器官,如冠状动脉,脑动脉,肝和肾动脉;

(3) 门静脉系栓子引起栓塞;

(4) 静脉系栓子从右心到左心,引起动脉系栓塞,称为交叉性栓塞;

(5) 大静脉栓子引起小静脉栓塞称为逆行性栓塞。

6. 弥散性血管内凝血(DIC)是指突然起病或隐匿发生的广泛的微循环内纤维蛋白血栓形成。这些血栓仅在显微镜下找见,可以引起脑、肺、心、肾等多器官的循环障碍。多量血栓的形成,伴随着血小板和凝血因子的快速消耗(也叫消耗性凝血病);同时,纤溶机制被激活,结果使起始的血栓性疾病变成了严重的出血性疾病。此时血小板、纤维蛋白原和凝血因子V,Ⅷ和X被迅速消耗;同时,因纤溶酶原纤溶酶系统激活,纤维素(纤维蛋白原)被降解,而产生抗凝作用。

7. 减压病发生于环境大气压突然改变时。使用水下呼吸器的深海潜水员,水下操作人员,以及未密封的飞行器内的人员在快速爬升时都有患该病的危险。当空气在高压状态吸入时(例如深海潜水时),通常气体(尤其是氮气)溶解于血液和组织中。如果潜水员上浮(减压)过快,氮气释放在组织中膨胀,在血液中则游离出来形成气体栓子。

在骨骼肌以及关节和周围支持组织内气泡快速形成时,会造成疼痛。气体栓塞还会造成一些组织的灶性缺血,包括脑和心。在肺,会出现水肿、出血、灶性肺不张和肺气肿,导致呼吸困难,即所谓的窒息。减压病的一种比较慢性的过程称为沉箱病,骨骼中的气体栓子持续存在导致多灶性的缺血性坏死,常见于股骨头、胫骨和肱骨。

8. 贫血性梗死与出血性梗死的区别见下表。

	贫血性梗死	出血性梗死
部位	实质器官	疏松组织、双重血供、有淤血时
	（心、脾、肾）	（肺、肠）
颜色	苍白	暗红
梗死与周围组织	分界清,有出血反应带	分界不清,水肿、淤血、出血

9. 血栓性静脉炎是由静脉的损伤或感染所致。在化脓性中耳炎时,感染可能发生在板障和硬膜的静脉;在产褥期败血症时,感染可能发生在子宫静脉;在骨髓炎时,感染可能发生在骨髓静脉。在无菌性血栓性静脉炎中,受累静脉内的血栓可发生机化,然后再通。在感染性血栓性静脉炎中,感染性血栓可能发生碎裂引起脓毒血症。

10. 闭塞性动脉内膜炎由细胞性结缔组织在血管内膜下层同心性增生引起动脉或小动脉管腔的缩窄,最后使该动脉官腔闭塞。正常情况下,闭塞性动脉内膜炎在发生于出生时的脐动脉,动脉导管和分娩后复原的子宫。病理情况下,闭塞性动脉内膜炎发生于慢性消化性溃疡基底部的血管,结核空洞的洞壁,梅毒或暴露于放射性射线的结果。

第四章　炎　　症

（一）选择题答案

1-E　2-C　3-C　4-D　5-A　6-B　7-A　8-C　9-D　10-E　11-C　12-D　13-B
14-E　15-A

（二）问答题答案

1. 炎症是机体对损伤(包括创伤、毒性物质和感染)的一种防御反应。其主要表现被古罗马的 Celsus 描述为红,热,痛,肿。此外,还有功能的丧失、全身白细胞增多和发热等。

2. 急性炎症历时短且组织破坏较小,容易愈合并恢复到正常状态。参与的炎细胞主要是中性粒细胞。慢性炎症有更多的组织破坏,参与的细胞主要是单核细胞,淋巴细胞,浆细胞和组织细胞。被破坏组织被肉芽组织取代,并通过纤维修复留下瘢痕。

3. 它们都属于单核-巨噬细胞系统,通常被认为有共同的起源且可相互转化。前体细胞在骨髓内,被称为幼单核细胞,进入血液成为单核细胞,单核细胞可能进入结缔组织,这时它们被称为组织细胞。它们表现出吞噬活性,被称为巨噬细胞。在肝内的库普费细胞、在肺内的肺泡巨噬细胞、排列在脾脏和淋巴结髓窦表面的巨噬细胞以及小胶质细胞都属于单核巨噬细胞系统。

4. 是指细胞向某种化学物质作定向运动,在急性炎症的情况下,可见中性粒细胞和组织细胞的趋化现象。

5. ①胺类:组胺、5-羟色胺;②补体系统;③激肽;④凝血系统;⑤花生四烯酸代谢产物;⑥白细胞;⑦氧自由基;⑧血小板活化因子;⑨细胞因子。

6. 肥大细胞见于机体任何部位的结缔组织中。它们的胞浆内含有异染颗粒,可以被甲苯胺蓝和吉姆萨染液染色。这些颗粒含有肝素和组胺,因此,肥大细胞可见于炎症和超敏反应中。

7. 葡萄球菌引起皮肤化脓性炎

（1）脓疱性皮炎:表现为表皮的浅表脓疱;

（2）毛囊炎:毛囊浅部的感染;

（3）疖:整个毛囊被感染,且形成脓肿;

（4）真皮的局限性脓肿;

（5）痈:境界不清的皮下化脓性病变,常形成数个脓肿的融合,具有多个排脓窦道。

8. 卡他性炎是黏膜的轻度炎症,黏膜渗出大量黏液和浆液,并向下流淌,一般没有明显的化脓性渗出。

9. 脓肿与蜂窝织炎的区别见下表。

	脓肿	蜂窝织炎
感染	金黄色葡萄球菌	链球菌
机制	血浆凝固酶	链激酶、透明质酸酶
组织	致密组织,实质脏器	皮下组织、肌肉、阑尾
病变	局灶性	弥漫性

10. 假膜性炎是发生在黏膜表面的纤维素性炎症,如白喉、菌痢。

11. 积脓或脓胸是胸膜腔的脓液积聚,因此提示感染是由化脓微生物引起。感染可来自

(1) 肺炎的肺部并发症;

(2) 胸壁损伤;

(3) 腹部,膈下脓肿;

(4) 食管穿孔或纵隔炎症;

(5) 血液播散(很少).

12. (1) 血流动力学作用和渗透压的改变。由于心衰或低蛋白血症如肝功能衰竭及营养不良;

(2) 炎症:浆液、浆液化脓性或出血性感染、菌血症;

(3) 肿瘤性,浆液或出血性渗出;

(4) 胸导管阻塞或撕裂引起的乳糜胸。

13. 慢性炎症刺激感染部位引流的淋巴结增生,淋巴窦扩张内含大量巨噬细胞,淋巴细胞,多型核细胞,这曾被描述为"窦性卡他"这是窦黏膜炎的表现。淋巴滤泡生发中心增生。皮肤损害的慢性刺激或肿瘤引起引流区域内淋巴结即使无转移亦可导致反应性增生。

第五章 肿 瘤

（一）选择题答案

1-C 2-A 3-D 4-D 5-E 6-D* 7-B 8-A 9-A* 10-D 11-B* 12-C
13-C 14-D 15-B 16-D 17-C 18-A 19-B* 20-A 21-E 22-D 23-C

（二）解释

6. 答案 D

间皮瘤发生于接触石棉之后。慢性铍中毒与支气管癌的发生呈双重相关,但与间皮瘤无关。慢性接触砷元素与肝血管肉瘤和肺癌发生增多有关。子宫内膜癌与长期雌激素治疗有关,而给孕妇用己烯雌酚治疗,与她们的女儿在十几岁时患阴道透明细胞腺癌有关。

9. 答案 A

很少有皮肤表浅部位的肉瘤,大部分肉瘤均位于真皮下深部区域,脂肪肉瘤更是如此。例外的有: Kapposis 肉瘤,见于艾滋病人皮肤上的紫红色结节。上皮样肉瘤,通常发生在上肢末端,包括手。血管肉瘤通常发生在老年人头颈部的皮肤,非典型性黄色纤维瘤,组织学上类似于恶性纤维组织细胞瘤,因为在皮肤表面,为良性的位于真皮浅层。

11-14. 答案 11-B, 12-C, 13-C, 14-D

前列腺癌和胃癌都是腺癌,而且它们在电镜下的结构相似。但是,这两种癌可通过免疫组化检测前列腺特异抗原来鉴别,前列腺特异抗原是识别前列腺癌的一个有价值的组织标记物。

电镜下可观察到癌细胞之间的连接(叫做细胞桥粒);淋巴瘤不显示这些超微结构。癌的免疫组化表现为细胞角蛋白阳性和白细胞抗原阴性,淋巴瘤则是细胞角蛋白阴性和白细胞抗原阳性。

电镜下见间皮瘤的微绒毛短而腺癌的微绒毛长。免疫组化分析常显示腺癌中的癌胚抗原,反之,多数间皮瘤不表达癌胚抗原。

不管来源如何,所有鳞状细胞的超微结构都类似。而且目前也没有特异的免疫组化标记物可以识别鳞癌的原发部位。

19-23 答案 19-B, 20-A, 21-E, 22-D, 23-C

N-myc 基因的增强与改善儿童成神经母细胞瘤的预后有关。*N-myc* 基因增强的病人其预后差于分期相同的肺腺癌病人和没有 *ras* 基因增强的病人。*C-erb B2* 基因过表达的乳腺癌妇女,其预后比该基因不表达者差。在伯基特淋巴瘤中发现 *C-myc* 基因,而 *Rb* 抑癌基因出现在视网膜母细胞瘤中。

(三)问答题答案

1. 增生是由于特定因素的过度刺激而引起的组织有限的生长。增生可以是生理性的、炎症性的、修复性。瘤形成是组织内细胞的过度生长,通常原因不明,良性肿瘤在一段时间后其过度生长可能停止;恶性肿瘤在原发和继发部位的过度生长呈相对无限制性。

2. 不典型增生是指组织的生长失调,特别是癌前病变中出现细胞学异常,即细胞不典型性、怪异和细胞极性紊乱,分为轻、中、重三级。上皮内瘤变 III 级中包括原位癌和不典型增生。

3. 错构瘤是指某个器官内发生的、由该器官或组织中分化良好的细胞组成的肿瘤,细胞生长紊乱,但其过度生长是有限度的。

4. 最初,肿瘤一词代表炎症性的、肿瘤性的或其他的任何肿块。现在它和"新生物"一词是同义词。通常被人们所接受的肿瘤的定义是 Willis 所阐述的,这个定义是:肿瘤是组织过度生长所形成的异常肿块,其生长与正常组织不协调,即使在引起病变的刺激因素去除后,仍能以同样方式持续生长。然而,在少数情况下,恶性肿瘤可以自行消退,如恶性黑色素瘤。

5.（1）焦油或页岩油含有的多环芳烃可导致皮肤癌,烟草燃烧的产物中也含有多环芳烃,可引起支气管肺癌。

（2）染料和橡胶工业中使用的苯胺染料可引起泌尿道上皮肿瘤;

（3）青石棉(石棉一种)可导致胸膜或腹膜的间皮肿瘤;

（4）木尘的吸入可引起鼻黏膜或鼻窦黏膜的腺癌;

（5）塑料工业中的氯乙烯,可引起肝的血管肉瘤;

（6）电离辐射,可导致身体多个部位的肿瘤;

（7）砷可导致皮肤癌;

（8）浅色皮肤的人,过量的紫外线照射可导致皮肤鳞癌或基底细胞癌,以及黑色素瘤;

（9）感染;

（10）病毒引起的恶性肿瘤在动物实验中已被证实,其与人类的关系还不清楚。人类恶性肿瘤中与病毒感染关系密切的有:①Burkitt 淋巴瘤;②鼻咽癌;③Kaposi 肉瘤。

（11）寄生虫如血吸虫,可引起膀胱癌。

6. 上皮来源的肿瘤,其细胞在形态上是恶性的,但未突破基底膜。例如皮肤上皮内癌(Bowen 病)。

7. 脱落细胞学是研究上皮或间皮表面脱落细胞或通过细针穿刺实体肿瘤所吸取的细胞的一门科学。通常的目的是检测或排除恶性肿瘤的存在。这种诊断方法最初用于子宫颈的检查。此外,对痰和尿液标本进行脱落细胞学检查可以排除或证实支气管或泌尿道恶性肿瘤的存在。胸水、心包积液或腹水的脱落细胞学检查可以证实导致这些渗出的恶性肿瘤细胞的存在。

8.（1）直接侵犯相邻组织器官,包括沿组织间隙、神经束衣扩散;

（2）转移①通过淋巴管;②通过血管;③通过体腔:胸腔、腹腔、脑室系统和蛛网膜下腔;④肿瘤种植 如 Krukenberg's tumor。

9. "胚胎性肿瘤"发生在婴幼儿和儿童。这些肿瘤好发于:①肾脏:肾母细胞瘤或 Wilm 瘤;②肾上腺或交感神经节:神经母细胞瘤;③小脑和第四脑室:髓母细胞瘤;④视网膜:视网膜母细胞瘤;⑤肝脏:肝母细胞瘤,非常罕见;⑥肺:肺母细胞瘤,非常罕见。

10. 这些肿瘤主要来源于生殖腺,少见于其发育过程中。这些肿瘤包括:①睾丸的精原细胞瘤和卵巢的无性细胞瘤;②畸胎瘤;③宫外绒毛膜癌;④卵黄囊瘤(发生在卵巢的内胚窦瘤和睾丸的睾丸母细胞瘤)。

11. 畸胎瘤由不同起源的多种组织组成。大部分发生在生殖腺,因而产生其为畸胎的概念,它们由卵子或精子单性生殖而来,但是也可出现在纵隔和骶骨。畸胎瘤可包含分化良好的上皮,间皮和内皮成分,产生诸如毛发,牙齿和胃肠道腺体的结构。如果仅含有上皮成分,畸胎瘤呈囊性,被称为皮样囊肿。卵巢的畸胎瘤大部分属于囊性,且为良性,而睾丸的畸胎瘤常常是实性,分化差且为恶性。

12. 它们是恶性肿瘤患者的一系列不相关的全身性表现,通常是由于激素的释放,但一般与肿瘤起源组织无关,副肿瘤综合征也可以由神经病变、脑病、肌病和血栓形成等引起。

13. 卵巢的继发性肿瘤,原发部位是胃肠道,穿破浆膜面进入体腔而种植于卵巢。组织学表现为:具有特征性的细胞基质背景上的大量印戒细胞,这种肿瘤是双侧性的。

14. 畸胎瘤。90%畸胎瘤患者血液中甲胎蛋白 (AFP) 和 β 绒毛膜促性腺激素(βHCG)水平升高。

15. 1775 年 Percival Pott 爵士描述了烟囱清洁工的阴囊皮肤癌。纺织厂工人腹股沟部位有相同的肿瘤(称为纺织工癌),与暴露于走锭织机使用的页岩油有关。

16. 白斑病是指口、喉、外阴或阴茎黏膜出现白斑。由多种原因引起,如吸烟刺激,原位癌,真菌感染或扁平苔藓,角化过度导致黏膜变白,现在认为该病为癌前病变。

17. 良恶性肿瘤鉴别见下表。

特征	良性	恶性
大体表现	膨胀,有包膜,界限清楚	浸润,无明显边界和包膜
组织分化程度	好	分化较差,不典型性异形细胞
有丝分裂数目	少	多
生长速度	慢	相对较快
生长方式	膨胀	浸润
继发改变	少	出血坏死
转移	无	常见
复发	少	常见
对机体的影响	压迫和阻塞	压迫、阻塞、出血、坏死、转移、感染、恶病质等

18. 癌和肉瘤的鉴别见下表。

	癌	肉瘤
组织学来源	上皮组织	间质组织
年龄	老	年轻
大体表现	质硬	质软,鱼肉状
组织学特征	巢状	弥漫
网状纤维染色	–	+
转移	淋巴道	血道
发病率	常见	少见

19. 癌前病变是指某些良性病变与随后发生的癌症有关。即一些临床疾病使发生恶性肿瘤的危险性增加,这些临床疾病就称为癌前病变。

常见的癌前病变有:

(1) 肝硬化-肝细胞肝癌;

(2) 伴恶性贫血的萎缩性胃炎-胃癌;

(3) 慢性溃疡性结肠炎-结肠癌;

(4) 口腔和生殖道黏膜白斑-鳞状细胞癌。

第六章　心血管疾病

（一）选择题答案

1-E　2-B　3-C　4-B　5-D　6-B　7-A　8-D　9-E　10-E　11-B　12-A
13-D　14-C　15-E

（二）问答题答案

1.（1）肺动脉瓣（或右心的漏斗部）狭窄；

（2）由于右心室压力的增大使右心室肥大；

（3）高位室间隔缺损，位于主动脉瓣和肺动脉瓣下方；

（4）主动脉向右骑跨，结果导致右心室减少的血流不能通过狭窄的肺动脉瓣射出，而是通过室间隔的缺损处射出，从而和左心室血流混合，然后通过主动脉瓣进入主动脉。不同程度紫绀的发生取决于以上4种异常情况的严重性。

2.动脉粥样硬化被世界卫生组织定义为在大、中型肌型动脉内层形成不同程度隆起的纤维脂质斑块。病变起源于内膜，并向中膜延伸。包括脂质、血液成分、纤维组织和钙盐的局灶性沉积。

3.（1）年龄：进展的有症状的病变通常出现在40岁以后；

（2）性别：女性动脉粥样硬化很少发生在绝经期前；

（3）环境因素：发展中国家此病的死亡率低于高度工业化的西方国家；

（4）高胆固醇血症，继发于糖尿病，黏液性水肿，肾炎综合征和家族性黄色瘤；

（5）高血压；

（6）吸烟及高度紧张的生活方式、A型血、肥胖、口服避孕药等。

4.由于组织器官血流的减少，动脉粥样硬化可导致相应临床症状的出现。血管阻塞程度的不同导致组织器官受到不同程度的影响。脑动脉受累导致脑萎缩，引起痴呆；肾动脉受累，肾脏纤维化导致高血压；冠状动脉受累，引发心肌纤维化和心绞痛；下肢动脉受累，引起下肢肌肉及皮肤缺血进而导致间歇性跛行，最后可发生坏疽。

5.动脉粥样硬化可以发生于动脉的几乎任何部位，但是更常见于动脉开口处和腹主动脉、冠状动脉、腹动脉、胸主动脉降支、颈内动脉和Wills环（发病频率依次降低）。

6.第Ⅰ阶段，脂纹，在内膜下聚集了吞噬有脂滴的平滑肌细胞和巨噬细胞。

第Ⅱ阶段，可见直径约几毫米的光滑的含有脂质的黄色斑块。在斑块外周，脂质位于细胞内，斑块中央区形成无结构的细胞外的无定形物质，此斑块由一层透明变的纤维组织与内皮分开。

第Ⅲ阶段，在斑块之间和周围有广泛的纤维组织增生，可导致不规则的内膜增厚。在晚期病变，内皮消失，使其下的脂质被暴露，留下粥瘤性溃疡，其上有附壁内血栓形成。钙化，尤其在主动脉远端斑块内的钙化，可发生在这一阶段。中膜变性导致受累血管动脉瘤形成。

7.小舞蹈症是指风湿病累及锥体外系，患儿出现肢体的不自主运动。

8.大动脉的退行性病变，主要但不总是发生在中老年人。与中膜的营养不良性钙化有关，内膜保持正常。血管变硬，管腔大小没有变化。

9.（1）风湿性心脏病时，主动脉瓣前叶增厚、收缩。（2）动脉粥样硬化。（3）Marfan综合征。（4）梅毒性主动脉炎，主要累及升主动脉。

10. 主动脉瓣狭窄可以是先天性的，也可以是后天性的。

（1）先天性主动脉瓣狭窄通常是由于三个瓣叶被一个带有一个中央孔的隔膜取代。少数情况是由瓣膜下隔膜。

（2）后天性主动脉瓣狭窄最常见于慢性风湿性心脏病，急性期形成的赘生物机化瓣叶粘连和瓣膜变形。极少见于先天性二尖瓣纤维化和钙化。

11.（1）先天性的。

严格地讲，先天性动脉瘤并不存在；但是动脉瘤这个词用来描述来源于 Willis 环及其分支的动脉瘤已经得到了普遍地认可。这种动脉瘤在出生时不表现出来，而是在后来形成。主要是由于中膜平滑肌先天的缺陷。

（2）获得性的。

1）退行性的-动脉粥样硬化-Erdheim 中膜变性。

2）感染性的-真菌-梅毒。

3）创伤性的-主要动脉的手术可能导致假性动脉瘤的形成，动静脉瘤性静脉曲张或曲张性动脉瘤。

4）曲张性的-这种类型发生在头皮且可能是先天性的，但通常是创伤性的。当被认为是先天性时则可能是产伤的结果。

12. 心瓣膜赘生物是由在心瓣膜上的血小板和纤维蛋白的沉积。发生于左心的瓣膜赘生物比发生于右心的多，且对二尖瓣的累及比对主动脉瓣的累及多。在急性风湿性心内膜炎时，其赘生物呈小疣状排列于受累瓣膜的闭锁缘，因而认为瓣膜闭锁缘心内膜的创伤导致溃疡形成，从而诱发了赘生物的形成。在急性和亚急性细菌性心内膜炎时，赘生物较大还含有细菌。

13. ①风湿性心脏病的急性或慢性期。急性期形成瓣膜赘生物；慢性期受累的瓣膜发生纤维化和变形。②急性感染性心内膜炎。③亚急性细菌性心内膜炎，毒力较低的细菌侵犯变形的瓣膜。④二尖瓣的粥样斑块形成，伴有纤维化和钙化有关的。⑤系统性红斑狼疮患者的 Libman-Sacks 心内膜炎。⑥不伴有动脉粥样硬化的主动脉瓣钙化。⑦类癌综合征时三尖瓣和肺动脉瓣的纤维化。⑧临终病人的消耗性心内膜炎。

14. 风湿热与 A 组乙型溶血性链球菌感染有关，细菌的外毒素刺激产生的抗体作为一种自身抗体攻击患者自身的心肌纤维，这种假说得到以下方面的支持：①从发生链球菌性咽喉炎到出现风湿热的间隔是 2~4 个星期。②风湿热患者的血清抗链球菌抗体滴度较高。③在心肌纤维中能找到链球菌抗原。这种假说不能解释所有的发病机制，尤其是心内膜和关节组织中胶原纤维的病变。风湿热常见于生活条件差的儿童。

15. 风湿热引起全心炎，包括心外膜炎、心肌炎和心内膜炎。

16. ①在心脏，可累及心内膜、心肌和心外膜。②皮下组织；③关节和腱鞘；④皮肤的皮疹，例如环形红斑；⑤累及心脏后引发的急性心力衰竭时，可以出现肺淤血和水肿。

17. ①心瓣膜病，导致狭窄和关闭不全或两者兼有。②心房纤颤，易在心房和心耳（通常是左心）中诱发血栓形成。可以产生"球瓣"血栓和栓塞。③由于心肌肥大和心排血量的减少引起心绞痛。④亚急性细菌性内膜炎。

18. Aschoff 小体是风湿小体。发生在风湿热时的心肌,最常见于室间隔、左心房和左心耳。

19. 风湿小体发生在心肌间质的小血管旁,中央是纤维素样坏死,邻近有少量的心肌纤维变性,病灶周围聚集了淋巴细胞、浆细胞、巨噬细胞和风湿细胞。风湿细胞是一种多形核的大细胞。愈合后留下小瘢痕。

20. 急性细菌性心内膜炎和致病力强的细菌如金黄色葡萄球菌引起的败血症有关,发生在无病变的心脏,好发于通过静脉吸毒者,体质差者,有脓毒性病灶的病人,大块质脆的赘生物发生在心瓣膜上,可以导致溃疡、穿孔、瓣膜变形,受累的瓣膜很快失去功能,如未经治疗可以导致功能受损,出现心力衰竭。相比较而言,亚急性心内膜炎是由致病力弱的细菌,例如草绿色球菌、大肠杆菌,偶尔真菌引起,在拔牙或导管插入术后,细菌进入血液,导致菌血症而不是败血症,定居在已有病变或患有先天性疾病的瓣膜上例如二叶式主动脉瓣,亚急性细菌性心内脉炎基本上是一种较轻的感染,在应用抗生素后可治愈,但瓣膜上已出现赘生物时则往往会导致瓣膜功能不全的结果。

21. 感染性心内膜炎分为急性和亚急性,其实它们之间有相当一部分重叠。急性是由毒力强的病原微生物引起的。溃疡,穿孔,瓣膜破坏导致死亡。亚急性大多数是发生在免疫力低下的病人,由条件致病菌或毒力弱的病原体引起,如草绿色链球菌或真菌等。亚急性心内膜炎通常为一些疾病的并发症,如慢性心内膜炎或一些先天性畸形例如二叶式主动脉瓣,室间隔缺损或动脉导管未闭。

22. ①猝死;②心绞痛;③心肌梗死;④心肌纤维化致心力衰竭;⑤束支传导阻滞导致心律不齐。

23. 心前区剧烈的疼痛,通常放射至左臂、颈部甚至下颌和牙齿。它通常由心肌缺血引起,休息或扩血管药物可缓解。

24. ①由于心衰和心源性休克引起的猝死;②由于心肌坏死导致心脏破裂,引起心脏压塞导致死亡;③心律不齐;④附壁血栓导致栓塞;⑤心肌纤维化导致慢性心衰;⑥室壁瘤;⑦恢复后遗留轻微的心绞痛或无任何症状。

25. 大约 8 小时。

26. (1) 风湿热 ;

(2) 感染性心内膜炎时瓣膜上的细菌蔓延,或败血症或脓毒血症时的血源性播散引起的化脓性心肌炎;

(3) 柯萨奇病毒 A 或 B 引起的病毒性心肌炎;

(4) 肉瘤样结节病;

(5) 梅毒螺旋体引起不同的心脏病变:①主动脉关闭不全;②冠状动脉口狭窄引起的心肌缺血;③如果梅毒树胶肿侵犯传导系统可引起传导阻滞;④先天性粟粒样梅毒树胶肿引起心肌纤维化;⑤由白喉,肺炎球菌肺炎,伤寒感染或其他败血症引起的中毒性心肌炎;⑥不明原因引起的孤立性心肌炎,与病毒性心肌炎相似。

27. 心肌病包括许多不明原因,且互不相关的慢性心脏病变。有四种类型:

(1) 肥大性:一些患者是常染色体显性遗传。心肌肥大,镜下心肌纤维呈典型的漩涡状排列,左心室肥厚影响心肌收缩,室间隔增厚阻碍血流自心室流出,对左心室影响较右心室大。这种类型可引起心绞痛或心衰。

（2）扩张性：心肌收缩力弱，心腔扩张。附壁血栓，心内膜及心肌间质纤维化。临床上病人产生不明原因的充血性心力衰竭。

（3）限制性：或称心内膜心肌弹性组织增生，较少见，发生于婴幼儿。心内膜下纤维弹力组织沉积，主要影响左心室。

（4）阻塞性：好发于非洲热带地区。乳头肌及肌腱的心内膜纤维化。

28.（1）急性心衰表现：①左心衰引起肺水肿；②心排血量下降可引起心源性休克；③右心梗死或肺栓塞可引起右心衰。

（2）慢性心衰：其症状取决于哪一侧心脏的病变。

1）左心：多数患者系由：①缺血性心脏病；②系统性高血压；③主动脉瓣及二尖瓣病变；④心肌病；⑤先天性心脏病引起。早期症状是呼吸困难，由劳力后呼吸困难逐步进展至休息时亦呼吸困难。

2）右心：普遍原因是①任何原因引起的肺动脉高压，例如二尖瓣狭窄，肺纤维化，血栓栓塞性疾病。②三尖瓣及肺动脉瓣狭窄。这些因素使右心肥厚，继之扩张。颈静脉怒张肝、脾肿大可及，淤血可诱发心房血栓形成及肺栓塞现象。

29.（1）由心肌和心包疾病引起：①缺血性心脏病引起的心肌纤维化；②心肌炎及心肌病；③心律不齐；④淀粉样变性；⑤心包积液或出血引起的心脏压塞。

（2）高血压和肺动脉高压。

（3）血容量增加。

（4）压力负荷增大：主动脉瓣狭窄或关闭不全引起左心室负荷过大。

（5）血流量增多：①由于房室间隔缺损或骨的 Paget 病时外周动静脉瘘引起心脏左右分流。②毒性甲状腺肿和维生素 B_1 缺乏病。

30.原发性高血压病因不明。继发性高血压病因大多数是慢性肾脏疾病。其次是原发性醛固酮增多症，Cushing 综合征或嗜铬细胞瘤。

31.（1）血管变化：①大动脉：出现动脉粥样硬化；②小动脉：早期变化包括血管平滑肌肥大和弹力纤维增生。后期纤维化使血管壁增厚，但机械强度下降；③细动脉硬化症：直径1mm 或更小的动脉变化依赖于高血压是良性还是恶性。前者内膜增厚，玻璃样变性。后者血管壁纤维化坏死伴血栓形成。

（2）累及脏器：①高血压性心脏病，左心室肥厚；②原发性固缩肾；③高血压脑血管血栓、栓塞和梗死，临床出现高血压危象。④视网膜相应变化。

32.（1）肾脏被膜下由于充血和出血可见暗红色区域；

（2）肾脏的部分弓状动脉出现动脉粥样硬化；

（3）小叶间动脉内膜由于结缔组织（主要是弹力蛋白）和平滑肌形成同心层状结构而增厚；

（4）终末小叶间动脉和入球动脉的血管壁发生纤维素样坏死，其后它们的管腔会被完全堵塞。肾小球也可发生相似的局部性坏死；

（5）在肾小球囊内可有血性渗出物；

（6）一些肾单位萎缩，它们的肾小球玻璃样变，而其他的肾小球扩张，肾小管膨胀，其内可有透明管型。

33.大脑中动脉,特别是其分支豆纹动脉,内囊为其供血区,中央前回运动细胞的轴突横过内囊到达脊髓,该动脉血栓形成破坏内囊的轴突和髓鞘,从而导致对侧肢体偏瘫,而感觉仍保存是因为感觉神经的传入纤维位于内囊较靠后的部位。

34.由血液或严重心包腔内浆液渗出或脓液引起的心脏窘迫。阻止心脏舒张,这种类似于缩窄性心包炎。

第七章　呼吸系统疾病

（一）选择题答案
1-B　2-B　3-B　4-C　5-D　6-C　7-B　8-D　9-E　10-D*　11-C*
12-E　13-D　14-B　15-A

（二）解释
10.答案 D

淋巴上皮瘤是上呼吸道的高度恶性的肿瘤;它发生在年轻人,尤其是亚洲人。可见EBV 感染。肿瘤由恶性上皮细胞和非肿瘤的淋巴细胞组成,它可能对恶性上皮成分有免疫反应。由于上皮成分生长迅速且有早期转移的倾向,因而可选用放射线治疗。用手术控制是不可能的。

11-15 答案 11-C, 12-E, 13-D, 14-B, 15-A

结核中常出现干酪样肉芽肿,而非干酪样肉芽肿出现于铍中毒和其他疾病中。单纯肺气肿有各种病因,如吸烟,但尘肺症中肺气肿的改变并不是单一的病变。胸膜钙化是石棉肺的典型表现,有极性的斑块状结节见于硅肺病。

（三）问答题答案

1.不是。肺不张是指出生后肺就未膨胀。肺萎陷是发生在先前扩张的肺,由于肺受压或气管阻塞。

2.大叶性肺炎从发病到治愈经过四个阶段,每个阶段和下一个阶段重合:

（1）充血水肿期:肺泡壁毛细血管充血。

（2）红色肝样变期:水肿液、红细胞和中性粒细胞从毛细血管进入肺泡腔,肺泡腔内有纤维素沉积。肺叶分界不清。

（3）灰色肝样变期:肺泡壁毛细血管被渗出物压迫,因而充血消失,巨噬细胞进入肺泡腔。

（4）溶解消散期:肺泡渗出物被崩解的炎症细胞释放的酶水解液化,并被咳出。巨噬细胞吞噬细胞碎屑和肺炎球菌。

3.(1) 从肺部播散的病原菌可引起化脓性胸膜炎或少见的化脓性心包炎;

（2）血源播散可以引起化脓性关节炎或脑膜炎;

（3）渗出物不能被及时吸收就会被机化。由于肺组织变成纤维化的实性肉样器官,称为肺肉质变。

4.大叶性肺炎好发于青壮年。90%是由于肺炎链球菌感染,而小叶性肺炎是由支气管或细支气管的炎症进展来的,更多发生在抵抗力低的个体如婴儿,老年人,恶性肿瘤或营养不良患者。小叶性肺炎由不同的病原菌引起,通常是来自上呼吸道的共生细菌,如金黄色葡萄球菌,化脓性链球菌,流感嗜血杆菌。大叶性肺炎可影响整个肺叶或数个肺叶。这些受感染的部位经历四个病理变化过程,铁锈色痰,而小叶性肺炎不同于大叶性肺炎,是以细支气管黏膜损害为开始,急性炎症波及这些细支气管所属的肺小叶。脓痰即使不进行药物治疗,大叶性肺炎通常可自行痊愈。偶尔死于呼吸衰竭,败血症或其他并发症。小叶性肺炎不予治疗可引起不同程度的肺纤维化。

5. 肺间质纤维化以及胸膜纤维斑块的形成。其次青石棉可以诱发胸膜或腹膜的间皮瘤,此外,对于吸烟的人来说,石棉还是一种潜在致癌物。

6. 肺气肿是肺气道的扩张伴肺泡壁破坏。而肺膨胀过度不伴有气道的破坏,因此是可逆的,但慢性化后可发展为肺气肿。

7. (1) 阻塞性:①小叶中央型;②全小叶型;③旁间隔型。

(2) 大泡性肺气肿:由前一种情况进展而来,青年患者可见单个大泡。如果破裂可引起自发性气胸或间质性肺气肿。

(3) 旁牵引性:当肺气肿发生在皱缩瘢痕或矽肺结节周围时。

(4) 代偿性:当一个肺叶或几个肺叶塌陷或被切除后。

(5) 老年性。

8. 慢性支气管炎临床定义:慢性咳嗽,咳痰每年发作 3 个月以上,超过 2 年。慢性支气管炎有以下组织学特征:(1) 支气管杯状细胞增多,纤毛上皮减少(黏液化生);(2) 黏膜下黏液腺肥大;(3) 非特异性炎症性变化;(4) 肺气肿,通常与慢性支气管炎有关。

9. 肺源性心脏病并不是一个精确的定义。它指由严重的肺疾病导致的心脏疾病,引起肺循环障碍,结果引起右心室肥大,如果治疗不成功,可引起心衰。

10. 新生儿肺透明膜病是由于早产儿缺乏 Ⅱ 型肺泡上皮产生的表面活性物质而发生的呼吸窘迫。覆盖于肺泡表面的透明膜由纤维蛋白和变性的细胞组成。吸入高浓度氧可能是诱因。表面活性物质是洗涤剂样的物质,可以减少表面张力,防止肺泡塌陷。

11. ①吸烟是最重要的因素。雪茄和烟斗由于影响范围较小,其影响还不明确。②接触青石棉。青石棉诱发肺癌的能力并不强,但它加重了吸烟致肺癌的危险性。③在过去,接触不同种类金属矿砂的矿工吸入了放射性粉尘与气体,也是肺癌好发的职业性因素,见于前捷克斯洛伐克和德国的萨克森州。

12. 肺癌主要分为支气管源性和继发于其他部位的转移肿瘤。肺的淋巴瘤及白血病多属于后者,尽管肺的原发性淋巴瘤也可发生。支气管源性肺癌在组织学上的分类有轻微差别,但基本上可分为以下几类:①鳞状细胞癌;②燕麦细胞癌(小细胞或小细胞间变性癌);③腺癌;④大细胞或大细胞间变性癌;⑤支气管-肺泡癌。最后一种可能是一种特殊类型的腺癌,大多数人认为其来源于肺泡上皮。因此和来源于支气管的肺癌相比,它们是真正的肺癌。

13. 燕麦细胞癌(小细胞癌)在电镜下可见神经内分泌颗粒,该肿瘤可引起类癌综合征。提示其来源于 APUD 细胞,类癌综合征主要和 5-HT 的分泌有关,此外,还可以分泌其他激素如 ADH,ACTH。

第八章 消化系统疾病

（一）选择题答案

1- A　2- C　3- E　4- C　5- B　6- A　7- D　8- C　9- D　10- E　11- D　12- E
13- A　14- D　15- C　16- D　17- D　18- E　19- C　20- B　21- D　22- E

（二）问答题答案

1. 门脉高压病人黏膜下静脉扩张。虽然这些静脉丛的血仍流入体循环静脉系统,但仍有小吻合静脉连接胃的门脉引流。门脉高压使血液通过吻合支进入食管静脉形成食管静脉曲张。

2. Barrett 食管是指食管末端具有分泌黏液的化生区域(原为鳞状上皮)。

3.（1）肿瘤;

（2）消化道狭窄;

（3）失迟缓症;

（4）少见病因包括:①进展性系统性硬化;②吞咽腐蚀性物质引起狭窄;③外部受压,常见原因是后纵隔的恶性淋巴结病或主动脉弓动脉瘤。④原虫感染,克氏锥虫引起的 Chagas 病,多见于南美洲,原虫释放毒素影响包括食道在内的全身的植物神经节。

4. ①鳞癌,起源于食管的鳞状上皮。环状软骨后区发生的鳞癌,女性患者更多见,是男性患者的 20 倍。②腺癌,起源于胃底贲门部位的肿瘤的直接延伸可引起食管末端腺癌。③未分化癌。④APUD 肿瘤。

5. 最常见的肉眼表现是黏膜表面隆起的结节,其中心可见溃疡形成。偶有环状生长,而弥漫性浸润引起广泛狭窄更少见。镜下表现:同一个肿瘤可有各种不同的分化类型,从有角化鳞癌细胞巢,到既无角化也无棘细胞的未分化类型。

6. ①3/4 食管癌患者发生于食管中 1/3 段。②女性鳞癌患者可在环状软骨后区,作为 Plummer-Vinson 综合征的一部分。

7. 食管癌扩散方式:①通过黏膜下淋巴管扩散至食管的其他部位,这对外科医生尤为重要,因为它不易在术中发现,只能在后来被病理医生的镜检证实。②经淋巴管到邻近淋巴结。③直接蔓延,穿破肌层后侵犯气管,支气管,肺或后纵隔。④经血道转移至肝,肺或肾上腺。

8. 糜烂:①经常为多灶性。②黏膜层缺损未达全层,残留基底部的腺体成分。③愈合后不留瘢痕。

溃疡:①是一种局限性病灶,黏膜全层缺损。②组织缺损可深达黏膜下、肌层。③愈合后留下瘢痕。

9. 黏膜缺损,缺损周围的黏膜显示慢性炎症反应。溃疡顶部有数量不等的坏死物,其中可找到多形核白细胞,溃疡底部是生长活跃的肉芽组织,或成熟的纤维结缔组织,这取决于溃疡处于活动期还是愈合期。肉芽组织含有内皮细胞肿胀的新生毛细血管,炎症细胞散在或聚集成巢。主要有淋巴细胞和浆细胞及一些多形核白细胞。肉芽组织或纤维组织可部分或全部取代溃疡底部胃壁原有的正常结构。愈合时形成瘢痕组织。

10.（1）穿孔,胃溃疡及十二指肠溃疡穿孔至腹腔可引起化学性腹膜炎。

（2）胃和十二指肠溃疡可"侵入"腔外组织,如胰腺。

（3）严重出血:胃溃疡可呕血,十二指肠溃疡有黑粪。

（4）过度纤维化：在十二指肠可引起幽门梗阻。

（5）胃溃疡有 1% 患者恶变，十二指肠溃疡不会癌变。

11.（1）饮食：——食物、水和食品防腐剂中的亚硝酸盐可转化为成亚硝胺类致癌物——烟熏、腌制的食物及蔬菜。——缺少新鲜水果和蔬菜。

（2）宿主因素：——慢性萎缩性胃炎及胃的肠化时的幽门螺旋杆菌（HP）感染，多数肠型胃癌患者伴有 HP 感染时出现的胃酸过少。——胃部分切除术导致胆汁反流——胃腺瘤是癌前病变。

（3）遗传因素：——A 型血人，某些种族以及胃癌病人的近亲。

12.“早期胃癌”是指胃的肿瘤局限于黏膜层或黏膜层与黏膜下层，即使原发肿瘤很小且很局限，但仍有局部淋巴结侵犯的可能。

13. 50% 胃癌发生于胃窦及幽门部，其余在贲门部。

14.（1）直接蔓延，侵犯黏膜下层及肌层，伴有纤维组织过度增生时可形成所谓的“革囊胃”，穿透浆膜层可累及胃肠道其他部位，主要是横结肠；

（2）通过淋巴管；

（3）通过血道；

（4）经腹腔引起种植性转移，可引起腹水并偶尔可继发卵巢肿瘤，称 Krukenberg 瘤。

15. 类癌主要发生在消化道，比如阑尾，极少发生在小肠，结肠和胃，类癌由 APUD 系统的细胞（嗜银细胞）组成，他们分泌 5-羟色胺。类癌只局部浸润很少远处转移。5-羟色胺及其他分泌物可引起类癌综合征。如阵发性面部潮红，腹泻，支气管痉挛，肺动脉狭窄，三尖瓣关闭不全。5-羟色胺转化成 5-羟基吲哚乙酸从尿排除。若类癌局限于肠道则类癌综合征不会发生，因为 5-羟基吲哚乙酸通过肝脏灭活。但若类癌出现肝转移或更远处转移时则肝脏灭活作用不会发生。类似的肿瘤也可在肺部发生，可能和高度恶性的肺小细胞癌有关。

16. 结肠“息肉”不是单一的病理变化。它仅仅是一种突出于黏膜的局限性肿块。息肉可以是无蒂或有各种长度的蒂。息肉有四种组织学类型：（1）肿瘤性（腺瘤或腺癌）；（2）错构瘤；（3）炎症性；（4）未分类。

17. 结直肠癌 Duke 分期表明了肿瘤的扩散。它是大肠癌预后的一个指标。虽然其他因素如组织学的分化也应考虑进去。A 期：肿瘤未突破黏膜固有层，无淋巴结转移；B 期：肿瘤进入结肠或直肠周围组织，但无淋巴结转移；C 期：肿瘤远处转移，不管直接蔓延的程度，无法治愈，仅 1/3 病人存活超过 5 年。

18. 血癌胚抗原（CEA）在水平升高最初被认为只与结肠癌有关。现在此结论已被进一步扩展。在其他肿瘤、肝硬化、肝炎病人 CEA 水平也可升高。但大肠癌切除术后 CEA 水平快速升高提示肿瘤复发。

19.（1）遗传因素：O 型血人群有较高患十二指肠溃疡的危险。同双卵双生相比，单卵双生有更高危险。

（2）酸浓度变化：慢性胃溃疡胃酸浓度正常或减少。而十二指肠溃疡患者胃酸分泌增高。尤其是夜间的胃酸分泌。Zollinger-Ellison 综合征患者高胃酸分泌导致严重溃疡。

（3）B 型胃炎患者有黏膜抵抗力受损。可能与 H.P 感染有关。90% 的胃溃疡患者可找到幽门螺杆菌。

（4）化生：十二指肠溃疡与十二指肠的胃上皮化生有关。

（5）相关疾病：十二指肠溃疡在酒精性肝硬化，慢性梗阻性肺疾病，慢性肾衰以及甲状旁腺功能亢进患者中更易发生。后二者与高钙血症有关，高钙血症可刺激胃泌素分泌，进而刺激分泌胃酸。

（6）其他因素包括吸烟及精神性因素。

20. 慢性胃炎有两种类型。

（1）自身免疫型胃炎（A 型胃炎）。这种类型胃炎中 90% 病人有壁细胞抗体。50% 病人有内因子抗体。后者可竞争维生素 B_{12} 结合位点，并引起恶性贫血。此型胃炎可伴有其他自身免疫性疾病，如桥本甲状腺炎及 Addison 病。疾病早期的胃黏膜活检显示黏膜的浆细胞和淋巴细胞浸润。后期胃萎缩，壁细胞被黏液分泌细胞所取代。

（2）幽门螺杆菌相关性胃炎（B 型胃炎）此型胃炎最常见，随着年龄增长发病率升高。病变主要在胃窦部。组织学表现为浆细胞浸润，另外在上皮层和固有层中有中性粒细胞浸润。HP 不侵犯黏膜，但在黏膜表面可找到 HP。两种胃炎均可恶变。

21. 确切机制仍不清楚。PH<4.0 时 HP 很容易被杀灭。但它可以在胃黏膜表面分泌的黏液层中生存。而且细菌可产生氨中和胃酸。体外培养时发现其可产生细胞外蛋白酶，它可降解胃黏液中的糖蛋白。因此推测，黏膜的抗酸保护作用被破坏。另外体外培养中发现该细菌可产生细胞毒性的外毒素。

22. 慢性肝炎指肝炎症状无缓解，持续超过 6 个月。除了乙型。丙型肝炎，慢性肝炎还可由酒精，长期胆道阻塞及代谢性疾病如 Wilson 病引起。慢性肝炎炎症大部分局限在门管区。病情更重时在门管区及其周围进行性纤维化，可引起肝硬化。此种形式可以是病毒感染，也可以是自身免疫反应，后者可由药物或其他未知因素诱发。临床上表现为不适、腹痛、肝肿大、血生化改变、终末期可出现肝衰竭。

23. 肝实质破坏和再生的过程形成了肝硬化的假小叶结节，伴随胶原纤维组织增生，形成纤维间隔包绕再生结节。再生结节失去了正常肝小叶的结构，肝细胞含有脂肪空泡，表明其受到持续的毒性损害。淋巴细胞浸润在汇管区和纤维间隔内。可以出现肝细胞性黄疸。肝脏可肿大和正常大小，但多数肝脏缩小。肝硬化是按病因学而非形态学，例如结节大小来分类的。

24. （1）散在肝细胞死亡属于凋亡。

（2）局灶性坏死：发生在化脓性门静脉炎、急性病毒性肝炎。急性药物性肝炎。这些病灶不位于肝小叶的特定部位。

（3）碎片状坏死：小叶界板虫蚀状破坏。

（4）桥接状坏死：发生于中央静脉到中央静脉区（C-C）、门管区到中央静脉区（P-C）、门管区到门管区（P-P）的坏死带。碎片状坏死和桥接状坏死均见于慢性肝炎中。

（5）带性坏死。按受累的小叶区域划分：①门脉周围坏死发生于磷中毒时；②中央小叶坏死发生于贫血、慢性肝淤血及酒精中毒时；③中央区坏死发生于黄热病。

（6）大块肝坏死（急性黄色肝萎缩）可由病毒性肝炎和药物对肝细胞的损害引起。如 CCl_4 导致大片不规则肝细胞坏死或重症肝炎。

25. 原发性胆汁性肝硬化较罕见且病因未明。女性发病率是男性的 8 倍。起先隐匿，出现不适和轻度黄疸。肝脏肿大，血清胆固醇增高并出现皮下黄色瘤。慢性病人可有吸收障碍。黄疸属阻塞性黄疸。组织学上,非化脓性炎症导致肝内胆管破坏。1/3 患者可出现肉瘤样肉芽肿,病灶区域的小胆管周围有大量淋巴细胞及浆细胞浸润。炎症向门管区周围延伸,破坏周围的肝细胞。门管区纤维化引起胆汁淤积。持续的肝细胞破坏及再生,以及纤维化导致小结节性肝硬化。

26.(1)恶性肿瘤

1)最常见的是继发性肿瘤。通常来自消化道、肺部或乳腺。

2)肝脏的原发性恶性肿瘤:①肝细胞性肝癌,可能是肝硬化的一种合并症。②胆管癌,和肝硬化无关,但是和肝吸虫感染有联系,因此在远东比较多见。

(2)良性肿瘤不常见:①肝腺瘤;②胆管腺瘤;③血管瘤,经常海绵状、紫黑色,肉眼观很容易与继发性黑色素瘤混淆。

27. Zollinger-Ellison 综合征是由于胰岛的 δ 细胞肿瘤导致胃泌素的过多分泌,60%为恶性,或是由于胃幽门胃泌素分泌细胞增生引起。导致盐酸高分泌,在十二指肠和空肠上段引起顽固性、多发性溃疡。胰腺分泌的碱性液体被中和,导致严重腹泻。胰酶被灭活导致脂肪痢。

第九章　造血及淋巴系统疾病

(一)选择题答案

1- D　　2- A

(二)问答题答案

1.①超敏反应,如花粉热,荨麻疹。②寄生虫感染。③某种慢性皮肤病,如天疱疮及类天疱疮。④结节性多动脉炎的部分患者。⑤霍奇金淋巴瘤的部分病例。

2.包括三种临床病理类型。病因不明,具有典型的巨噬细胞肿瘤样增生,但并不是肿瘤。

(1)Letterer-Siwe 病:多见于儿童,短期内死亡。是由于骨髓被不含脂质的巨噬细胞取代。

(2)Hand-Schüller-Christian 病:也可见于成人但大多数见于儿童。巨噬细胞含脂质,主要是胆固醇。患者可存活至 10 岁。脂质沉积不是疾病的原因,因此并不是一种脂质沉积病。

(3)骨的嗜酸性肉芽肿,是孤立的病灶,也可能是一种惰性的 Letterer-Siwe 病。巨噬细胞增生伴有嗜酸粒细胞的聚集。多见于青少年和年轻成人。

3.除胸腺瘤,白血病以外淋巴组织的恶性肿瘤。可以原发于一个或一组淋巴结、脾脏、胸腺或有淋巴组织的任何部位,如骨髓或胃肠壁。淋巴瘤也可原发于皮肤——蕈样霉菌病。这个疾病最终可变为多灶性,恶性淋巴细胞广泛侵犯人体。非霍奇金淋巴瘤可侵入血液系统引起淋巴细胞性白血病。

4.有多种分类方法,但对临床而言,下面的分类方法较实用。级别越低,恶性程度越低。

低级:①小淋巴细胞。②滤泡性,小透明细胞为主。③滤泡性,小透明细胞和大细胞混合。

中级:①滤泡性,大细胞为主;②弥漫性,小透明细胞;③弥漫性,大、小细胞混合;④弥漫性,大细胞。

高级:①大细胞免疫母细胞性;②淋巴母细胞性;③非透明小细胞性;④混合性。

5. R-S 细胞是霍奇金淋巴瘤的主要特征,直径大于 40μm,有双叶核,并有丰富的嗜酸性胞浆,有时呈空泡状。

6. Ann Arbor 系统分期法:Ⅰ期:一个或一组淋巴结受累;Ⅱ期:受累淋巴结全在横膈以上或全在横膈以下;Ⅲ期横膈上下的淋巴结均受累,伴或不伴其他组织的侵犯;Ⅳ期:广泛侵犯一个或多个非淋巴组织,伴或不伴淋巴结受累。其意义对治疗和预后都很重要,单个或单组淋巴结受累(Ⅰ和Ⅱ期)可给予局部放射治疗,其他则要化疗。和组织学类型一样,分期也影响到预后,级别越高,预后越差。

7. 目前,就组织学而言,WHO 分型法得到全世界公认,霍奇金淋巴瘤分为二型:结节淋巴细胞为主型霍奇金淋巴瘤(NLPHL)和经典型霍奇金淋巴瘤。后者又可分为以下 4 个亚型:

(1) 淋巴细胞为主型:大部分是淋巴细胞,R-S 细胞也较多,嗜酸粒细胞稀少。

(2) 淋巴细胞消减型:较多的 R-S 细胞,数量不等的嗜酸粒细胞,可以有弥漫性纤维化,淋巴细胞稀少。

(3) 结节硬化型:淋巴结被膜纤维性增厚,并向淋巴结实质伸出小梁。

(4) 混合细胞型:R-S 细胞、巨噬细胞、中性粒细胞、嗜酸粒细胞、淋巴细胞及浆细胞均可见。有弥漫性的胶原纤维(不同于结节硬化型)。

15%的霍奇金淋巴瘤为淋巴细胞为主型和淋巴细胞消减型;结节硬化型和混合细胞型各占 30%~40%,Ⅰ期的结节硬化型预后最好,其次是淋巴细胞为主型,混合细胞型预后较差,淋巴细胞消减型预后最差。虽然预后与分型有关,但治疗仅由分期决定。NLPHL 发展慢,预后好。

8. 发生在皮肤的 T 细胞恶性淋巴瘤:真皮上部可见巨噬细胞,淋巴细胞,网状细胞,浆细胞和嗜酸粒细胞的浸润。表皮可见淋巴细胞浸润和 Pautrier 脓肿。

第十章 免疫性疾病

(一) 选择题答案

1- B 2- B 3- C 4- C 5- E 6- D* 7- B 8- A 9- D 10- D 11- D*

(二) 解释

6. 答案 D

迪乔治(DiGeorge)综合征是由于无胸腺和甲状旁腺发展而来的。甲状旁腺组织的缺陷引起低钙血症和手足抽搐。迪乔治综合征中 B 细胞是完好的,所以浆细胞的数量正常。无胸腺导致 T 细胞免疫缺失。

11. 答案 D

Sjögren 综合征的特点包括有泪腺和唾液腺的增大;组织学上有淋巴浆细胞的浸润,腺泡组织萎缩,导管阻塞;形成肌上皮岛。病变常与风湿性关节炎有关。一些患有 Sjögren 综合征的病人有发展为淋巴瘤的风险。Sjögren 综合征本身并不是恶性的,所以,不会发生局部淋巴结的转移。

(三)问答题答案

1. 在免疫缺陷的个体,由腐生或共生的微生物所致的严重感染,主要影响呼吸系统。主要病原体包括:(1) 原虫和蠕虫,如隐孢子虫病和弓形虫病。(2) 真菌,如白色念珠菌和曲霉菌。(3) 细菌,如分枝杆菌,放线菌属和沙门菌属。(4) 病毒,如巨细胞病毒。

2. Kaposis 肉瘤是一种来源不明的恶性肿瘤,可能来源于异常的原始间充质。包括四种类型:

(1) 经典型,据报道在北欧犹太人中常见,在下肢皮肤产生红色或紫色的斑块或结节。很少导致死亡。

(2) 非洲型 Kaposis 肉瘤,与欧洲发现的肿瘤相似,但多见于儿童,且与淋巴结肿大有关。

(3) 移植相关型,免疫抑制停止后此型常消退。

(4) 艾滋病相关型,可早期扩散,但对细胞毒性药物和 α-干扰素敏感。大约 1/3 的此型 Kaposis 肉瘤可继发其他恶性肿瘤,常见的有淋巴瘤、白血病和骨髓瘤。

组织学上,所有 Kaposis 肉瘤的表现是特征性的,由梭形细胞和含有红细胞的裂隙组成。这样的表现提示血管源性,但是偶尔可见纯细胞型或间变性 Kaposis 肉瘤。

3. 人类免疫缺陷病毒(HIV 病毒)是一种反转录病毒,和其他反转录病毒的感染相似,从病毒感染到出现临床表现有一段较长的潜伏期(7~10 年)。感染的结果是严重的免疫抑制,这可使 HIV 病毒感染者易发生机会性感染、肿瘤和神经系统症状。即艾滋病临床表现。

4. (1) Kaposis 肉瘤,间质细胞源性肿瘤,可以在严重的免疫缺陷发生以前形成。(2) Burkitt 淋巴瘤,发生于大约 3% 的感染者。此肿瘤几乎均是 B 细胞来源的,有侵袭性,常发生于脑。(3) 宫颈癌。尤其是伴有人类乳头状瘤病毒感染的艾滋病患者,人类乳头状瘤病毒和宫颈的不典型增生,原位癌以及鳞癌有关。

5. 移植物抗宿主反应发生于含有供体淋巴样细胞的组织或血液输入免疫缺陷或免疫抑制的宿主体内时。这种情况下移植的淋巴细胞可存活并产生对抗宿主组织的免疫应答。移植物抗宿主反应有两种形式:(1) 急性型:在移植后 3 个月内发生,如骨髓移植。表现为剥脱性皮炎,腹泻,小肠吸收不良,胆汁淤积性肝病。(2) 慢性型:多在 15 个月内发生。症状与进行性系统性硬化症相似,在各种组织产生广泛的纤维化。如累及食管可引起吞咽困难,累及小肠可致吸收不良。至少有半数病人死于累及肾脏引起的肾功能衰竭。

6. (1) 超急性型:供体肾使宿主致敏产生大量移植抗体。(2) 急性型:这种反应常在移植手术后一年内发生,受者会出现发热、少尿、受累肾区触痛。(3) 慢性型:在数月或数年后移植物失去功能,这种情况常伴有高血压、蛋白尿、在尿液中有纤维蛋白降解产物。

7. 病变发生在肾动脉和肾实质。由于间断性血小板聚集形成血栓,并与动脉内膜融合导致了小叶间动脉和弓状动脉内膜增厚,在肾实质、肾小球基底膜和肾小管上皮增厚。免疫荧光显示 IgM、IgG 和补体呈现细颗粒状沉积肾小球基底膜和肾小管。

8. Down 综合征的发生是由于在卵子生成期 21 号染色体分离失败,最后导致在受精卵中出现了三条这样的染色体。因此,在典型的 Down 综合症患儿的体内染色体的组成是 47,XX,+21 或 47,XY,+21。这种组合方式说明了在男性或女性体内有一条多余的 21 号染色体,这种基因型称为 21 三体。Down 综合征多见于高龄产妇。Down's 综合征有一种罕见的形式与母亲年龄无关,而是 46 条染色体。这其中有一条大的染色体由 21 号和 15 号染色体通过易位组成。这样的情况实际上是隐匿性的三体。

9. 巨细胞病毒是一种疱疹病毒,主要经胎盘途径感染新生儿。在许多组织可发生病变,由于核内出现病毒包涵体而使细胞核膨胀,包涵体也可见于胞浆内。在新生儿,病因是脑炎,存活的儿童会出现智力发育迟缓或发展成脑积水。在成人,血清学证明是感染者的,可以只表现类似传染性单核细胞增多症的轻微症状或亚临床表现。这种病毒可引起任何年龄的免疫缺陷患者发生机会性感染。

10. Sjögren 综合征的基本病理改变是腮腺,泪腺的破坏,伴有淋巴细胞浸润而引起的肿大。此病女性多于男性。临床上这些腺体破坏可导致口干,进食困难,干燥性角结膜炎。淋巴样组织也可发生这样的病变。腺体中存在抗自身微粒体的抗体。

第十一章 泌尿系统疾病

(一) 选择题答案

1-B 2-D 3-A 4-A 5-C 6-B 7-C 8-E 9-A

(二) 问答题答案

1. 肾小球肾炎是一组肾脏疾病,其主要病理改变是在肾小球增生为主的炎症改变,机制是Ⅲ型或Ⅱ型超敏反应。通过光学显微镜观察可以进行分类。

2. 肾小球肾炎可以是弥漫性的,影响所有的肾小球,也可以是局灶性的,只影响一部分肾小球。局灶性损伤通常呈节段性,如一部分肾小球毛细血管丛损伤比其他部分更严重。弥漫性损伤通常累及整个肾小球。镜下肾小球的变化,归纳起来包括增生(细胞数量增加)和细胞外物质增加(如毛细血管基底膜和/或系膜基质),具体分类:

(1) 弥漫性膜性肾小球肾炎:细胞数正常,基底膜均匀增厚。

(2) 弥漫性系膜增生性肾小球肾炎:毛细血管正常但系膜基质和系膜细胞数量增加。

(3) 弥漫性毛细血管内增生性肾小球肾炎:内皮细胞和系膜细胞数量增加,使肾小球肿胀,毛细血管腔闭塞,可见多形核白细胞浸润。

(4) 弥漫性系膜毛细血管性肾小球肾炎:系膜细胞增生,系膜基质增加,毛细血管袢管壁增厚,管腔闭塞。

(5) 局灶节段性增生性肾小球肾炎:部分毛细血管丛细胞数增加,基质增多,有时伴有坏死,背景出现弥漫性系膜细胞增生。

(6) 弥漫性毛细血管外增生性肾小球肾炎:壁层上皮增生形成"新月体"。

3. 弥漫性毛细血管内和弥漫性系膜增生性肾小球肾炎通常会消退,后者除非进展否则并不严重。1/4 膜性肾病会自发性缓解,剩余的病例经过 5~10 年从肾病综合征发展到慢性肾衰竭。系膜毛细血管性肾炎很少缓解,很快发展到慢性肾衰。新月体的广泛形成说明了肾功能在几个月内很快丧失,其表现重叠了弥漫性毛细血管内、局灶节段性、系膜毛细血管性肾小球肾炎。

4. 许多肾小球肾炎病因不明,因此是特发性的,能引起肾小球肾炎的全身性疾病是系统性红斑狼疮、亚急性感染性心内膜炎和血小板减少性紫癜。它们引起一系列的病变,轻者是弥漫性系膜增生性肾炎,稍严重的是局灶节段性肾炎,最严重的是弥漫性毛细血管外(新月体)肾炎。结节性多动脉炎和 Wegener 肉芽肿病也可以引起肾炎,但是血管炎性,而不是过敏性。膜性和系膜毛细血管性肾小球肾炎主要是特发性的,尽管前者可能与恶性肿瘤、肉样瘤病、乙型肝炎表面抗原、用青霉素和金治疗类风湿性关节炎有关。系膜毛细血管性肾小球肾炎常继发于系统性红斑狼疮、血小板减少性紫癜、亚急性感染性心内膜炎、感染性房室分流。类似于弥漫性毛细血管内增生性肾炎，它也可以发生于链球菌感染后。弥漫性系膜增生性肾炎很少是特发的，除了全身性疾病外，还可见于 IgA 肾病，一种以复发性血尿为主要表现的自限性的疾病。SLE 可引起各种类型肾病。

5. 通过免疫荧光和电子显微镜，它们位于光学显微镜所观察到的病变处。①在膜性肾小球肾炎，复合物线状排列于肾小球毛细血管基底膜外。②在弥漫性系膜性肾小球肾炎，复合物沉积在系膜区。③在系膜毛细血管性肾小球肾炎，复合物沉积在系膜和毛细血管内侧。在许多病例中复合物的成分是特异的，IgG 和 G3 存在于膜性肾小球肾炎，C3 存在于系膜毛细血管性肾小球肾炎，IgA 存在于 IgA 肾病，但是在 SLE 中无论形态学上如何，其免疫复合物是混合的。

6. 轻微病变性肾炎是一种除了肾小球上皮细胞足突消失以外没有其他病变的肾炎，这种改变在电镜下才能观察到。所以在光学显微镜下肾脏组织是正常的。此病好发于儿童，主要表现为选择性蛋白尿而导致肾病综合征的表现。它对皮质激素治疗敏感，停药后病情仍可持续缓解。

7. 该病通常出现在弥漫性毛细血管外增生性肾炎。免疫荧光显示 IgG 沿着毛细血管基底膜呈线性沉积，因为这种综合征是抗基底膜抗体引起的 Ⅱ 型超敏反应。在其他的肾小球肾炎免疫荧光呈颗粒状。

8. (1) 肾实质肿瘤。

1) 良性：常见，但没有重要的临床意义。它们包括腺瘤，黄色的境界清楚的圆形肿瘤，球旁细胞肿瘤来源于球旁细胞，是一种少见但重要的肿瘤，因为它们分泌肾素，因此是引起高血压的罕见原因。

2) 恶性：占所有恶性肿瘤的 1%。①肾母细胞瘤，常在 7 岁以前发生。②肾腺癌。

3) 肾盂的来源于泌尿道移行上皮的肿瘤，多为恶性。

4) 结缔组织肿瘤，包括：平滑肌瘤、纤维瘤、脂肪瘤，这些肿瘤是良性的，但少见。

9. 肾腺癌起源于肾皮质，体积小的肿瘤通常突出于肾脏的上、下极，切面呈黄色。陈旧性的出血区呈棕色，坏死区呈灰白色。肿瘤可通过直接蔓延侵犯肾静脉腔。镜下：瘤细胞呈小梁状排列或呈腺管、乳头状。大部分这种肿瘤由特征性的透明细胞和颗粒细胞组成，透明细胞含有脂肪和糖原，在切片制作的过程中被溶解。

10. 肾母细胞瘤大约占儿童肿瘤的 1/3。大部分在 3 岁时发病，很少见到大于 7 岁的患者。肾母细胞瘤切面呈白色或灰白色，由于出血或胶样变性可出现囊腔。镜下可见由梭形细胞组成的特征性的间质，其内是原始、低分化的肾小球和肾小管。肿瘤经常向邻近组织蔓延，血行转移主要到肺、骨和肝。

11. 肾盂肾炎是肾盂、肾盏、肾间质的细菌感染性炎症，经常由下尿道的大肠杆菌逆行感染引起。可以是急性的也可以是慢性的，累及单侧或双侧。这种病女性较男性多见是因为前者膀胱炎发生率高。在女性这也是引起慢性肾功能衰竭的重要原因。

12. (1) 性别　肾盂肾炎在女性较常见，这是因为女性尿道短且在性交过程中容易发生损伤，因此下尿路感染常见。修女相比性生活较多的女性其尿路感染的发生率很低。怀孕时由于激素引起输尿管松弛和扩张可致尿液停滞，从而导致上尿路的急性细菌性感染。

（2）尿路阻塞。尿路阻塞时引起感染的原因是：①滞留的尿液是肠道细菌良好的培养基。②膀胱颈部的阻塞造成膀胱-输尿管反流。③反流的压力降低了肾脏对感染的抵抗力。④慢性阻塞引起的肾衰竭降低了整个机体对于感染的抵抗力。

13. 肾脏体积增大、水肿。在肾髓质可见放射状的黄色脓液形成的条纹,在肾皮质可形成小的黄色脓肿。肾盂黏膜增厚、充血、表面有渗出。镜下肾盂黏膜下层可见化脓性炎症,肾小管和组织间隙也可见脓细胞。

14. 慢性肾盂肾炎常继发于慢性膀胱-输尿管流及下尿路阻塞。肾实质不规则变薄导致肾脏萎缩,表面变形。镜下可见脓肿,在肾小管和肾盂黏膜可见化脓性病变。所有病例的肾小球硬化,被玻璃样变性的胶原纤维所取代,间质大量炎症细胞渗出。在病变晚期整个肾脏纤维化时,炎症反应逐渐消失。形成宽阔 U 形瘢痕。

15. 膀胱泌尿道上皮来源的肿瘤可以呈外生性乳头状生长,或呈实性使膀胱壁增厚,并形成不同程度的溃疡。

16. 膀胱肿瘤的镜下表现有赖于分化程度的高低,主要是移行细胞癌。低度恶性的高分化肿瘤由大小形态一致、排列整齐的细胞组成,形成乳头状的突起;随着分化程度下降,细胞侵犯膀胱壁,形态大小不一,核深染、核分裂象多见。

第十二章　生殖系统和乳腺疾病

（一）选择题答案

1-D　2-C　3-D　4-C　5-D　6-D　7-C　8-C　9-D　10-D　11-C　12-D　13-B　14-D　15-B　16-E　17-D　18-C　19-E　20-A

（二）问答题答案

1. 子宫内膜异位症是正常子宫内膜（包括腺体和基质）出现在子宫外,如卵巢、输卵管、大肠、脐部皮肤、腹部瘢痕、腹腔浆膜面。子宫腺肌病一度被作为一种特殊的子宫内膜异位症,是指正常子宫内膜深入子宫肌层内部。

2. (1)与宫颈癌不同,此病在绝经后的女性常见。(2)在未产妇多发。(3)一些病例与高雌激素刺激有关。(4)可局灶性或弥漫性累及子宫内膜。在穿透子宫肌层时所有的改变都属晚期。可直接侵犯到盆腔,然后累及盆腔外淋巴结和远处器官。(5)腺癌中可以出现鳞状上皮化生。如果鳞化很明显,则称为腺棘皮癌。也可出现有恶性鳞状上皮成分的腺鳞癌,预后不良。(6)早期诊断,预后较好,5 年存活率为 66%。

3. 几乎所有的子宫颈恶性肿瘤都是癌。90% 是鳞癌,其余是腺癌。鳞癌与过早性行为和性生活紊乱、早孕、多产有关。疱疹病毒、包皮垢、精子的 DNA 被怀疑是致癌物。在犹太人女性中这种病不常见,很可能是因为她们男性性伴侣行了包皮环切术而不是因为基因的关系。腺癌多发生于未产妇,与上述因素无关。易发生于年轻女孩,特别是当她们的母亲怀孕时接受了雌激素治疗的。未发现其他病因。

4. 通过脱落细胞学检查、活检或同时使用两种方法可以检测出宫颈癌的早期征兆,即鳞状上皮不典型增生。在一些病例中可发展至原位癌,最后成为浸润癌,这个过程需要大约15 年,不典型增生可自发性逆转,但所有的不典型增生都具有潜在恶变倾向,现在被归为宫颈上皮内瘤变(CIN),并被分为 1 到 3 级。最高级也就是严重的不典型增生,有时就是原位癌。要判断哪些 CIN 病例会成为恶性还不可能。宫颈炎伴有不典型增生是个复合的诱因。

5.（1）复层的鳞状上皮细胞不能分化成扁平、角化、含糖原的成熟细胞。（2）基底细胞增生成多层。（3）正常时扁平排列的上皮细胞失去极性。（4）细胞增大且大小不一。（5）核深染，核分裂象多见。

6. 卵巢肿瘤种类很多。很多种类都有良、恶性之分。

（1）普通上皮性肿瘤。90% 是恶性。许多为囊性。囊壁实性或呈乳头状常提示为恶性。①浆液性囊腺瘤：有良、恶性之分。②黏液性囊腺瘤：有良、恶性之分。③Brenner 瘤，常为良性。

（2）性索间质肿瘤：①颗粒细胞瘤：低度恶性，分泌雌激素。②卵泡膜细胞瘤：良性，分泌雌激素。③性腺母细胞瘤，由支持细胞、间质细胞或两者混合组成，大多数为良性，且产生雄性激素（有时为雌激素）。

（3）生殖细胞肿瘤：①无性细胞瘤，与精原细胞瘤在组织学、恶性度、对放射线敏感性等方面相似。②内胚窦瘤（卵黄囊瘤）。③卵巢的绒毛膜癌。④畸胎瘤：恶性畸胎瘤和成熟畸胎瘤（良性），后者在以前称为皮样囊肿。

（4）其他肿瘤，如纤维瘤、脂肪瘤、平滑肌瘤、恶性淋巴瘤。

（5）继发性肿瘤，来源于乳房、子宫、胃、大肠。

7. 由卵巢纤维瘤引起的腹水和胸腔积液。这是良性肿瘤，切除后可痊愈。

8.（1）葡萄胎：来源于局限于子宫内膜的绒毛。这种肿瘤常为良性但有向绒毛膜癌转变的可能。（2）侵袭性葡萄胎。5% 的葡萄胎的绒毛可以侵袭甚至穿透子宫肌层。所形成的栓子可转移到远处器官。这是良性的，胎块切除转移组织就逐渐消失。发展成绒毛膜癌的可能性并不比葡萄胎大。（3）绒毛膜癌。1/2 的绒毛膜癌继发于葡萄胎，1/4 发生于流产后，1/4 发生于正常妊娠后的妊娠产物残留，这是一种高度恶性的肿瘤，过去死亡率很高，应用细胞毒性药物治疗后 80% 病例可以治愈。（4）胎盘部位滋养细胞肿瘤（PSTT）。

9. 胎盘组织的肿块，其绒毛高度水肿形成水泡状外观。这是由滋养层细胞增生形成的，受精时由于卵子死亡，带有 X 染色体的精子细胞复制成二倍体，细胞分裂直到产生胎块。事实证明，胎块细胞含有两条 X 染色体，且都来源于父亲。尽管认为这是一种良性肿瘤，但有 5% 可发展为高度恶性的绒毛膜癌。

10.（1）脂肪坏死，由外伤引起。

（2）炎症（乳腺炎）：①脓肿；②结核病；③浆细胞性乳腺炎（腺泡或扩张的导管破裂）；④真菌病、寄生虫病（少见）。

（3）乳腺不典型增生（纤维囊性病）。

（4）原发性肿瘤：1）良性：①纤维腺瘤；②腺瘤（少见）；③导管内乳头状瘤；④叶状瘤，也叫叶状囊性肉瘤或巨大纤维腺瘤，20% 为恶性；⑤脂肪瘤。2）恶性：①癌；②肉瘤、白血病和淋巴瘤，少见。

（5）继发性肿瘤少见。

11. 这是一种上皮成分和结缔组织混合生长的肿瘤，叫做纤维腺瘤，单纯腺瘤很少见。与恶性肿瘤的好发人群相比，纤维腺瘤的发病年龄较轻。它们与周围乳腺组织境界清楚，从肿瘤中间切开后可见肿瘤组织突出来。在镜下，它们由纤维性间质中分化良好的腺体组成，其表现不易与癌相混淆。可分为小管内和小管周围两种类型。但是多数为混合性的,所以这种分类方法无临床意义。

12. 病因尚不清楚。乳腺癌在未产妇较多产妇多见。哺乳次数的多少并不重要但初次怀孕较早似乎可起到保护作用。在小鼠体内未发现与乳腺癌相关的病毒或遗传因素。

13. (1) 原位癌:①导管内原位癌;②小叶内原位癌。

(2) 浸润性癌:①浸润性导管癌;②浸润性小叶癌;③混合存在并非罕见。

(3) 不常见的类型:①黏液癌(胶样癌);②鳞癌;③梭形细胞癌;④大汗腺癌;⑤髓样癌,有大量的淋巴样细胞浸润。

14. 这是临床上用来描述一种生长快、扩散快的乳腺癌,常在妊娠或哺乳期发生。肿瘤表面的皮肤呈红色且水肿,因此命名。其在所有乳腺癌中不到2%。

15. 在临床上是慢性乳头湿疹可累及乳晕及周围皮肤。组织学上除了非特异性慢性炎症细胞浸润真皮层,在增厚的真皮层中可见典型的 Paget 细胞。这是一种体积大、淡染、有明显核仁的细胞,单个或聚集成群。皮肤可形成溃疡。真皮层病灶下方是乳腺导管癌,为原位癌或浸润癌,这种癌很小,需要组织学检查才能发现,Paget 细胞起源于此。

16. 雌激素受体是位于细胞内或细胞表面的蛋白质,雌激素与其结合,从而导致这种细胞增殖。因而他们会出现在雌激素作用下的靶器官的细胞上。这包括正常乳腺上皮。乳腺癌细胞上有数量不等的雌激素受体。乳腺癌细胞上具有相当数量的雌激素受体首先提示它们分化较好;其次,也表明肿瘤对抗雌激素治疗(药物或内分泌腺切除)反应良好。

17. 约有1%乳腺癌发生在男性。他们在组织学上与女性相似。在所有男性恶性肿瘤中不到1%。在男性其病因是 Klinefelter 综合征,这种病中出现2~4条 X 染色体。1000 名男性之中有 2 名基因型可表现为 XXY。

18. 可以是男性乳房发育、炎症或肿瘤。男性乳房发育是男性乳房肿大最常见的原因,可出现全乳弥漫性增大,但经常表现为不对称或呈结节状,所有的乳房肿瘤中有 1/1000 发生于男性乳房。

19. 男性乳房发育一般认为是由于雄激素/雌激素比例失调所致的乳腺肥大。可以在青春期和更年期自发产生。或者直接通过雌激素起作用,这种情况发生在肝硬化时对正常产生的雌激素灭活下降。男性乳房发育也可发生于患有分泌雌激素的肿瘤的男性、用雌激素治疗前列腺癌和工作时通过皮肤吸收雌激素时。不论何种原因引起,其组织学上表现相似。导管数目增多。导管上皮细胞层次增多,有时与导管内肿瘤相似,有乳头状突起,基质包绕这些导管形成特征性的水肿样外观。无恶变倾向。

第十三章 内分泌系统疾病

(一) 选择题答案

1- B   2- A   3- C

(二) 问答题答案

1. (1) 弥漫性非毒性甲状腺肿   患者可以是甲状腺功能正常。

(2) 弥漫性毒性甲状腺肿,功能亢进,浸润性眼球突出和水肿样纤维化。

2. 结节性甲状腺肿含有数量不等的结节,由局灶增生引起。结节之间有胶原纤维束分割。部分结节中出现胶样变性,而其他部位发生出血导致坏死和囊性变。在变性的结节中可发生纤维化和钙化。

3. 单纯性甲状腺肿由广泛扩张的甲状腺腺体组成,甲状腺无功能亢进或低下的表现。组织学上单纯性甲状腺肿由增大的滤泡组成,其内充满了胶质,被覆有扁平上皮。

4. ①饮食中缺碘。②甲状腺素需要量增加,如妊娠时的生理性甲状腺肿。③先天性酶缺乏,阻碍了甲状腺摄碘或甲状腺素的合成。④化学物质干扰甲状腺素合成,如:对氨基水杨酸、硫尿嘧啶、卡比马唑、芥类蔬菜(甘蓝、萝卜)中的物质。

5. 在未治疗的毒性甲状腺肿,甲状腺滤泡被高度增生的上皮覆盖,该上皮形成内折突入滤泡形成乳头。这些细胞比正常细胞大,胶质减少。在滤泡边缘的淡染的胶质中可见空泡,形成特征性的贝壳状表现。在用碘治疗后,胶质被再次充满,但如果用抗甲状腺素药物治疗如给卡比马唑治疗,增生和折叠的上皮就会增加。通常会有一些淋巴样细胞弥漫浸润,但有时为局灶性。

6. 桥本甲状腺炎中的甲状腺对称性或非对称性增大。表面光滑,腺体呈灰白色,切面呈均质状,主要特征是腺体缺乏血管。镜下:最突出表现是淋巴细胞和浆细胞的大量浸润。局部聚集可形成淋巴滤泡。在晚期,残留的甲状腺滤泡变小,只含有少量的胶质。滤泡上皮细胞增生、形成体积大、形态不规则,胞浆嗜酸性的细胞,称为 Askanazy 细胞。

7. 甲状腺肿瘤

(1) 良性:①胚胎性腺瘤;②胎儿型腺瘤;③Hürthle 细胞腺瘤;④单纯型腺瘤;⑤胶样腺瘤;⑥不典型腺瘤。

(2) 恶性:少见,占癌症死亡总数的 0.3%。①乳头状癌;②滤泡性癌;③间变性癌;④髓样癌;⑤鳞状细胞癌;⑥其他肿瘤,包括恶性淋巴瘤和畸胎瘤。

8. (1) 肿瘤孤立,包膜完整。

(2) 镜下:肿瘤由大量滤泡和数量不等的细胞团块组成。透明细胞和嗜酸性细胞(Hürthle 细胞)呈片状排列,形成了肿瘤的大部分。

(3) 发现包膜和/或血管侵袭可证实其为恶性。

9. ①很少有完整包膜;②在 20% 病例中肉眼可见多个肿瘤病灶;③肿瘤可含有砂粒体;④镜下,在充满胶质的滤泡中可见乳头状突起;⑤肿瘤很少经血道扩散,但可侵犯邻近的淋巴结。

10. (1) 20% 的患者是家族性的,属于多发性内分泌性肿瘤(MEN)Ⅱ型综合征。

(2) 肿瘤起源于分泌降钙素的滤泡旁细胞(C 细胞)。

(3) 散发性肿瘤常为单侧,在家族性病例中常为双侧且多发。

(4) 肿瘤为散在的,色灰白。

(5) 镜下:肿瘤由小的未分化细胞和含有淀粉样物质的基质组成。

(6) 肿瘤转移至局部淋巴结,然后转移至骨、肝、肺。

11. 糖尿病的并发症有高血压、动脉粥样硬化、肾盂肾炎。这种糖尿病性肾小球肾炎是最严重的损害,在儿童病死率很高是由于糖尿病性肾小球硬化。该病中在肾小球小叶系膜区有嗜酸性透明物质沉积,沉积物可呈结节状或弥漫分布,沉积物呈弥漫分布地表现与其他弥漫性肾小球肾炎相似。

12. 引起肾上腺急性损伤的原因有:细菌或病毒感染、妊娠、严重的创伤、弥散性血管内凝血。在感染化脓菌性脑膜炎时有典型的症状——沃-弗(Waterhouse-Friderichsen)综合征。急性损伤可致严重低血压、发绀、死亡。慢性肾上腺损伤原因为结核杆菌、真菌感染、继发性肿瘤、自身免疫病、与类风湿性关节炎相关的淀粉样变。慢性损伤导致 Addison 病。

13. Addison 病是因为各种原因引起的肾上腺皮质慢性损伤。主要表现为疲劳、肌力低下、腹部不适、颊黏膜和暴露在光线下的皮肤褐色素沉着,是由于垂体产生过量的促肾上腺皮质激素导致黑色素细胞被激活。皮质醇不足引起细胞内、外水和钠离子失平衡最终可引起低血压。

14. (1) 男性化引起男孩性早熟、女孩假两性畸形。

(2)女性化导致女孩性早熟,男孩女性化。

(3) 醛固酮增多症。

(4) Cushing 综合征:肥胖、满月脸、水牛背、蛋白丢失、腹部皮肤变薄、紫纹,许多病人可出现骨质疏松、多尿症。

15. Cushing 综合征因为肾上腺皮质腺瘤、癌或肾上腺皮质增生分泌过量的皮质类固醇,而 Cushing 病是由于垂体腺瘤分泌过量的 ACTH,刺激肾上腺分泌可的松。

16. 原发性醛固酮增多症是由于肾上腺皮质分泌过量的醛固酮,或由于皮质增生、皮质腺瘤或癌引起。生化异常包括:低血浆肾素、低血钾、高血钠、糖耐量降低。临床表现为多尿、多饮、周期性肌力下降。

17. 这种综合征以一个以上内分泌腺增生或形成瘤为特征。可分为 3 型,都明显为常染色体显形遗传。MEN I (Werner 综合征)由垂体、胰岛和甲状旁腺腺瘤组成,尽管甲状旁腺只表现主要细胞增生。肾上腺皮质腺瘤和甲状腺腺瘤也可见。MEN II (Sipple 综合征)主要是甲状腺髓样癌、嗜铬细胞瘤、甲状旁腺主细胞增生。MEN III (MEN II B or Gorlin 综合征)由甲状腺髓质癌、嗜铬细胞瘤、黏膜的神经瘤(尤其在唇部),骨骼畸形、Marfanoid 样体形。

第十四章　神经系统疾病

(一) 选择题答案

1- D　2- D　3- C　4- B

(二) 问答题答案

1. 流行性脑脊髓膜炎和流行性乙型脑炎的区别见下表。

	流行性脑脊髓膜炎	流行性乙型脑炎
季节	冬春季	夏秋季
病因	脑膜炎双球菌	乙型脑炎病毒
感染途径	呼吸道	虫媒叮咬入血
病变部位	脑脊髓膜	脑实质
病变性质	化脓性炎	变质性炎

2. Wallerian 变性描述的是一种当神经纤维与神经细胞分离时产生的改变。12 小时内的轴突断裂可以被观察到,随后,髓鞘和轴突形成的卵形体被增生的施万细胞所包绕。变性的速度取决于:①髓鞘形成　粗的有髓纤维变性快于无髓纤维。②功能　感觉纤维变性速

度快于运动纤维。随着髓鞘和轴突的变性,巨噬细胞、成纤维细胞、施万细胞形成融合体,称为 von Bungner 带,这好比是建筑上的脚手架,变性的轴突在其中生长。同时这些改变也发生在断裂的远端,神经细胞核周发生中心尼氏体溶解。最后神经细胞内只剩下外周很少的尼氏体。这种改变不是退行性变,而只是神经细胞再生之前的反应。

3. 脑出血常发生在:①豆状核,出血来自大脑中动脉的豆纹动脉分支。②脑桥。③小脑白质。主要诱因有:①高血压造成动脉粥样硬化的血管或微动脉瘤的破裂。②原先存在的大脑损伤,如原发性或继发性肿瘤,或脓毒性病灶。出血在大脑皮质形成血肿或出血破入脑室可以导致死亡。

4. ①先天性血管中层的缺陷导致颅内小动脉瘤(Berry)的发生。尽管血管中层结构薄弱经常可见,但是引起动脉瘤却很少发生。这种动脉瘤经常发生在大脑中动脉起始处或其分支处。②动脉粥样硬化。③高血压。④真菌病,发生于亚急性细菌性心内膜炎的患者。

5. (1) 原发性肿瘤

1) 神经源性肿瘤在儿童多见,且为恶性:神经母细胞瘤,髓母细胞瘤,视网膜母细胞瘤。

2) 神经胶质肿瘤都是恶性的,种类较多。①组织分化良好的胶质瘤,生长缓慢。依据起源细胞命名,包括星形细胞瘤;少突神经胶质瘤;室管膜瘤。②间变性胶质瘤,如多形性胶质母细胞瘤多为高度恶性。

3) 脑膜瘤,多为良性。

4) 神经鞘和神经根肿瘤,都是良性。①神经鞘瘤(听神经瘤)。②创伤性神经瘤。③神经纤维瘤,多发时可以变成恶性(von Recklinghausen 病)。

5) 不常见的肿瘤和囊肿:①血管瘤,一种发育畸形。②血管母细胞瘤,是恶性的。③表皮样囊肿。④畸胎瘤,恶性或良性(皮样囊肿)。⑤颅咽管瘤(小脑囊肿),良性。

(2) 继发性肿瘤很常见,可以继发于身体各个部位的肿瘤,有时以神经系统症状为首发症状。

6. 来自施万细胞的肿瘤,可以发生于颅神经或脊神经。颅内常见的原发部位是第八对颅神经,肿瘤一般位于内耳道听神经的内侧。肿瘤一般实性,神经鞘瘤中心会发生液化性坏死。镜下肿瘤由交织成网状的梭形细胞组成,相邻细胞平行排列形成"栅栏状"。

7. 脑(脊)膜瘤来源于蛛网膜细胞。它们经常发生在上矢状窦,也可在椎管。脑膜瘤生长缓慢,形成光滑的或结节状的、易碎的、有包膜的、白色的肿瘤,肿瘤可以侵犯其上方的骨组织。镜下表现多样,最常见的是合胞体型,由无明显界限的多角形细胞组成。少见的是过渡型,由同心圆层状排列形成漩涡的细胞巢组成,细胞巢可钙化形成砂粒体。恶性的很少见。

第十五章　传染病和寄生虫病

(一) 选择题答案

1- E　　2- A　　3- A　　4- E

(二) 问答题答案

1. 在男性,感染部位是尿道,前列腺,精囊腺和副睾。在女性,感染通常不严重,感染部位有尿道,宫颈,宫腔和盆腔腹膜。在青春期前的女性,由于阴道的中性 pH 容易发生淋球菌性阴道炎。在成熟女性,由于雌激素的分泌,阴道 pH 呈酸性,因此具有抗菌作用。

2. 在感染部位,中性粒细胞首先出现,且很快被巨噬细胞和淋巴细胞取代。随着病变进展,从中央到周边区域形成一个结构清晰的结节:①结节中央的干酪样坏死区,可发现结核杆菌。②由巨噬细胞构成的区域,包含有和皮肤的棘细胞有一定相似性的细胞,被称为上皮样细胞,其中散在分布有多核巨细胞,称为朗汉斯细胞。结核杆菌最可能在这个区域被发现。③淋巴细胞,其外围有肉芽组织或纤维结缔组织,这取决于病灶的新旧,组织损伤的程度及愈合的阶段。

3. 原发性和继发性结核都好发于相同的部位,最常见的是肺和肠。但原发性结核病往往自发愈合。继发性结核病在没有治疗的情况下,受累组织往往进展形成空洞。如果原发性结核和继发性结核病都发生进展,则以相似的方式播散,但是,原发性结核引起引流区域的淋巴结肿大往往比较明显,在易感机体内结核杆菌经血源性播散引起的粟粒性结核病在原发性结核病中更为常见。

4. 来自感染的原发灶,如肺,肠或皮肤(罕见)的结核杆菌可以经淋巴管播散到邻近的淋巴结,然后经血流播散到脑,脑膜,泌尿生殖道,骨和关节。如果原发灶是肺,当痰被吞咽后可能感染肠,或者当被咳出时可能感染气管,声带或舌。

5. 肾结核可由有或无临床表现的身体任何部位结核病灶中的结核分枝杆菌经血源播散而引起。

6. 梅毒瘤(梅毒树胶肿)是第三期梅毒的典型病变。它是几乎可发生在任何器官的凝固性坏死,并最终发生纤维化而似橡胶一般硬。病灶局部由于对梅毒螺旋体的超敏反应而发生缺血性梗死。尽管坏死类似于干酪样坏死,但是组织发生了干尸化,而不像干酪样坏死那样彻底崩解,因此,它的原始结构仍然依稀可辨。病灶中可见大量炎症细胞,包括淋巴细胞,浆细胞,组织细胞,偶见巨细胞。成纤维细胞产生胶原。好发部位是肝,睾丸,皮下组织和骨。

7. 由于这段主动脉有丰富的淋巴管。此淋巴管为梅毒螺旋体提供了从纵隔淋巴结到血管壁的通道。基本病变是血管外膜分支状滋养动脉的动脉炎。

8. 受感染的肠壁上皮变得粗糙并可形成溃疡。在晚期肠壁纤维化,也可钙化。在肠壁可见多核虫卵。

9. 阴茎的硬下疳由梅毒螺旋体引起。初起是位于阴茎冠状沟的硬结。其后出现表浅或较深的溃疡,30~60天可自愈,在所有病例中都有显著的腹股沟淋巴结肿大。镜下,首先出现多形核白细胞的浸润,但很快被淋巴细胞和浆细胞取代,炎症细胞浸润多见于血管周围。

10. (1) Milroys 病 :淋巴管先天性缺乏或发育不良。

(2) 肿瘤性渗透。

(3) 慢性淋巴腺炎。

(4) 班氏丝虫对淋巴管的侵袭,或成虫阻塞淋巴管,尤其是引流双下肢和外生殖器的淋巴管。

Answers and Explanations for All Chapters

Chapter 1   Cell and Tissue Adaptation and Injury

Answers and Explanations for Choose Tests
1- C   2- E

Answers and Explanations for Questions

1. Atrophy is usually considered to be pathological although it may be argued whether the atrophic changes of old age constitute a pathological state. Involution is physiological and is exemplified by branchial cleft disappearance during embryogenesis and the uterus reverting to normal size postparmm.

2. The term hydronephrosis implies that the pelvis and calyces of the kidney have become grossly dilated. If the dilated pelvis is intrarenal, marked atrophy of the renal tissue occurs due to a reduction in the renal blood flow causing is chaemic destruction of the nephrons; first of the tubules and later of the glomemli. When the pelvis is extrarenal it may dilate considerably with the renal parenchyma remaining intact for a relatively long time. Hydronephrosis occurs as the result of chronic obstruction of the urinary tract at any level from the pelvi-ureteric junction to the external urethral meatus.

3. A fistula is an abnormal communication between the lumena of two hollow viscera or between the lumen of a viscus and the exterior. Examples are the vesico-colic fistula complicating colonic diverticulitis and fistula-in-ano.

4. An ulcer is a break in the continuity of an epithelial or endothelial surface.

5. In both cases, the organ or tissue is enlarged due, in the case of hypertrophy, to an increase in size of the constituent cells and, in hyperplasia, to an increase in the number of cells.

6. Amyloid stains red with congo red which is apple green colour in polarised light and immunohistochemically use monoclonal antibodies to detect specific type of amyloidosis.

7. Amyloidosis is a condition in which one of several varieties of abnormal glycoprotein is deposited in the tissues, it is most commonly an idiopathic condition but it may be secondary to: ①rheumatoid arthritis,②myelomatosis,③chronic sepsis, e.g. chronic osteomyelitis or bronchiectasis. Death from amyloidosis frequently occurs as a result of renal or cardiac failure caused by its deposition in these organs.

8. Hepatocytes, myocardial fibres and renal tubular epithelial cells.

9. ①Pyknosis,②Karyorrhexis,③Karyolysis.

10. Pathologically, gangrene is huge tissues necrosis with secondary corrupt bacteria infection and deck colour. There are three types. ①dry gangrene, the organ or limb becomes mummified in the absence of infection. ②wet gangrene, necrosis and putrefaction occur due to superadded infection. ③gas gangrene, due to gas bacillus infection which produce gas in the necrosis tissue.

11. Pathologic calcification is the deposition of calcium salts in tissues other than osteoid or teeth.There are two types: ①dystrophic calcification when calcification occurs in dead or dying tissue, ②metastatic calcification in which calcification occurs in normal tissue due to hypercalcaemia from any cause.

12. Metaplasia is a change from one type of differentiated tissue to another. Examples are:

(1) The respiratory epithelium which is normally composed of pseudostratified columnar epithelium may change to a squamous epithelium as a result of smoking or the inhalation of dust or into an epithelium predommantly composed of goblet cells in chronic bronchitis.

(2) The transitional epithelium lining the urinary tract may change to stratified squamous in the presence of stones.

(3) The glandular epithelium of the gall bladder may become squamous when calculi are present .

(4) Metaplasia can occur in connective tissues, e.g. osseous or cartilaginous metaplasia in fibrous tissue.

13. See Table.

	Coagulation necrosis	Apoptosis
Stimuli	Hypoxia, toxins	Physiologic and pathologic factors
Histologic appearance	Cellular swelling	Single cells chromatin condensation
	Coagulation necrosis	Apoptotic bodies
	Disruption of organelles	
DNA breakdown	Random diffuse	Internucleosomal
mechanisms	ATP depletion membrane injury	Gene activation
	Free radical damage	Endonucleases proteases
Tissue reaction	Inflammation	No inflammation, Phagocytosis of apoptotic bodies

14. The morphologic alterations in aging cells include irregular and abnormally lobed nuclei , pleomorphic vacuolated mitochondria, decreased endoplasmic reticulum, and distorted Golgi apparatus. Concomitantly , there is a steady accumulation of the pigment lipofuscin.

Chapter 2   Repair for injury

Answers and Explanations for Choose Tests
1- D

Answers and Explanations for Questions
1. Not, as was previously thought, due to the contraction of collagen laid down by the fibroblasts but due to the removal of oedema and contraction of granulation tissue before it develops into a collagenous scar. Fibroblasts or myofibroblasts in the granulation tissue are responsible for its contraction.

2. ①Haematoma forms at the broken ends of the bone. ②Acute inflammation occurs. ③Granulocytes and histiocytes remove the debris, i.e. the haematoma and any necrotic tissue including fragments of bone.④Granulation tissue forms between and around the bone ends after removal of the debris. ⑤Cartilage and bone are laid down in this granulation tissue which becomes

hard and is consequently called callus. The cartilage ossifies and the bone laid down is known as woven bone because of the lack of normal lamellar organisation. It occupies the original marrow cavity as well as bridging the compact bone ends. ⑥The woven bone is resorbed and replaced by lamellar bone.⑦During ⑥, remodelling occurs simultaneously so that, in a properly reduced fracture, no deformity remains.

3. A fibrocyte is a mesenchymal cell, elongated in shape with a thin nucleus, which is quiescent. A fibroblast is its active counterpart, larger in size,which produces collagen.

4. Granulation tissue consist of proliferative fibroblasts and mumerous new capillaries, and loose ECM contain inflammatory cells. The effects of it is ①anti-infection and protecting raw surface,②supply wound of entry and loss of tissues, ③organize and encapsulate the necrotic tissues, thrombus, inflammatory effusion and other extraneous substance.

Chapter 3   Local Fluid and Hemodynamic Derangements

Answers and Explanations for Choose Tests
1- D   2- D

Answers and Explanations for Questions
1. Oedema is the accumulation of excessive fluid in the interstitial tissues although in the case of pulmonary oedema the fluid is in alveolar spaces. Generalised oedema is frequently associated with pleural, pericardial and peritoneal effusions.

2. The formation in the circulating blood of a solid mass composed of the constituents of the blood, chiefly fibrin and platelets with an admixture of erythrocytes and leucocytes.

3. ①Damage to, or destruction of endothelium or endocardium. ②Changes in blood flow caused by: a. slowing of the blood stream b. eddy currents c. increase in blood viscosity. ③Alterations in the constituents of the blood: a. thrombocytosis b. increase in clotting factors c. hyperlipidaemia.

4. ①Thrombi from the pelvic or iliac veins or deep veins of the leg. ②Tumour, derived from primary tumors elsewhere in the body. ③Fat, following fractures or merely trauma. ④Amniotic fluid, follwing childbirth.

5. The kinds of embolus inclind solid, liquid, and gaseous mass, such as:thrombus, fat embolus, air embolus, nitrigen embolus, amniotic fluid embolus, tumor embolus, parasitic embolus, and so on.

They are major five pathways of embolism:

(1) Venous embolus may cause pulmonary embolization and infarction.

(2) Arteria embolus can embolize the important organs of body, such as coronary, cerebal, liver and kidney vessles.

(3) Portal vein embolus may cause embolism.

(4) Venous embolus from right heart to left heart cause arteria systemembolism, known as crosses embolism.

(5) Large venous embolism may cause small venous known as retrograde emblism.

6. Disseminated intravascular coagulation (DIC) is the sudden or insidious onset of widespread fibrin thrombi in the microcirculation. While these thrombi are not usually visible on gross inspection, they are readily apparent microscopically and can cause diffuse circulatory insufficiency, particularly in the brain, lungs, heart, and kidneys. With the development of the multiple thrombi, there is a rapid concurrent consumption of platelets and coagulation proteins (hence the synonym consumption coagulopathy); at the same time, fibrinolytic mechanisms are activated,

and as a result an initially thrombotic disorder can evolve into a serious bleeding disorder with the development of the multiple thrombi, there is rapid consumption of platelets, prothrombin, fibrinogen, and factors V, VIII and X; at the same time, the plasminogen-plasmin system is activated, and fibrin(cogen) degradation are formed having an anticoagulation effect.

7. Decompression sickness occurs when individuals are exposed to sudden changes in atmospheric pressure. Scuba and deep sea divers, underwater construction workers, and individuals in unpressurized aircraft in rapid ascent are all at risk. When air is breathed at high pressure (e.g., during a deep sea dive), increased amounts of gas (particularly nitrogen) become dissolved in the blood and tissues. If the diver then ascends (depressurizes) too rapidly, the nitrogen expands in the tissues, and bubbles out of solution in the blood to form gas emboli.

The rapid formation of gas bubbles within skeletal muscles and supporting tissues in and about joints is responsible for the painful condition called the bends. Gas emboli may also induce focal ischemia in a number of tissues, including brain and heart. In the lungs, edema, hemorrhages, and focal atelectasis or emphysema may appear, leading to respiratory distress, the so-called chokes.

A more chronic form of decompression sickness is called caission disease, in which persistence of gas emboli in the bones leads to multiple foci of is chemic necrosis; the more common sites are the heads of the femora, tibiae, and humeri.

8. See Table.

	Anemic infarcts	Hemorrhagic infarcts
tissue	solid organs	loose tissues,dual circulations and previously congestion
	(heart,spleen,kidney)	(lung, intestine)
colour	white or pale	red, or dark red
margins	spared margins	indistinct margins

9. Thrombophlebitis is caused by injury or infection of a vein. Infection may occur in the veins of the diploë and dura during the course of suppurative otitis media, in the uterine veins in puerperal sepsis and in the veins of the bone marrow in osteomyelitis. In aseptic thrombophlebitis the thrombus within the affected vein becomes organised and later recanalised. In infective thrombophlebitis pyaemia.

10. Endarteritis obliterans consists of the narrowing of arterial or arteriolar lumena by concentric subintimal laminae of cellular connective tissue which finally obliterate them. It occurs normally at birth in the umbilical arteries, in the ductus arteriosus and in the involuting post-partum uterus. It occurs pathologic ally in vessels in the base of chronic peptic ulcers, in the walls of tuberculous cavities, in syphilis and as a result of irradiation.

Chapter 4   Inflammation

Answers and Explanations for Choose Tests

1- E   2- C   3- C   4- D   5- A   6- B   7- A   8- C   9- D   10- E   11- C   12- D
13- B   14- E   15- A

Answers and Explanations for Questions

1. Inflammation is a defence mechanism of the body to a variety of injuries, including trau-

ma, toxic substances and infections. The cardinal signs were described by Celsus(a Roman living in Provence in the 1st century AD) as rubor, calor, dolor and tumor, in other words inflammation forms a red, hot, painful, swelling. Besides, loss of function and generalised leukocytosis are also associated with inflammation.

2. Acute inflammation is of short duration and destruction of tissue is minimal, permitting resolution; a virtual return to normal. The inflammatory cell involved is predominantly the neutrophil granulocyte. In chronic inflammation, more tissue is destroyed and mononuclear cells, lymphocytes, plasmacytes and histiocytes also take part. The destroyed tissue is replaced by granulation tissue and healing is by fibrosis leaving a scar.

3. They are cells of the mononuclear phagocyte system, and are generally considered to have a common origin and to be interconvertible. The precursor cell is in the bone marrow. This produces the promonocyte which, in turn, produces the monocyte which enters the bloodstream. Monocytes may then migrate into the connective tissues when they are called histiocytes, meaning 'tissue cells'. Showing phagocytic properties, they may also be called macrophages. The Kupffer cells in the liver, the alveolar macrophages in the lung, the macrophages lining the sinusoids of the spleen and lymph nodes and possibly the microglial cells all belong to the mononuclear phagocyte system.

4. It is the directional movement of a cell in response to a chemical substance and, in the context of acute inflammation, it is applied to the neutrophil granulocytes and histiocytes.

5. ①Amines: histamine and 5-HT.②Certain products of the complement system. ③Kinins system. ④Clotting system. ⑤Arachidonic acid metabolites. ⑥Lysosomal constituents of leukocytes. ⑦Oxygen-derived free radicals. ⑧Platelet activating factor(PAF). ⑨Cytokines.

6. Mast cells are found in the collagenous connective tissues anywhere in the body. They are recognised by their intracytoplasmic granules which stain metachromatically with stains such as toluidine blue and Giemsa. The granules consist of heparin and histamine and the cells, therefore, are important in inflammatory and anaphylactic responses.

7. Staphylococci cause abscess formation in skin. ①Impetigo, presents as superficial pustules in the epidermis. ②Folliculitis, when the superficial part of a hair follicle is infected. ③Furuncles, when the whole shaft and root of the hair follicle is infected and an abscess forms. ④A localised suppurative abscess may occur in the dermis. ⑤Carbuncles, when an ill-defined, subcutaneous, suppurative process occurs usually producing several confluent abscesses with multiple discharging sinuses.

8. Catarrhal inflammation is a mild inflammation of a mucous membrane in which there is an outpouring of mucus and serous exudate without frank suppuration.

9. See Table.

	abscess	cellulitis
infection	staphylococcus	streptococci
pathologenesis	topspin	hyaluronidase
tissues	skin,lung,brain,liver	connective tissue appendic
lesions	localization	diffuse

10. Fibronous inflammtion happens in mucous surface such as diphtheria, bacillary dysen-

tery.

11. Empyema or pyothorax is pus in the pleural cavity and therefore implies infection by a pyogenic organism. Infection may occur from:

(1) the lung as a complication of pneumonia.

(2) the chest wall following injury.

(3) the abdomen-extension of a subphrenic abscess.

(4) a perforated oesophagus and mediastinitis.

(5) blood spread (rarely).

12. (1) Haemodynamic and osmotic;due to heart failure or hypoproteinaemia as in liver failure or malnutrition.

(2) Intfammatory; serous, sero-purulent and haemorrhagic effusions and empyema.

(3) Neoplasms; serous or haemorrhagic effusions.

(4) Obstruction to or tearing of the thoracic duct; chylothorax.

13. Enlargement due to stimulation as a result of lymph draining into it, usually from a chronically infected part. The sinuses may be distended by lymph containing numerous macrophages as well as lymphocytes and possibly polymorphs. These appearances are described as ' sinus catarrh'. The lymphoid follicles including their germinal centres are hyperplastic. Chronic irritation as a result of an itchy skin lesion or even drainage from a cancer, without metastasis being present in the node, may cause reactive hyperplasia.

Chapter 5   Tumor

Answers and Explanations for Choose Tests

1- C   2- A   3- D   4- D   5- E   6- D* 7- B   8- A   9- A* 10- D   11- B* 12- C
13- C   14- D   15- B   16- D   17- C   18- A   19- B* 20- A   21- E   22- D   23- C

Explanations

6. The answer is D

Mesothelioma follows exposure to asbestos. Chronic berylliosis is associated with a twofold increase in the incidence of bronchogenic carcinoma, but it is not linked to mesothelioma. Chronic exposure to ar- senical products has been associated with an increased incidence of hepatic angiosarcoma and lung cancer.Endometrial cancer has been linked to long-term estrogen therapy and diethylstilbestrol (DES) therapy during pregnancy has been linked to the later development of clear cell adenocarcinoma of the vaginain the teenage daughters of these women.

9. The answer is A

There are very few superficial sarcomas; most of them are deep to the subcutaneous region, as is particularly true of liposarcoma. The exceptions include the following: Kaposi's sarcoma, the purplish nodules seen in patients with AIDS; epithelioid sarcoma, a tumor that commonly affects the upper extremities,including the hand; angiosarcoma, which occurs on the skin of the head and neck of the elderly; and the atypical fibroxanthoma, a lesion histologically similar to malignant fibrous histiocytoma (MFH), but with a benign course due to its superficial cutaneous location.

11- 14. The answers are: 11- B, 12- C, 13- C, 14- D

Both prostate cancer and gastric cancer are adenocarcinomas; and, structurally, they appear similar under the electron microscope (EM). However, the two cancers can be distinguished by immunohistochemical (IHC) testing for prostatic-specific antigen, a tissue marker that is valuable in identifying prostatic cancer.

Carcinomas reveal cell-to-cell junctions (called desmosomes) when viewed with an EM; lymphomas do not demonstrate these ultrastructural components. The IHC profile of a carcinoma is cytokeratin (CK) positive and leukocyte common antigen (LCA) negative, whereas a lymphoma is CK negative and LCA positive.

EM examination reveals long microvilli in a mesothelioma and short microvilli in an adenocarcinoma. IHC analysis usually reveals the presence of carcinoembryonic antigen (CEA) in adenocarcinomas, whereas most mesotheliomas do not express CEA.

All squamous cell carcinomas (SCC), regardless of origin, look alike ultrastructurally. Unfortunately, no markers currently used in IHC can help to identify the primary site of an SCC.

19- 23. The answers are: 19- B, 20- A, 21- E, 22- D, 23- C

Amplification of n-myc oncogene is associated with improved prognosis in childhood neuroblastoma. Patients who have adenocarcinoma of the lung with amplification of ras oncogene fare less well than patients with a similar tumor stage but without ras amplification. Women who have breast cancers that overexpress c-erb B2 have poorer prognoses than women whose breast cancers do not. The oncogene c-myc is found in Burkitt's lymphoma, and the Rb suppressor gene was identified from retinoblastomas.

Answers and Explanations for Questions

1. Hyperplasia is a limited overgrowth of a tissue as a result of the excessive action of a specific stimulus. It may be considered physiological, inflammatory and repairing proliferation. Neoplasia is an excess growth of cells in a tissue, commonly for no known reason, which may stop after a time in the case of benign neoplasms or continue unabated at the primary and secondary sites in the case of malignant neoplasms.

2. Dyspasia arises from a disordered growth in a tissue, especially dysplasia, mean cytologic abnormalities. The term is also applied to individual cells having an atypical or bizarre appearance. It covers mild, moderate and severe. The term "intraepithelial neoplasia" is used to embrace both carcinoma in sita and dysplasia.

3. A hamartoma is a disorderly but limited over growth in an organ or tissue of well-differentiated cells which are normally present in that organ.

4. Originally a tumour meant any lump, inflammatory, neoplastic or otherwise. Nowadays it is synonymous with 'neoplasm' or 'new growth'. The commonly accepted definition of a neoplasm is that of Willis who stated that a tumour is an abnormal mass of tissue the growth of which exceeds and is uncoordinated with that of the normal tissues and which persists in the same excessive manner after the cessation of the stimuli which evoked the change. However, on rare occasions, malignant neoplasms have been known to regress spontaneously e.g. malignant melanoma.

5. (1) Polycyclic hydrocarbons found in tar or shale oil, cause skin cancer and, from tobacco smoke, bronchial cancer.

(2) Some aniline dyes used in the dyestuffs and rubber industries; urothelial tumours.

(3) Crocidolite, one of the three varieties of asbestos; mesotheliomata of the pleura or peritoneum.

(4) Wood dust when inhaled; adenocarcinoma of the nasal mucosa or paranasal sinuses.

(5) Vinyl chloride, in the plastic industry; angiosarcoma of the liver.

(6) Ionising irradiation; neoplastic changes in various sites.

(7) Arsenic; skin cancer.

(8) Ultraviolet light in fair-skinned individuals may cause squamous or basal cell carcinoma and melanoma.

(9) Infections.

(10) Viral cancer is well-recognised in animals, in man the association is less clear but examples in which viruses are important in man include: ①Burkitt's lymphoma, ②nasopharyngeal cancer, ③Kaposi's sarcoma.

(11) Metazoan parasites such as Schistosoma causing cancer of the bladder.

6. A neoplasm of epithelial origin, the cells of which are morphologically malignant but which have not breached the basement membrane. An example is intra-epithelial cancer of the skin, Bowen's disease.

7. Exfoliative cytology is the study of cells shed from epithelial or mesothelial surface. S or cells obtained by fine needle aspiration of solid tumors. The purpose, nearly always, is to detect or exclude the presence of a malignant neoplasm. This diagnostic tool was developed originally for the investigation of the cervix uteri. However, sputum and urine specimens are commonly examined in order to exclude or confirm the presence of bronchial or urothelial cancers. Examination of pleural, pericardial or ascitic fluid may also reveal the presence of the malignant cells which cause these effusions.

8. (1) By direct invasion of adjacent structures, including tissue interstitial perineural spread.

(2) Matastansis, ①By lymphatic vessels, ②By blood vessels, ③Across body cavities; pleural, peritoneal, the ventricular system of the brain and the subarachnoid space. and ④By implantation.

9. "Embryonic tumors" occur in infancy and childhood. They occur in: ①the kidney, the nephroblastoma or Wilm's tumour, ②the adrenal or sympathetic ganglia, the neuroblastoma, ③the cerebellum and 4th ventricle, the medullo blastoma, ④the retina, the retinoblastoma, ⑤the liver, the hepatoblastoma, very rare, ⑥the lung, pulmonary blastoma, very rare.

10. These tumors arise in the gonads and rarely during their development. They are: ①seminoma of testis and dysgerminoma of the ovary, ②teratoma, ③choriocarcinoma (extrauterine), ④yolk sac tumour (endodermal sinus tumor when in ovary and orchioblastoma in testis).

11. Teratomata Consist of multiple tissues foreign to the pan from which they arise. Most occur in the gonads which led to the concept that they were monsters which developed parthenogenetically from an ovum or sperm but they can also arise in the mediastinum and sacrum. Such tumours may contain well-differentiated epithelial, mesothelial and endothelial elements producing such structures as hair, teeth and gastrointestinal glands. If only epithelial structures are involved the tumours are cystic and classified as dermoids. Whereas many teratomata of the ovary are cystic and benign, testicular teratomata are more usually solid, poorly-differentiated and malignant.

12. They are a variety of unrelated systemic conditions occurring in patients suffering from malignant disease, commonly due to the excretion of hormones not usually associated with the tissue of tumour origin. Paraneoplastic syndromes not caused by hormone secretion include neuropathies, encephalopathies, myopathies and thrombotic conditions.

13. A secondary carcinoma in the ovary which has spread by the transcoelomic route from a gastric or colonic primary. Histologically it is composed of signet ring cells in a very cellular stroma which is characteristi. These tumors are frequently bilateral.

14. Teratomata. Raised levels of alpha-fetoprotein (AFP) and beta human chorionic gonadotrophin (βHCG) are found in the blood of 90% of patients suffering from teratomata.

15. Carcinoma of the skin of the scrotum in chimney sweeps, described by Sir Percival Pott in 1775. The same tumour (known as mule spinner's cancer) was also observed to occur in the groin region in men exposed to the shale oil which is sprayed from the spinning mule.

16. Leukoplakia is a clinical term indicating the presence of white patches in the mucosa of the mouth, larynx, vulva. or penis. There are a variety of causes, irritation due to smoking, carcinoma in situ, fungal infection or lichen planus. The whiteness of the mucosa is due to hyperkeratosis.How this condition is recognized as preneoplastic lesion.

17. See Table.

Feature	benign	Malignant
Gross appearance	Circumscribed or well-define capsule	Infiltrating the borders of the lesions without discrete and no capsule
Histologic differentiation	good	poorer, atypia pleomorphic cells
Mitotic figures	less	more
Growth speed	slow	relatively rapid
Growth pattern	expansion	Infiltration
Secondary change	A few	Bleeding and necrosis
Metastasis	no	Often
Recurrent	A few	Often
Effects to host	Compressing and obstruction	Compressing, obstruction, bleeding, necrosis, infection , cachexia.etc

18. See Table.

	carcinoma	Sarcoma
Histologic origin	Epithelial tissue	Mesenchymal tissue
age	old	young
Gross appearance	hard	Fish flesh like and soft
Histologic character	Nest like	Diffuse
Net fibro stain	–	+
metastasis	Lymphatic	Blood vessel
ratio	More often	less

19. Certain benign tumors are also associated with the subsequent development of cancer. Certain clinical conditions are associated with an increased risk of developing cancers, these condition are referable to precancerous lesions.

(1) Cirrhosis of the liver-hepatocellular carcinoma.

(2) Atrophic gastritis of pernicious anemia-stomach cancer.

(3) Chronic ulcerative colitis-carcinoma of the colon.

(4) Leukoplakia of the oral and genital mucosa-squamous cell cancers.

Chapter 6   Diseases of the Heart and Blood Vessles

Answers and Explanations for Choose Tests

1- E   2- B   3- C   4- B   5- D   6- B   7- A   8- D   9- E   10- E   11- B   12- A   13- D   14- C   15- E

Answers and Explanations for Questions

1. ①Stenosis of the pulmonary valve (or infundibular part of right ventricle). ②Rightventricular hypertrophy clue to increased pressure in that chamber. ③A high interventricular defect just below the aortic and pulmonary valves. ④Overriding of the aorta to the right (dextroposi-

tion) so that the reduced blood from the right ventricle, which cannot be ejected through the stenosed pulmonary valve, passes through the interventricular defect to mix with left ventricular blood and thence through the aortic valve to the aorta. A variable degree of cyanosis occurs, depending on the severity of the above abnormalities.

2. Atherosclerosis is defined by the World Health Organization as a focal intimal fibrofatty plaques, in which variable changes develop in the internal layers of large to medium sized muscular arteries. These changes which originate in the intima and extend into the media, consist of focal accumulations of lipids, complex carbohydrates, blood and blood products, fibrous tissue and calcium salts.

3. ①Age: progressive symptomatic disease is only common after 40 years of age. ②Sex: in females atherosclerosis rarely occurs in the premenopausal period. ③Environment; the mortality from this disease is much lower in developing countries than in the highly industrialized western world. ④A high serum cholesterol, such as occurs in diabetes, myxoedema, the nephrotic syndrome and familial xanthosis. ⑤Hypertension. ⑥Smoking, secondary or high-style, type A personality, obesity and otal contraceptives.

4. Atherosclerosis causes symptomatic disease by depriving tissues or organs of blood. The effects of gradual occlusion differ according to the tissue or organ affected, e.g. involvement of the cerebral arteries causes cerebral atrophy followed by dementia; of the renal arteries, renal scarring causing hypertension; of the coronary arteries, myocardial fibrosis associated with angina; of the lower limb arteries; ischaemia of the muscles and skin causing claudication and finally gangrene.

5. Atherosclerosis can occur at almost any part of an artery but it is commoner around the ostia of arterial branches and in the abdominal aorta, coronary arteries, arteries cruralis, descending thoracic aorta, interal carotid arteries, and circle of Wills (in descending order of frequence).

6. Stage I, a fatty streak composed of smooth muscle cells and macrophage, which containing fat develops immediately beneath the intima. Stage II, confluent smooth yellowish plaques several millimetres in diameter, which are composed of lipid can be seen. At the periphery of such a plaque the lipid is intracellular but in the centre it forms a structureless extrscellular amorphous mass, The plaque is separated from the endothelium by a layer of hyaline fibres. Stage III. Around and in between the plaques widespread proliferation of fibrous tissue occurs causing irregular thickening of the intima. In advanced disease the endothelium disappears leaving the underlying lipid exposed, producing the atheromatous ulcer upon which mural thrombosis may develop. Calcification, particularly in plaques in the distal aorta, occurs at this stage. Degeneration of the media leads to aneurysmal dilatation of the affected vessel.

7. Chorea minor is a cndition when rheumatism involves extracorticospinal tract, and the patients, usually baby child, show involuntary movement of their limbs.

8. A degenerative disease of the large arteries chiefly, but not alwsys, occurring in the elderly and associated with dystrophic calcification of the media, the intima remaining normal. The vessel becomes rigid without any reduction in the size of the lumen.

9. ①Rheumatic heart disease in which the aortic cusps become thickened and contracted. ② Atherosclerosis. ③Marfan's syndrome. ④Syphilitic aortitis which specificially affects the ascending part of the aorta.

10. Aortic stenosis may be congenital or acquired.

(1) Congenital aortic stenosis is most commonly due to the replacement of the three valve cusps by a single diaphragm-likc membrane with a central foramen. Less commonly it is due to a subvalvular membrane.

（2）Acquired aortic stenosis is most commonly seen in chronic rheumatic heart disease when organisation of the vegetations formed in the acute stages produce adhesions between cusps and deformity of the valve. Less commonly it results from the fibrosis and subsequent calcification of congenitally bicuspid valves.

11. （1）Congenital. Strictly, congenital aneurysms do not occur but the term has gained general acceptance to describe those aneurysms which arise on the circle of willis and its branches. Such an aneurysm is not present at birth but develops later because of a congenital deficiency of the smooth muscle of the media.

（2）Acquired: ①degenerative-atherosclerosis-Erdheim's medial degeneration ②infective-mycotic-syphilitic. ③traumatic-surgery to a major artery may lead to the development of a false aneurysm, an aneurysmal varix or varicose aneurysm. ④cirsoid-this variety occurs on the scalp and may be congenital but is usually traumatic. While considered congenital, it may be the result of a birth injury.

12. Valvular vegetations are formed by deposits of platelets and fibrin on the cusps of the valves of the heart. They occur more commonly in the left side of the heart than the right and affect the mitral more frequently than the aortic valve. In acute rheumatic endocardifis the vegetations are small excrescences in the line of apposition of the affected cusps, hence it is believed that trauma on valve closure leading to ulceration of the endocardium precedes the development of the vegetations. In acute and subacute bacterial endocarditis, the vegetations is larger and also contain micro-organisms.

13. ①Rheumatic heart disease in the acute or chronic stage. In the acute stage vegetations develop on the valve cusps and in the chronic stage scarring and deformity of the affected valves occur. ②Acute infective endocarditis. ③Subacute bacterial endocarditis, an infection of deformed valves by organisms of normally low pathogenicity. ④Atheroma of the mitral valve associated with fibrosis and calcification. ⑤Libman-Sacks endocarditis occurring in patients with systemic lupus erythematosus. ⑥Calcification of the aortic valve not associated with atherosclerosis. ⑦Fibrosis of the tricuspid and pulmonary valves in association with the carcinoid syndrome. ⑧Marantic endocarditis occurring in terminally ill patients.

14. Rheumatic fever is caused by Streptococcus haemolyticus, Lancefield Group A. It is believed that antibodies stimulated by the exotoxin of this bacterium act as auto-antibodies against the patient's own myocardial fibres. This hypothesis is supportetl, by: ①the time lapse of 2—4 weeks between the onset of the streptococcal throat infection and rheumatic fever. ②patients developing rheumatic fever, have a higher titre of streptococcal antibodies than those who do not. ③ streptococcal antigens can be found in the myocardial fibres. This hypothesis cannot explain all aspects of the disease since collagen, particularly of the endocardium and periarticular tissues is also affected. The disease is commoner in children living in poorer social conditions.

15. Rheumatic fever causes a pancarditis; the pericardium, myocardium and endocardium being involved.

16. ①In the heart, the endocardium, myocardiumand pericardium. ②The joints and tendon sheaths. ③The subcutaneous tissues. ④The skin causing rashes, e. g. erythema marginatum. ⑤Acute congestion and pulmonary oedema caused by the acute heart failure, secondary to the myocardial involvement.

17. ①Valvular heart disease, causing stenosis incompetence or both. ②Atrial fibrillation which predisposes to thrombus formation in the atria （usually left）and their appendages. This may give rise to a ' ball-valve' thrombus or emboli. ③Angina pectoris due to myocardial hypertrophy and decreased cardiac output, both caused by the valve disease. ④Subacute bacterial endo-

carditis.

18. An aschoff body is a rheumatic body, which occurs in the myocardium in acute rheumatic fever. It is most commonly found in the interventricular septum, the left atrium and the left auricular appendage.

19. Aschoff bodies develop in the connective tissue septa adjacent to the small blood vessels within the myocardium. Each consists of a focus of fibrinoid necrosis in the collagen associated with degeneration of a few myocardial fibres in the immediate vicinity. The cellular aggregation around each lesion chiefly consists of lymphocytes, plasmacytes and macrophages together with Aschoff cells. The last are large cells containing up to three pleomorphic nuclei. The lesion heals leaving a small scar.

20. Acute bacterial endocarditis is a fulminating condition associated with septicaemia caused by highly pathogenic organisms such as staphylococcus aureus, occuring in an individual with a normal heart prior to the onset of the disease.It frequently occurs in addicts receiving their drugs by the intravenous route, in debilitated patients and in patients with a septic focus. Large friable vegetations develop on the heart valves which soon become ulcerated, fenestrated and distorted. The rapid destruction of the affected valve or valves, if unchecked, interferes with their function causing heart failure. In contrast subacute bacterial endocarditis is caused by organisms of low pathogenicity including streptococcus viridans, escherichia coil, enterococci and occasionally fungi. The organism enters the bloodstream e.g. following tooth extraction or catheterisation, causing a bacteraemia rather than a septicaemia, and settles on valves already abnormal due to disease or suffering some congenital defect, e.g. a bicuspid aortic valve. Subacute bacterial endocarditis essentially presents as a low grade infection in which cure can nearly always be obtained by the administration of the correct antibiotic. If, however, vegetations have formed on the valves dysfunction nearly always results.

21. Infective endocarditis is divided for descriptive purposes into acute and subacute types although there is considerable overlap between them. The acute type is caused by virulent pathogenic organisms during the course of a septicaemia. Ulceration, fenestration and destruction of valves causes death. The subacute variety is most commonly caused by commensals or weak pathogens, classically streptococcus viridans or by fungi in immunosuppressed patients. Subacute endocarditis is superimposed upon pre-existing disease, either chronic endocarditis or some congenital malformation such as a biscuspid aortic valve, a septal defect or a patent ductus arteriosus.

22. ①Sudden death. ②Angina pectoris. ③Myocardial infarction. ④Cardiac failure due to myocardial fibrosis. ⑤Arrhythmias due to bundle branch block.

23. "Anguish in the chest". A very severe pain in the chest usually on the left side, frequently radiating into the left arm, neck or even into the jaws and teeth. It is the result of myocardial ischaemia and may be relieved by rest or vasodilator drugs.

24. ①Immediate death due to heart failure due to cardiogenic shock. ②Early death due to rupture of the necrotic myocardium (myomalacia cordis), causing a haemopericardium. ③An arrhythmia. ④A mural thrombus leading to embolic phenomena. ⑤Chronic heart failure due to myocardial fibrosis. ⑥Cardiac aneurysm. ⑦Recovery followed by mild angina pectoris or no symptoms at all.

25. About 8 hours.

26. (1) Rheumatic fever.

(2) Suppurative myocarditis caused either by extension of a bacterial infection from the valves in an infective endocarditis or by haematogenous spread in the course of a septicaemia or pyaemia.

（3）Viralmyocarditis caused by the Coxsackie A or B viruses.

（4）Sarcoidosis.

（5）Syphilitic, the spirochaeta pallidum may cause a variety of cardiac lesions: ①aortic incompetence. ②myocardial ischaemia from narrowing of the coronary ostia. ③gumma of the myocardium which may cause heart block if the conducting system is involved ④fibrosis of the myocardium due to miliary gummata in congenital syphilis.

（6）Toxic myocarditis resulting from an infective fever such as diphtheria, pneumococcal pneumonia or typhoid or any septicaemia.

（7）Isolated myocarditis for which there is no known cause, but it resembles viral myoarditis.

27. The term cardiomyopathy embraces many unrelated chronic conditions of the myocardium whose causes are unknown. There are four types: ①hypertrophic: in some patients this condition is inherited as an autosomal dominant gene. The myocardium is hypertrophied; microscopically the myocardial fibres are arranged in a typical whorled pattern. The thickening of the left ventricle interferes with systole and the thickened interventricular septum obstructs the outflow from the ventricles, affecting the left rather than the right. This type presents with angina or heart failure. ②congestive; the myocardium is flabby and the various chambers of the heart dilated. Mural thrombi, together with endocardial and interstitial fibrosis may be present. Clinically the patient presents with congestive heart failure for which no cause can be found. ③restrictive or endomyocardial fibro-elastosis; this is a rare condition occurring in infancy in which, a thick subendocardial layer of fibroelastic tissue develops, chiefly in the left ventricle. ④obliterative; this condition occurs chiefly in adults in tropical Africa. The endocardium is very fibrosed in the region of the papillary muscles and chordae tendineae.

28.（1）An acutely failing heart may present as: ① pulmonary oedema, due to left ventricular failure. ②cardiac shock due to a low output state. ③right heart failure in a right-sided infarction or pulmonary embolism.

（2）Chronic heart failure. The presentation of chronic heart failure depends upon the side of the heart which is affected:

1）left sided; in most patients it is due to: ①ischaemic heart disease ②systemic hypertension ③aortic and mitral valve disease ④cardiomyopathies ⑤congenital heart disease.An early sign is dyspnoea, on exertion progressing to dyspnoea at rest.

2）right sided; the common causes are: ①pulmonary hypertension from whatever cause, e.g. mitral stenosis, pulmonary fibrosis and thrombo-embolic disease ②tricuspid and pulmonary stenosis. These conditions produce hypertrophy followed by dilatation of the right side of the heart. The neck veins become dilated and there is evidence of venous congestion of the liver and spleen which may become palpable. Stasis predisposes to atrial thrombosis and pulmonary embolic phenomena.

29. (1) Causes in the myocardium and pericardium: ①myocardial fibrosis caused by ischaemic heart disease. ② myocarditis and the cardiomyopathies. ③ arrhythmias ④ amyloidosis, ⑤cardiac tamponade due to pericardial effusion or haemopericardium. ⑥constrictive pericarditis.

（2）Systemic and pulmonary hypertension.

（3）Increase in blood volume.

（4）Pressure overload: a stenotic or incompetent aortic valve causes left ventricular overload.

（5）Increase in blood flow: ①shunt between the left and right sides of the heart caused by atrioventricular septal defects or peripheral arteriovenous shunts as in Paget's disesse of bone.

②thyrotoxicosis and beri-beri.

30. In primary (essential or idiopathic hypertension), there is no known cause. In secondary, in the majority of patients the cause is chronic renal disease. Less common causes include primary aldosteronism, Cushing's syndrome or a phaeochromocytoma.

31. (1) Vascular changes in: ①the large arteries: Occur atherosclerosis; ②the small arteries: The earliest change consists of hypertrophy of the smooth muscle and elastic fibres. Later fibrosis occurs so that the vessel wall is weakened although thickened luminal narrowing; ③arteriolosclerosis: The changes in the smaller arteries of 1 mm or less in diameter depend upon the type of hypertension, i.e. whether it is benign or malignant In the former, gross intimal thickening develops together with a lesser degree of medial thickening and hyaline degeneration. In the latter, fibrinoid necrosis of the wall together with superadded thrombosis occurs.

(2) Organs change in: ①hypertensive heart disease: Left ventricular hypertrophy and heart failure. ②Primary contracted kidney. ③Brain vessels form thrombosis, embilism, infarction, hemorrhage, aneurysm. Clinically, hypertensive crisis may develop. ④Relinal relativity changes.

32. ① The subcapsular surface of the kidneys is spotted with dark red areas due to congestion and haemorrhage. ②The renal, segmental and arcuate arteries are atherosclerotic. ③ The intima of the interlobular arteries is thickened by concentric layers of connective tissue (notably elastin) and smooth muscle cells. ④Fibrinoid necrosis of the wall of the terminal portions of the interlobular arteries and the afferent arterioles occurs and their lumena may be completely blocked. Similar focal necrosis occurs in the glomeruli. ⑤ A bloody exudate occurs in the capsular space of glomeruli. ⑥Some nephrons atrophy and their glomeruli become hyalinised while others enlarge and their tubules dilate and may contain hyaline casts.

33. The middle cerebral, in particular the lenticulo-striate branch which supplies that part of the internal capsule which is traversed by the axons of the motor cells in the precentral gyrus as they pass to the cord. Thrombosis of this artery destroys the axons and myelin sheaths in the affected part of the internal capsule resulting in a contralateral hemiplegia. Sensation is preserved because the afferent fibres are situated further back in internal capsule.

34. Embarrassment of the heart's action by blood or other substance such as serous effusion or pus in the pericardial sac. This prevents diastolic filling .The condition is similar to constrictive pericarditis.

Chapter 7　Diseases of the Respiratory System

Answers and Explanations for Choose Tests

1- B　2- B　3- B　4 - C　5- D　6- C　7- B　8- D　9- E　10- D*　11- C*　12- E
13- D　14- B　15- A

Explanations

10. The answer is D

Lymphoepithelioma is a highly malignant tumor of the upper respiratory tract; it occurs in young adults, particularly those of Asian heritage. A link to Epstein-Barr virus (EBV) infection has been noted. The tumor consists of both malignant epithelial cells and nonneoplastic lymphoid cells, which probably represent an immune response to the malignant epithelial component. Radiotherapy is the treatment of choice since the epithelial component grows rapidly and tends to metastasize early. Surgical control is virtually impossible.

11—15. The answers are:11- C,12- E, 13- D, 14- B, 15- A.

Caseating granulomas are found in tuberculosis, whereas noncaseating granulomas are seen in berylliosis as well as many other diseases. Simple emphysema has a variety of causes, such as smoking, but the emphysematous changes seen in the pneumoconioses are not simple. Pleural calcifications are typical of asbestosis, and nodules with polarizable silica are seen in silicosis.

Answers and Explanations for Questions

1. No. Atelectasis means that the lung has never expanded from birth. Collapse occurs in a previously expanded lung and may be due to pressure on the lung (pressure collapse) or obstruction of a bronchus (absorption collapse).

2. Classically from the onset of the disease to healing, lobar pneumonia passes through four stages, each stage blending into the next. ①Congestion. The alveolar capillaries are distended with blood. ②Red hepatization. Oedema fluid, erythrocytes and pus cells pass from the capillaries into the alveolar spaces in which fibrin is deposited. The lobe is consolidated. ③Grey hepatisation. The congestion disappears partly due to capillary compression by the intense cellular infiltration, which now includes macrophages, into the alveoli. ④Resolution. The alveolar exudate is liquefied by enzymes liberated from the lysed inflammatory cells and is expectorated. Macrophages appear and engulf cellular debris and pneumococci.

3. ①Direct spread of the organism from the lung causing either a pleural effusion followed by an empyema or more rarely suppurative pericarditis. ②Haematogenous spread leading to suppurative arthritis or meningitis. ③Failure of resolution followed by organization of the exudate. This process is known as carnification because of the solid, fleshy appearance of the fibrosed lung tissue.

4. Lobar pneumonia usually occurs in otherwise healthy young adults and in 90% of cases is caused by Streptococcus pneumoniae whereas bronchopneumonia, due to the extension of a bronchitis or bronchiolitis, is most frequent in individuals whose resistance to infection has been reduced, e.g. in infancy, by old age or by a debilitating condition such as malignancy or by malnutrition. In bronchopneumonia, a variety of organisms is responsible, usually commensals from the upper respiratory tract, such as the staphylococcus aureus, streptococcus pyogenes and haemophilus infiuenzae. Lobar pneumonia may affect a part of a lobe, an entire lobe or several lobes, the affected areas passing through four distinct pathological changes clinically rusty-coloured sputum whereas bronchopneumonia, otherwise known as lobular pneumonia, begins with mucosal damage in the small bronchioles and the acute inflammatory process affects the lobules they supply. Clinically purulent sputum. Even before chemotherapy lobar pneumonia usually resolved spontaneously with no residual damage. Occasionally death due to respiratory failure, septicaemia or complications would occur. Untreated bronchopneumonia may result in varying degrees of fibrosis of the lung.

5. Interstitial fibrosis of the lungs associated with the development of fibrous pleural plaques. Less common is the induction of pleural and sometimes peritoneal mesotheliomata by blue asbestos (crocidolite). Asbestos also potentates the carcinogenic effect on the lung of cigarette smoking, but alone it is only a mild lung carcinogen.

6. Emphysema is an enlargement of the air spaces of the lung accompanied by destruction of alveolar walls. In overinfiafion there is no destruction and this condition is therefore reversible although it will progress to emphysema if it becomes chronic.

7. (1) Generalized: ①centriacinar (also called centrilobular or bronchiolar, the respiratory bronchiole being involved). ②panacinar. ③paraseptal.

(2) Bullous emphysema is applied to advanced cases of (1) But an occasional single bulla may be present in young people. If it ruptures, spontaneous pneumothorax or interstitial (surgical) emphysema may occur.

(3) Paratractional, when the emphysema occurs round shrunken scars or silicotic nodules.

(4) Compensatory, in a lobe or lobes when another lobe or a lung has collapsed or has been excised.

(5) Senile.

8. Chronic bronchitis has a clinical definition (chronic cough with sputum production on most days during a 3-month period of the year for at least 2 years in succession). The following are likely to be seen in the bronchi histologically: ①an increase in the bronchial goblet cells at the expense of the ciliated epithelium (mucous metaplasia). ②hypertrophy of the submucosal mucous glands. ③ the changes of non-specific acute bronchitis. ④ emphysema, which is frequently associated with chronic bronchitis.

9. Cor pulmonale is not a precise term. It means heart disease due to advanced lung disease, which causes obstruction of the pulmonary circulation. The resuit is right ventricular hypertrophy followed, if treatment is unsuccessful, by heart failure.

10. A condition leading to respiratory distress in premature infants due to lack of surfactam, a lipoprotem produced by type II pneumocytes. The hyaline membrane which lines the alveolar walls is composed of fibrin and degenerating cells. Exposure to high oxygen concentrations may be a contributory factor. Surfactant is decreasing surface tension, normally prevents alveolar collapse.

11. ①Cigarette smoking is the most significant factor. ②Exposure to crocidolite, one of the three types of asbestos. Alone the inhalation of crocidolite causes only a modest increase in the incidence of lung cancer but it potentates the carcinogenic effect of cigarette smoking considerably. ③In the past the inhalation of radioactive dusts and gases by the miners of various metal ores in former Czechoslovakia and Saxony was an important occupational hazard.

12. Lung cancers may be primary bronchogenic carcinomata or secondary (metastatic) growths from elsewhere. Lymphomata and leukaemias are included in the latter although primary lymphomata of lung do occur. Bronchogenic carcinomata are classified histologically. Histological classifications vary slightly but most can be placed in one of the following categories (mixtures occur): ①squamous (epidermoid) carcinomata, ②oat cell (small cell or anaplastic) carcinoma, ③ adenocarcinoma, ④anaplastic (large cell anaplastic) carcinoma, ⑤broncho-alveolar carcinoma. The last may be a variety of adenocarcinoma or, as some consider, they may be derived from the alveolar epithelium, in which case they are lung, rather than bronchogenic, carcinoma.

13. The cells of an oat cell (small cell) carcinoma usually contain neurosecretory granules as shown by the electron microscope and the tumour sometimes produces the carcinoid syndrome which suggests that the origin of the growth is from APUD (Feyrter) cells. Although this accounts for 5-HT secretion by some of these tumors, others appear to secrete different hormones, e. g., ADH and ACTH.

Chapter 8   Diseases of the Digestive System

Answers and Explanations for Choose Tests

1- A   2- C   3- E   4- C   5- B   6- A   7- D   8- C   9- D   10- E   11- D   12- E
13- A   14- D   15- C   16- D   17- D   18- E   19- C   20- B   21- D   22- E

Answers and Explanations for Questions

1. Dilatations of submucosal veins which develop in patients suffering from portal obstruction. Although these venous plexuses normally drain into the systemic venous system, there are small anastomotic veins connecting them with the portal drainage of the stomach. High pressure

in the portal system forces blood through the anastomoses into the systemic oesophageal veins which become dilated and varicose.

2. A Barrett's oesophagus is one where the lower end has an area of metaplastic mucous-secreting epithelium (instead of stratified squamous).

3. (1) Carcinoma.

(2) Peptic stricture.

(3) Achalasia.

(4) Rarer causes include: ①progressive 'systemic' sclerosis. ②strictures caused by swallowing corrosives. ③external compression due most commonly to malignant lymphadenopathy within the posterior mediastinum or an aneurysm of the aortic arch. ④Chagas' disease caused by a protozoon, trypanosoma cruzi, common in South America. This parasite exerts a toxic effect on the autonomic ganglia in various sites including the oesophagus.

4. (1) Squamous carcinoma which arises from the stratified squamous epithelium lining the oesophagus, Lesions of this type in the post cricoid region are some twenty times more common in women than in men.

(2) Adenocarcinoma occuring at the lower end of the oesophagus due to direct extension of tumours originating in the cardiac end of the stomach.

(3) Undefferentiated carcinoma.

(4) APUD tumor.

5. The commonest macroscopic appearance is of a raised nodule on the mucosa in the centre of which a variable degree of ulceration has occurred. Occasionally an annular growth occurs and even more rarely diffuse infiltration produces a long stricture, Microscopically the same tumour may have all grades of differentiation from a keratinising squamous carcinoma exhibiting cell nests to an undifferentiated tumour in which neither keratin nor prickle cells are present.

6. ①Three-quarters of all squamous carcinoma of the oesophagus arise in the middle third. ②In women, a squamous carcinoma may arise in the post-cricoid region as part of the Plummer-Vinson (Patterson-Kelly) syndrome.

7. Carcinoma of the oesophagus spreads: ①within the submucosal lymphatics to other parts of the oesophagus. This is particularly important to the surgeon because it may be unrecognised at operation only to be identified later at microscopy by the pathologist. ②via the lymphatics externally to the regional lymph nodes. ③direct spread, after the muscular coats are breached, to involve the trachea, bronchi, lungs or posterior mediastinum. ④by the bloodstream to produce metastatic disease in the liver, lungs or adrenal glands.

8. Erosions: (1) are frequently multiple;

(2) result from a loss of less than the full thickness of the mucosa leaving some basal gland elements;

(3) usually heal without scarring whereas an ulcer: ①is a circumscribed lesionin which the full thickness of the mucosa is lost; ②has variable degress of penetration of the underiying submucosa, muscularis mucosa and muscular layers; ③heals with scarring.

9. By definition there is absence of the mucosa at the ulcer and the surrounding mucosa shows chronic inflammatory changes. The floor of the ulcer contains indeterminate necrotic material among which polymorphs may be recognized. Deep to this, the base of the ulcer, there is either active granulation tissue or mature collagen with fibroblasts, depending on the stage of activity or healing. The granulation tissue consists of newly developed capillaries lined by plump endothelial cells and contains inflammatory cells, scattered and in foci these are mainly lymphocytes and plasma cells with some polymorphs. This granulation or fibrous tissue replaces all the normal

coats of the stomach wall beneath the ulcer down to and including the muscularis propria, partly or entirely. Heals with scarring.

10. ①Perforation; both gastric and duodenal ulcers may perforate into the peritoneal cavity causing chemical peritonitis. ②Posterior gastric and duodenal ulcers may 'invade' extramural tissues, e.g. the pancreas. ③Severe bleeding causing, in the case of gastric ulceration, haematemesis and in the case of duodenal ulceration, melaena. ④Extensive fibrosis, in the stomach producing an 'hour glass' stomach or in the duodenum pyloric stenosis. ⑤Gastric ulceration may account for some 1% of gastric carcinoma. Duodenal ulceration is never associated with malignant change.

11. ①Diet: —nitrites in food, water and nitrate preservatives in food are converted to nitrosamines and nitrosamides which are considered to be the carcinogens-smoked and salted foods and pickled vegetables-lack of fresh fruit and vegetables. ②Host factors: —infection by H pylori which occurs in chronic atrophic gastritis and intestinal metaplasia. Hypochlohydria favours colonisation by H pylori which are present in most cases of intestinal type carcinoma-partial gastrectomy predisposes to alkaline reflux-gastric adenomas are likely to be precancerous. ③Genetic-slight increased incidence in people with blood group A, in some racial groups and in close relatives of patients with gastric cancer.

12. The term "early gastric cancer" defines a gastric neoplasm which is confined to the mucosa or mucosa and submucosa. Lymphatic drainage from these may result in invasion of regional nodes even though the primary carcinoma seems small and localised.

13. Fifty per cent of all carcinoma of the stomach arise in the antrum and pyloric region. The rest arise in the cardia.

14. ①By direct spread, within the submucosa and muscle coats, occasionally accompanied by extensive fibrosis producing the condition known as "linitis plastica" or "leather bottle" stomach. Penetration of the serosa leads to the direct involvement of other parts of the gastrointestinal tract, notably the transverse colon. ②By the lymphatics. ③By the bloodstream. ④Via the peritoneal cavity to produce peritoneal seedlings and ascites and occasionally secondary tumors of the ovaries known as Krukenberg tumors.

15. Carcinoid tumors arise chiefly in the alimentary tract, usually in the appendix when they are inactive; less commonly in the small intestine, colon and stomach. The tumors are composed of cells of the APUD (Amine Precursor Uptake and Decarboxylation) system, the argentaffin cells, which contain silver-staining granules. They secrete 5-hydroxytryptamine (5-HT). The tumors are locally invasive and seldom metastasize. 5-hydroxytryptamine and other mediators cause the carcinoid syndrome which is characterised by paroxysmal facial flushing, diarrhoea, bronchospasm and occasionally pulmonary stenosis and tricuspid incompetence. 5-HT is excreted in the urine as 5-hyroxyindole acetic acid (SHIAA). If the tumour is confined to the gut the carcinoid syndrome does not occur because the 5-HT is inactivated by the liver but if the tumour metastasises to the liver and beyond, such inactivation cannot occur. Similar tumors occur in the lung where they are possibly related to the highly malignant small cell (oat cell or round cell) carcinoma.

16. The term 'polyp' is devoid of pathological significance. It merely indicates the presence of a circumscribed tumour which projects from the mucous membrane. A polyp may be sessile or, possessing a stalk of variable length, pedunculated. There are four main histological types: ①neoplastic (adenomatous or malignant), ②hamartomatous, ③inflammatory, ④unclassified.

17. Duke's classification of colorectal cancers defines the degree of spread of a tumour. It is one guide to prognosis although other factors such as the degree of histological dedifferentiation

should also be taken into account. Duke's A. The tumour has neither spread beyond the muscularis propria nor spread by the lymphatics. Duke's B. The tumour has spread through the muscularis propria into the pericolic or perirectal tissues although no lymphatic involvement is present.Duke's C. The tumour is associated with metastases irrespective of the degree of direct spread. Cure is impossible and only one-third of patients in this group survive for more than five years.

18. A raised carcinoembryonic antigen (CEA) level in the blood was initially considered to be associated only with carcinoma of the colon. This has now been disproved and it has been shown that CEA may be raised in other tumors, in cirrhosis of the liver and in viral hepatitis, However, a rapid rise in the CEA following the removal of colorectal cancer indicates recurrent tumour.

19. ①Genetic factors. There is a relatively higher incidence of duodenal ulceration in people with blood Group O and a higher concordance in monozygotic as compared with dyzygotic twins. ②Alterations in acid concentration. In chronic gastric ulceration acid production is normal or reduced, whereas in duodenal ulceration hypersecretion is common, particularly during the nocturnal phase of secretion. In the Zollinger-Ellison syndrome hypersecretion of acid leads to severe ulceration. ③Impaired mucosal resistance as in type B gastritis, possibly related to infection with H.pylori which can be found in 90% of patients suffering from chronic gastric ulceration. ④Metaplastic changes. Duodenal ulceration is commonly associated with metaplastic gastric epithelium in the duodenum. ⑤Associated disease.Duodenal ulceration is more frequent in alcoholic cirrhosis, chronic obstructive pulmonary disease, chronic renal failure and hyperparathyroidism. The last two are associated with hypercalcaemia which itself stimulates the secretion of gastrin and thus of acid. ⑥Miscellaneous causes include smoking and psychogenic factors.

20. There are two major types of chronic gastritis.

(1) Autoimmune-associated gastritis (type A). In this form of gastritis antibodies to parietal cells are present in 90% of cases and to the intrinsic factor in 50%, the latter blocks vitamin B_{12} binding sites and causes pernicious anaemia. This type of gastritis is frequently associated with other manifestations of autoimmune disease such as Hashimoto's thyroiditis and Addison's disease.Early in the course of the disease, biopsies of the gastric mucosa show mucosal infiltration by plasma cells and lymphocytes. Later, complete gastric atrophy occurs with the loss of the parietal cells of the stomach which are replaced by mucin-secreting cells.

(2) Helicobacter-associated gastritis (type B). This is the commonest type of gastritis and occurs increasingly with advancing age. The changes are mainly confined to the antral area of the stomach and the predominant histological picture is an intense plasma cell infiltration. In addition neutrophils are present in the superficial epithelium and the lamina propria. Helicobacter do not invade the mucosa but are seen lying on the surface.Both types of gastritis may result in the development of carcinoma of the stomach.

21. The precise mechanism by which it causes peptic ulceration is as yet undetermined. The organism itself is readily destroyed by exposure to a pH below 4.0 but it lives a protected existence in the mucous layer overlying the gastric mucosa. Furthermore the organism produces ammonia which neutralizes the surrounding acid. Isolates cultured in vitro produce an extracellular protease whose action breaks down the glycoproteins in gastric mucus. Presumably the protective effect of the mucus against acid erosion of the mucosa is removed. In addition a cytotoxic exotoxin has also been identified in tissue culture.

22. Chronic hepatitis is an inflammatory condition of the liver continuing without remission for at least 6 months. Apart from viral infections, especially with HBV and HCV, chronic inflammation of the liver can be caused by alcohol, long-standing biliary obstruction and by metabolic

disorders such as Wilson's disease.Chronic hepatitis in which inflammation is largely confined to the portal areas, which is more aggressive and in which portal and periponal areas show progressive fibrosis causing cirrhosis. That may follow a viral infection or it may be an autoimmune response. The latter could be drug-induced or of unknown aetiology. Clinical conditions are associated with malaise, abdominal pain, enlargement of the liver and biochemical changes in the blood. In the end-stages signs of liver failure appear.

23. Cirrhosis consists of pseudolobule nodularity of the whole liver caused by a process of destruction and regeneration of the parenchyma with the formation of bands of collagenous fibrous tissue which separate the nodules. The regenerated nodules have lost the normal hepatic architecture, hepatocytes may show fatty vacuolation, indicating continuing toxic onslaught. There is a variable lymphoid cell infiltrate in portal tracts and in the collagen bands, and hepatocellular jaundice may be present. The liver may be enlarged or of normal size but it usually becomes small in time. The classification of the various forms of cirrhosis is by aetiology rather than liver morphology, such as the size of the nodules.

24. (1) Scattered hepatocytes may die: apoptosis.

(2) Focal necrosis: this occurs in portal pyaemia and acute viral or drug-induced hepatitis. Such foci are not situated in any particular part of the liver lobules.

(3) Piecemeal necrosis a "moth-eaten" distroy to the limiting plate.

(4) Pridging necrosis linking portal-central, portal-portal, central-central necrotic areas. Both (3) and(4) are the characteristic feature of chronic hepatitis.

(5) Zonal necrosis, according to the zone of the lobule affected: ①periportal necrosis occurs in phosphorus poisoning. ②central zonal (centrilobular) necrosis occurs in anaemia, chronic venous congestion and alcoholic poisoning. ③midzone necrosis occurs in yellow fever.

(6) Massive hepatic necrosis (acute yellow atrophy) may be caused by viral hepatitis or exposure to hepatotoxic drugs such as carbon tetrachloride causes large irregular necrotic areas.

25. Primary biliary cirrhosis is uncommon and its aetiology is unknown. It is eight times commoner in women. The onset is insidious with ill health and mild jaundice at first. The liver is enlarged and serum cholesterol is increased thus predisposing to subcutaneous xanthelasmata. Malabsorption occurs in chronic cases. The jaundice is obstructive. Histologically, the intrahepatic bile ducts are destroyed by non-suppurative inflammation. Lymphocytes and plasma cells are present in large numbers round the smaller bile ducts where sarcoid-like granulomata develop in a third of cases. The inflammation extends periportally to some extent destroying adjacent hepatocytes, and the portal tracts eventually become fibrosed which causes cholestasis, Continuing hepatocyte destruction with regeneration and fibrosis results in a micronodular cirrhosis.

26. (1) Malignant

1) the most common are secondary carcinoma from almost any primary, usually of alimentary, pulmonary or breast origin.

2) primary malignant tumors of liver: ①hepatocellular carcinoma, which may be a complication of cirrhosis.②cholangiocarcinoma, not related to cirrhosis but associated with liver fluke infestation and hence commoner in the Far East.

(2) Benign are uncommon ①liver cell adenomata. ②bile duct adenomata. ③haemangiomata, usually cavernous and dark purple; they may be mistaken for secondary melanomata by the naked eye.

27. The Zollinger-Ellison syndrome is caused by the excessive secretion of gastrin by delta cell tumors of the pancreatic is lets, 60% of which are malignant, or by hyperplasia of the gastrin-secreting ceils of the pylorus of the stomach. This causes hypersecretion of hydrochloric acid re-

sulting in intractable multiple peptic ulcers in the duodenum and upper jejunum. The alkaline secretion of the pancreas is neutralized causing severe diarrhoea and the inactivation of the pancreatic enzymes leads to steatorrhea.

Chapter 9   Disorders of Hematopoietic and Lymphoid System

Answers and Explanations for Choose Tests
1- D   2- A

Answers and Explanations for Questions

1. ①Hypersensitivity states such as hay fever and urticaria. ②Infections by animal parasites, notably helminths such as trichinella and schistosoma. ③Certain chronic skin diseases; pemphigus and pemphigoid. ④Some patients with polyarteritis nodosa.⑤Some cases of Hodgkin's lymphoma.

2. Three clinical and pathologic conditions fall into this category. They are of unknown aetiology and are typified by neoplastic-like proliferations of macrophages but are not considered neoplasms. ①Letterer-Siwe disease, which is rapidly fatal and affects children. It is essentially due to marrow replacement by macrophages which do not contain lipid. ②Hand-Schüller-Christian disease sometimes affects adults but mostly occurs in children and the macrophages contain lipids, mainly cholesterol. The patient may survive up to 10 years. Lipid accumulation is not the cause of this disease and it is therefore not a lipid-storage disease.③Eosinophil granuloma of bone. This is a solitary lesion and possibly represents an indolent variety of Letterer-Siwe in which eosinophils accompany the collections of macrophages. It occurs in adolescents and young adults.

3. A malignant condition of lymphatic tissue excluding thymoma and leukaemia.It may present primarily in a lymph node or group of nodes or in the spleen,thymus,or indeed,any site where lymphoid tissue is present,e.g. marrow or the wall of the stomach or intestine. Lymphoma may also arise primarily in the skin——mycosis fungoides. The disease eventually becomes multifocal or at least the malignant lymphocytes invade the body widely and, in the case of non-Hodgkin's lymphoma, may spill into the blood stream to cause lymphatic leukaemia.

4. There are various classifications but for clinical purposes, the following is most useful.

The lower the grade, the less malignant they are low grade: ①small lymphocytic. ②follicular, mainly small cell. ③follicular, mixed small and large cell.

Intermediate grade:①follicular,mainly large cell. ②diffuse, small clear cell. ③diffuse,mixed small and large cell. ④diffuse, large cell.

High grade: ①large cell immunoblastic. ②lymphoblastic. ③small non-clear cell. There is also a miscellaneous group.

5. The Reed-Sternberg cell is an essential feature of Hodgkin's disease.It is large,40 μm or more in diameter,and characteristically has a bilobed nucleus and abundant eosinophilic cytoplasm which is sometimes vacuolated with large, round, prominent nucleoli.

6. The Ann Arbor system of staging. Stage I: one node or a group of nodes is affected. Stage II: the affected nodes are either all above or all below the diaphragm. Stage III: nodes both above and below the diaphragm are affected with or without lesions in other tissues. Stage IV: there is widespread involvement of one or more non-lymphoid tissues with or without nodal involvement. The importance is for treatment and prognosis. A single node or group (Stages I and II) is treated by local radiotherapy. Otherwise chemotherapy is given. As well as the histological type the stage affects, the prognosis; the higher the stage, the poorer the outlook.

7. By histological appearances and, at present, the WHO classification is internationally agreed. HL is divided into two types: nodular lymphocyte predominant HL (NLPHL) and classical HL, the latter including four subgroups. ①Lymphocyte-predominant, where most ceils are lymphocytes, Reed-Sternberg cells arc frequent and eosinophils are very scanty. ②Lymphocyte-depleted. Many Reed-Steinberg cells with variable eosinophils are present. Fibrosis may be prominent but is diffuse. Lymphocyte are sparse. ③Nodular sclerosing in which the lymph node capsule is thickened by collagen which sends trabeculae through the node.④Mixed cellularity. Reed-Sternberg cells, macrophages, neutrophils, eosinophils, lymphocytes and plasmacytes are all present. There may be diffuse (unlike 3) collagen. 15% of cases of Hodgkin's disease fall into each of groups 1 and 2 and 30%~40% into each of 3 and 4. Nodular sclerosis in Stage I of the disease has the best prognosis. Otherwise lymphocyte predominant has the best prognosis, mixed cellularity is worse and lymphocyte-depleted the worst. The disease tends to progress in the order of the last three. Although prognosis is related to the above types, treatment is determined by the stage only. NLPHL develops slowly with well prognosis.

8. This is a malignant T cells lymphoma which occurs in the skin. The upper dermis is infiltrated by macrophages, lymphocytes, reticulum cells, plasma cells and eosinophil leucocytes. Collections of lymphocytes, the Pautrier's abscesses, are found in the epidermis.

Chapter 10   Diseases of Immunity

Answers and Explanations for Choose Tests
1- B   2- B   3- C   4- C   5- E   6- D*   7- B   8- A   9- D   10- D   11- D*

Explanations
6. the answer is D

DiGeorge syndrome is caused by failure of the thymus and parathyroid glands to develop. The defect in parathyroid tissue leads to hypocalcemia and tetany. The B-cell areas are intact in DiGeorge syndrome; thus, plasma cells are present in normal numbers. The absence of thymus leads to absence of T-cell immunity.

11. The answer is D

Characteristics of Sjögren's syndrome include enlargement of lacrimal and salivary glands; histoiogic evidence of lymphoplasmacytic infiltration, acinar tissue atrophy, and ductal destruction; and formation of epimyoepithelial islands. The disorder frequently is associated with rheumatoid arthritis. Some patients with Sjögren's syndrome appear to be at increased risk for development of lymphoma. Sjögren's syndrome itself is not a malignant condition, hence, metastases to regional lymph nodes would not occur.

Answers and Explanations for Questions
1. In immunodeficient individuals, infection by saprophytic or commensal organisms may cause severe disease affecting chiefly the respiratory system. The main infective agents are: ①protozoal and helminthic, e.g. cryptosporidiosis and toxoplasmosis. ②fungal, e.g. Candida albicans and Aspergillus fumigatus. ③baterial, e.g. Mycobacteria, Nocardia and Salmonella. ④viral, e.g. cytomegalic virus.

2. Kaposi's sarcoma is a malignant tumour of undetermined origin, possibly arising from the abnormal primitive mesenchyme. Four different varieties have been described. ①A classic type, reportedly more common in Ashkenazi Jews, producing red or purple plaques, or nodules m the skin of the lower extremities. It rarely causes death. ②African Kaposi, similar to the tumors found in Europe but especially common in children and associated with lymph node enlargement.

③Transplant associated, often regressing when immunosuppression is discontinued. ④AIDS-related tumors which disseminate early but respond to cytotoxic drugs and α-interferon approximately one-third of AIDS related Kaposi's sarcomata develop a second malignant tumour, commonly lymphoma, leukaemia or myeloma. Histologically the appearances of all Kaposi's sarcomas are characteristic, consisting of spindie cells with slits containing erythrocytes. Such an appearance suggests tissue of vasoformative orgin but occasional pure cellular or anaplastic types are seen.

3. The HIV virus is a human retrovirus. In common with other retroviral infections, a long incubation period (7~10 years) occurs between infection and the development of clinical manifestations. The pathological consequences of infection are the development of severe immunosuppression which later predisposes the infected individual to opportunistic infections, neoplasms and neurological manifestations. The clinical consequences of these complications constitute AIDS.

4. ①Kaposi's sarcoma, a tumour of fibroblastic cells which may develop prior to the onset of severe immunodeficiency. ②Burkitt's lymphoma, which occurs in about 3% of all affected individuals. The tumour is almost exclusively of B cell origin, is aggressive and commonly found in the brain. ③Carcinoma of the cervix. There is a greatly increased prevalence of infection with the Human Papilloma Virus in AIDS, a virus known to be associated with cervical dysplasia, carcinoma-in-situ and squamous cell carcinoma of the cervix.

5. The graft versus host reaction occurs when a tissue graft or blood, containing donor lymphoid cells, is injected into an immunodeficient or immunosuppressed host. In such a situation the graft lymphocytes may survive and mount a response against host tissues. Two forms of GVH reaction are recognized: ①an acute form occurring within 3 months of grafting, e.g. a bone marrow transplant, Characteristically, exfoliative dermatitis, diarrhoea, intestinal malabsorption and cholestatic liver disease develop. ②a chronic form occurs and usually develops within 15 months. In this condition symptoms similar to those of progressive systemic sclerosis develop a condition in which excessive fibrosis occurs in various tissues. For example, involvement of the oesophagus can cause dysphagia and of the small bowel malabsorption. In at least half the cases, death occurs due to renal failure by involvement of the kidneys.

6. ①Hyperacute：when the donor kidney has been sensitized to a large number of transplantation antibodies. ②Acute：such reactions commonly occur within one year of transplantation. The recipient develops a fever, oliguria and tenderness over the affected kidney. ③Chronic：when the graft ceases to function after a period of months or years. This event is accompanied by hypertension, proteinuria and the appearance of fibrin degradation products in the urine.

7. Lesions develop in both the arteries and renal parenchyma. Gross intimal thickening occurs in the interlobular and arcuate arteries due to the intermittent aggregation of platelets to form thrombi and their incorporation into the wall of the artery. In the renal parenchyma the basement membranes of the glomemlar and tubular epithelia become thickened. Immunoffuorescent studies demonstrate fine granular deposits of IgM, IgG and complement fractions which outline the capillary walls of the glomemli and the basement membranes of the tubules.

8. Down's syndrome is caused by the failure of chromosome 21. to separate during oogenesis with the result that three of these chromosomes are present in a fertilized ovum. Thus the chromosomal composition of a typical Down's baby is 47,XX, +21. or 47,XY, +21, this formula indicating the presence of a male or female with an additional 21. chromosome, a genotype known as trisomy 21. This type of Down's syndrome is commonest in women who bear children towards the end of their reproductive life. A rarer form of Down's syndrome, not related to maternal age, is associated with 46 chromosomes. One of these is large and is composed of 21. attached to 15, constituting a translocation. Thus the normal complement of chromosomes is present and the tri-

somy is latent.

9. The cytomegalovirus is a herpesvirus chiefly affecting newborn babies via the transplacental route. Changes develop in many tissues, the colonized cells becoming greatly enlarged due to distension of the nucleus by inclusion bodies which may also be intracytoplasmic. In infants, death is the result of an encephalitis and children who survive may be mentally retarded or develop hydrocephalus. In adults, many of whom have serological evidence of infection, only a mild or subclinical disease mimicking infectious mononucleosis may occur. This virus is one cause of opportunistic infection in individuals of all ages who are immunodeficient.

10. The fundamental pathological feature of Sjögren's syndrome, which is commoner in women than in men, is destruction of the salivary and lacrimal glands, with enlargement due to lymphocytic infiltration. Clinically the destruction of these glands results in dryness of the mouth causing difficulty in eating, and kerato-conjunctivitis sicca, associated with these changes may be lymphadenoid goitre. Auto-antibodies to the microsomal fraction of all these glands may be present.

Chapter 11   Diseases of the Kidney and its collecting System

Answers and Explanations for Choose Tests
1- B   2- D   3- A   4- A   5- C   6 - B   7- C   8- E   9- A

Answers and Explanations for Questions

1. Glomerulonephritis is the term applied to a group of renal diseases where the predominant pathologicai changes are in the glomeruli with inflammatory proliferation changes and the mechanism is that of either a type III or type II hypersensitivity reaction. They are classified by their light microscopical appearances.

2. Glomemlonephritis is either diffuse, affecting all glomeruli, or focal affecting only some. Focal lesions often show a segmental pattern as well i.e. part of the glomerular tuft being more severely affected than the rest. Diffuse lesions tend to affect the whole glomerulus. Glomemlar reactions by light microscopy are, in broad terms, mixtures of proliferation (increased cellularity) and an increase of extracellular material (i.e, capillary basement membrane and/or mesangial matrix). Hence: ① diffuse membranous: the cellularity is normal and basement membranes are uniformly thickened. ②diffuse mesangial proliferative: capillaries are normal but there is an increase in mesangial matrix and cells. ③ diffuse endocapillary proliferative: there is a great increase in endothelial and mesangial cells which swell the glomerulus and obliterate capillary lumina in some of which polymorphs are seen. ④diffuse mesangiocapillary: increased mesangial cells and matrix with thickening of capillary loops leading to their obliteration. ⑤focal segmental proliferative: there are increased cells and matrix in parts of the tuft, sometimes with necrosis and usually against a background of diffuse mesangial proliferation. ⑥diffuse extracapillary: parietal epithelial cells proliferate to form "crescents".

3. Diffuse endocapillary and diffuse mesangial proliferative will usually resolve, the latter not being serious unless it progresses. A quarter of membranous cases will remit spontaneously and the remainder progress through the nephrotic syndrome to chronic renal failure (CRF) slowly, usually over more than 5 or even 10 years. Mesangiocapillary rarely remits and results in CRF more rapidly. Widespread crescent formation is indicative of rapid loss of renal function probably over months and can be seen superimposed on diffuse endocapillary, focal segmental and mesangiocapillary glomemlonephritis.

4. Most cases of glomerulonephritis have no known cause and are therefore idiopathic. Sys-

temic diseases which cause glomemlonephritis are systemic lupus erythematosus, subacute bacterial endocarditis and Henoch-Schönlein purpura. They give rise to a range of changes, the mildest being diffuse mesangial proliferative; the next most severe, focal segmental and the most serious, a superimposed diffuse extracapillary (crescentic) pattern. Polyarteritis nodosa and Wegener's granulomatosis also follow this scheme but are vasculitides, not hypersensitivity, reactions. Membranous and mesangiocapillary glomemlonephritis are predominantly idiopathic though the former may be associated with malignancy, sarcoidosis, hepatitis B surface Antigenemia and penicillinase or gold treatment for rheumatoid arthritis. Mesangiocapillary glomemlonephritis is sometimes secondary to systemic lupus erythematosus, Henoch-Schönlein purpura or infections such as subacute bacterial endocarditis and infected ventriculo-atrial shunts. Like diffuse endocapillary proliferative, it may also be a post-streptococcal phenomenon. Diffuse mesangioproliferative is rarely idiopathic, and, in addition to the systemic diseases, is seen in IgA nephropathy, a syndrome of recurrent haematuria which is usually serf-limiting. SLE can cause any picture.

5. By immunofluorescence and electron microscopy. They are found where changes are seen on routine light microscopy: ①in membranous glomerulonephritis complexes are seen in a row outside the glomerular capillary basement membrane. ②in diffuse mesangial glomemlonephriris in the mesangium. ③in mesangiocapillary glomemlonephritis in the mesangium and on the inside of capillary loops. The components in most diseases are usually specific, IgG and C3 in membranous, C3 in mesangiocapillary and IgA in IgA nephropathy respectively, but in systemic lupus erythematosus the immunology is mixed whatever the morphology may be.

6. A glomemlar disease characterised by no other changes than obliteration of the foot processes of glomemlar epithelial cells which can only readily be seen by electron microscopy. The kidney is thus normal by routinemicroscopy. Predominantly a disease of children, it may give rise to a selective proteinuria heavy enough to cause the nephroric syndrome. This responds to steroids and usually continues in remission on their withdrawal.

7. This most commonly takes the form of a diffuse extracapillary proliferation. Immunofiuorescence reveals linear deposition of IgG along the capillary basement membrane because this syndrome is a type II hypersensitivity reaction due to anti-basement membrane antibodies. Immunofluorescence in all other glomerulonephritides is granular.

8. Tumors of the renal parenchyma.

1) Benign: These are common but seldomclinically important. They include adenomata, forming well-defined rounded tumors yellowish in colour, and juxtaglomerular tumors arising from the juxtaglomemlar apparatus. The last are rare but important since they secrete renin and thus are a rare cause of hypertension.

2) Malignant. These form 1% of all malignant tumors: ①nephroblastoma, usually occurring before 7 years of age.②renal adenocarcinoma (hypernephroma).

3) Urothelial tumors arising from the transitional epithelium of the renal pelvis are always malignant.

4) Connective tissue tumors including leiomyomata, fibromata and lipomata are benign and rare.

9. Renal adenocarcinomata arise from the cortex and, if small, tend to project from the upper or lower pole of the affected kidney. The cut surface is usually yellow in colour. Old haemorrhages cause brown patches; necrosis, light grey areas. The tumour tends to invade the lumen of the renal vein by direct spread. Microscopically the tumor cells are arranged in solid trabeculae or in a tubular or papillary fashion. Most of these tumours are composed of characteristic clear cells and granular cells. The clear cells are due to their content of fat and glycogen dissolving out on

histological processing.

10. Nephroblastoma account for approximately one-third of all childhood tumors. The maximum age incidence is 3 years and they are seldom encountered after the age of seven. The cut surface of a nephroblastoma is white or greyish white in colour. Cystic spaces may develop as a result of haemorrhage and gelatinous degeneration within the tumour. Microscopically there is a characteristic mesenchymal stroma composed of spindle cells within which there are primitive, poorly differentiated glomeruli and tubules. Direct spread to adjacent structures is common and blood spread is mainly to lungs, bone and liver.

11. Pyelonephritis is a bacterial-induced inflammation of the renal pelvis, calyces and renal mesenchymal. It is most commonly caused by E. coli ascending from the lower urinary tract. It may be acute or chronic and affect one or both kidneys. The condition is commoner in females than males because of the greater incidence of cystitis in the former. In females it is also an important cause of chronic renal failure.

12. (1) Sex. It is presumed that pyelonephritis is much commoner in females because infection of the lower urinary tract is commoner in them due to the shorter urethra and trauma to it during sexual intercourse. Nuns have a very low incidence of urinary tract infection compared with sexually active women. Pregnancy may lead to acute bacterial infection of the upper urinary tract due to hormonally induced ureteric atony and dilatation causing urinary stasis.

(2) Urinary tract obstruction. This causes infection because: ①Stagnant urine is a suitable culture media for enteric bacteria. ②Obstruction of the bladder neck predisposes to vesico-ureteric reflux. ③Back-pressure lessens the natural resistance of the kidneys to infection. ④Renalfailure caused by chronic obstruction lowers the general resistance of an individual to infection.

13. The kidneys are enlarged and oedematous. Radially arranged yellow streaks of pus develop in the medulla and small yellow abscesses eventually occur in the cortex. The pelvic mucosa is thickened, congested and coated with exudate. Microscopically suppurative inflammation is seen in the pelvic submucosa with pus cells in tubules as well as interstitially.

14. Chronic pyelonephritis commonly follows Chronic vesico-ureteric reflux and obstructive lesions of the lower urinary tract. The kidneys become shrunken and the surface. deformed as the thickness of the renal parenchyma irregularly reduced. Microscopically, pyogenic-abscesses, pus in the tubules and suppuration of the pelvic mucosa may be present. In all cases the glomeruli are sclerosed and replaced by hyalinised collagen. An interstitial chronic inflammatory cell exudate is present but inflammatory changes gradually diminish at the end stage of the disease when the kidney becomes fibrosed, often broad, u-shaped scars.

15. Urothelial tumors of the bladder form either exophytic papillary growths or solid thickening of the wall with a variable degree of ulceration.

16. The microscopic appearance of a vesical tumour depends upon the degree of differentiation. The most common is transitional cell carinoma. Highly differentiated tumors of low malignant potential consist of papillary projections formed of cells of uniform size and shape which are very regularly arranged. With increasing dedifferentiation, the cells forming the fronds invade the wall and become increasingly irregular in shape and variable in size. Nuclei are hyperchromatic and show numerous mitoses.

Chapter 12　Diseases of the Genital System and Breast

Answers and Explanations for Choose Tests
1- D　2- C　3- D　4- C　5- D　6- D　7- C　8- C　9- D　10- D　11- C　12- D
13- B　14- D　15- B　16- E　17- D　18- C　19- E　20- A

Answers and Explanations for Questions

1. Endometriosis is the presence of normal endometrium (glands plus stroma) in extrauterine sites such as the ovaries, uterine tubes, large bowel, the umbilical skin or abdominal scars and on the serosa of the peritoneal cavity. Adenomyosis, once considered a variety of endometriosis, refers to normal endometrium which is situated deeply in the myometrium.

2. ①It is commoner in. post-menopausal women, unlike cervicai carcinoma. ②It occurs more often in nulliparous women. ③In some cases, hyperoestrinism is responsible. ④There may be focal or diffuse involvement of the endometrium. Both varieties are late in penetrating the myometrium. Spread is directly to the pelvis and later to the extra-pelvic lymph nodes and distant organs. ⑤It is an adenocarcinoma which may show evidence of squamous metaplasia, If the last is marked, the growth is described as an adenoacanthoma. A true adenosquamous carcinoma with a malignant squamous cell element is recognised and has a poor prognosis. ⑥ With early diagnosis the prognosis is reasonably good, resulting in a 5-year survival rate of 66% .

3. Nearly all are carcinoma. Nine-tenths are squamous and the remainder adenocarcinomata. Squnmons carcinomata are associnted with early and promiscuous sexual activity, early pregnancy and multiple pregnancies. Herpes virus, smegma and DNA from sperm are suspeced carcinogens. The disease is uncommon in Jewish women most probably due to circumcision of their male partners rather than to genetic factors. Adenocarcinomata do not appear to be associated with the above causes since they occur more frequently in nulliparous women. They are liable to occur in young girls whose mothers, while bearing them, were treated with oestrogens. Otherwise no other aetiological factors have been identified.

4. The earliest sign of cervical carcinoma is dysplasia of the squamous epithelium as assessed by exfoliative cytology, biopsy or both. In some cases this progresses to carcinoma-in-situ and eventually invasive cancer, a process which can take up to fifteen years. Conversely the dysplasia may reverse spontaneously, but since all cases of dysplasia are potentially malignant, the condition is currently described as Cervical Intraepithelial Neoplasia (GIN) and graded I to III, the last being very severe dysplasia, possibly carcinoma-in-situ. The identification of those cases of CIN which are to become malignant is impossible. Dysplasia caused by cervicitis is a complicating factor.

5. ①The stratified squamous epithelial cells show lack of maturation to flat, cornified, glycogencontaining cells. ②The basal cells form several layers instead of one. ③There is loss of polarity of the cells which are normally parallel to the surface. ④The cells become large and variable in size. ⑤Nuclei become hyperchromatic and show increased mitotic activity.

6. A large number of tumors occur in the ovary and since the common ones vary in their benign or malignant behaviour, classification does not depend on this.

(1) Common epithelial tumors. Nine-tenths are malignant. Many are cystic. Solid or papillary areas in the cyst wall suggest malignancy. ①Serous cystadenomata; benign and malignant varieties. ②Mucinous cystadenomata; benign and malignant varieties. ③Brenner tumors; nearly always benign.

(2) Tumors of sex cord-stromal origin. ①Granulosa cell tumors, of low grade malignancy and oestrogen secreting. ② Theca cell tumors, benign and oestrogen secreting. ③ Androblastomata, composed of Sertoli or Leydig cells or a mixture of these. Most are benign and most produce virilising (occasionally oestrogenising) hormones.

(3) Germ cell tumors. ①Dysgerminoma-very similar in histology, malignancy and radio-sensitivity to the seminoma. ②Endodermal sinus tumour (yolk sac tumour). ③Choriocarcinoma of ovary.④Teratoma; malignant and mature (benign) varieties, the latter described as a dermoid cyst in the past.

(4) Miscellaneous tumors, e.g. fibromata, lipomata, leiomyomata and malignant lymphomata.

(5) Secondary growths, usually from breast, uterus, stomach and large intestine.

7. Ascites and pleural effusions associated with a fibroma of the ovary. This tumour is benign and on its removal, complete cure occurs.

8. ①Hydatidiform mole. The villi are confined to the endometrium. These tumors are benign but liable to become choriocarcinomata. ②Invasive mole.This complicates 5% of hydatidiform moles when the villi penetrate the myometrium and even beyond. Emboli of the mole may spread to distant sites. This is benign, the disseminated tissue regressing on excision of the mole. There is no greater chance of choriocarcinoma developing than in a hydatidiform mole. ③Choriocarcinoma. Half of these occur following a mole, a quarter after an abortion and a quarter after a normal pregnancy following the retention of products of conception. This is a highly malignant growth and was invariably fatal until the introduction of cytotoxic drugs which now cure 80% of cases. ④Placental site trophoblastic tumor (PSTT).

9. A mass of placental tissue whose villi are exceedingly oedematous thus resembling hydatid cysts. It is the result of trophoblastic proliferation following fertilisation when the ovum later dies. The sperm nucleus with the X chromosome replicates to become diploid and cell division continues to produce the mole. This is borne out by the fact that the mole cells always have two X chromosomes and both are of paternal origin. Although considered benign neoplasms, 5% become highly malignant choriocarcinomata.

10. (1) Fat necrosis caused by trauma.

(2) Inflammation (mastitis): ①pyogenic abscess, ②tuberculosis, ③plasma cell mastitis (rupture of a cyst or ectatic duct), ④fungal and parasitic diseases (rare).

(3) Mammary dysplasia (fibrocystic disease).

(4) Primary tumors:

1) Benign: ①fibroadenoma,②adenoma (rare),③intraduct papilloma, ④phyllodes tumour, also known as cystosarcoma phyllodes or giant fibroadenoma, 20% of which are malignant,⑤lipoma.

2) Malignant: ①carcinoma, ②sarcomas, leukaemias and lymphomas are rare.

(5) Secondary tumors are rare.

11. This is a mixed epithelial and connective tissue growth and is therefore described as a fibroadenoma. Pure adenomata occur but are rare. Fibmadenomata occur in women younger than those liable to develop carcinoma: They are well demacated from the surrounding breast from which they pout when cut across. On microscopy they consist of well, differentiated glandular structures in a fibrous stroma and have characteristic appearances which cannot be confused with carcinoma. Two varieties, the intracanalicular and pericanalicular are described but many are mixed and there is no clinical significance in this classification.

12. The cause or causes are unknown. Breast cancer is, however, more common in nulliparous than multiparous women. The number of lactations or breast feeding are not important but

early maternal age at first pregnancy appears to be protective. There is no evidence for a viral or genetic factor as has been found in mice,

13. (1) in situ carcinoma:①intraduct,②intralobular.

(2) infiltrating carcinoma:①infiltrating duct,②infiltrating lobular,③mixture of duct and lobular, is not uncommon.

(3) unusual forms:①mucoid (colloid) carcinoma, ②sqamous carcinoma, ③spindle cell carcinoma,④apocrine carcinoma,⑤medullary carcinoma, has a heavy lymphoid cell infiltrate.

14. This is a clinncal term used to describe a very fast-growing and rapidly-disseminating cancer of the breast which usually develops during pregnancy or lactation. The skin overlying the tumour is red and oedematous hence the name. Accounts for less than 2% of all breast cancer cases.

15. Clinically, it is a chronic eczema of the nipple which may include the areola and surrounding skin. Histologically, as well as a non-specific chronic inflammatory cell infiltrate in the dermis, typical Paget's cells are seen in the thickness of the dermis. These are large, pale cells with prominent neucleoli occurring singly or in small groups. The epidermis may ulcerate.Underlying the dermal lesion there is a ductal carcinoma of breast, in situ or invasive, which may be so small as to require histological examination for detection and from which the Paget's cells are derived.

16. Oestrogen receptors are proteins in or on cells to which oestrogens attach themselves thereby inducing the proliferation of these cells. They are therefore present in the cells of organs which are under oestrogen control. This includes normal breast epithelium. Breast carcinoma cells contain variable amount of receptors and if they are present in appreciable quantities it signifies, firstly, a better prognosis presumably indicating better differentiation and secondly, that the tumours are liable to respond better to antiestrogen therapy (drugs and endocrine ablation).

17. About 1% of all breast cancers arise in males. They have the same histological appearances as in women. Of all male malignancies, less than 1% are breast cancers. A predisposing factor in the male is Klinefelter's syndrome where 2 to 4 X chromosomes are present. XXY males occur in 2 per 1000 male births.

18. Gynaecomastia, inflammation or carcinoma are the most likely. Gynaecomastia, the commonest swelling in the malee breast, may present as diffuse enlargement of the whole breast but is frequently asymmetrical and nodular. One per cent of all mammary carcinomata arise in the male breast.

19. Gynaecomastia, hypertrophy of the male breast, is considered to be due to androogen/oestrogen imbalance. It may thus occur spontaneously at puberty and the climacteric. Otherwise, it is caused by the direct action of oestrogens as is liable to occur in cirrhosis of the liver when normally present oestrogens are not metabolized. Gynaecomastia may also occur in males with oestrogen-producing tumors, in patients treated by oestrogens for prostatic carcinoma and in men who absorb the hormone from skin while working with it. The histology is the same whatever the cause. There is an increase in the number of ducts, the epithelial lining of which shows cellular multilayering, sometimes with papillary, projections simulating intraduct carcinoma the stroma immediately surrounding these ducts has a characteristic oedematous appearance. There is no risk of malignancy.

Chapter 13   Disorders of the Endocrine System

Answers and Explanations for Choose Tests

1- B   2- A   3- C

Answers and Explanations for Questions

1. ①Diffuse nontoxic goiter are more commonly diffuse enlarged gland. The patient may be euthyroid. ②Diffuse toxic goitres may be over-active with infiltrative ophthalmopathy and edematous dermopathy.

2. A nodular goitre consists of numerous nodules, which are the result of foci of hyperplasia, separated by bands of collagen. Some of these foci undergo colloid change whereas in others haemorrhage occurs leading to necrosis and cyst formation. Both fibrosis and calcification can occur in the degenerate nodules.

3. A simple goitre consists of a generalized enlargement of the thyroid gland without evidence of under-or over-activity. Histologically a simple goitre is composed of enlarged vesicles filled with colloid and lined by a flattened epithelium.

4. ①A dietary deficiency of iodine. ②An increased demand for thyroid hormones, e.g. in pregnancy, producing a physiological goitre.③A congenital enzyme defect which either interferes with the uptake of iodine by the gland or the synthesis of thyroxine. This is a dyshormogenic goitre. ④Chemical agents which interfere with thyroxine synthesis, e.g. para-aminosalicylic acid, thiouracil, carbimazole and substances occurring in vegetables of the brassica family (cabbage and turnips).

5. In an untreated toxic goitre the thyroid follicles are lined by a hyperplastic epithelium which produces papillary infoldings into the follicles. The cells are larger than normal and the amount of colloid is reduced. Clear spaces are seen in the watery pale, staining colloid at the margin of the follicle giving it a characteristic scalloped appearance. Following treatment with iodine the colloid stores are replenished but if anti-thyroid drugs, such as carbimazole, are administered, the hyperplasia and infolding of the epithelium increases. Commonly there is some degree of lymphoid infiltration of the thyroid, usually diffusely scattered throughout the gland but sometimes focal.

6. The thyroid in Hashimoto's disease is enlarged symmetrically or asymmetrically. The surface is smooth. The gland is greyish white in colour and the cut surface is uniform. One striking feature is the avascularity of the gland. Microscopically the most distinctive feature is the intense lymphocytic and plasma cell infiltration. Foci of these may contain lymphoid follicles, In the late stages, remaining thyroid follicles are small and contain only minimal quantities of colloid. The follicular epithelial cells become large and irregular with eosinophilic cytoplasm and are known as Askanazy cells.

7. Tumors of the thyroid may be:

(1) Benign: ①embrynal adenoma ②fetal adenoma ③Hürthle cell adenoma ④simple adenoma ⑤colloid adenoma ⑥atypical adenoma.

(2) Malignant: these are rare, accounting for 0.3% of all cancer deaths: ①papillary carcinoma ②follicular carcinoma ③anaplastic carcinoma ④medullary carcinoma ⑤squamous cell carcinoma ⑥miscellaneous tumors including malignant lymphoma and teratoma.

8. ①The tumor is commonly solitary and well encapsulated. ②Microscopically the tumour consists of numerous follicles and a varying number of solid masses of cells. Clear cells and oxyphilic (Hürthle) cells forming solid sheets make up a large part of the tumour.③The diagnosis of malignancy is confirmed by finding capsular and/or vascular invasion.

9. ①It is rarely encapsulated. ②Multiple foci of tumor are visible to the naked eye in 20% of cases. ③The tumour may contain psammoma bodies. ④Microscopically, papillary projections are seen in the colloid-filled follicles. ⑤The tumour rarely spreads via the bloodstream but may be found in adjacent lymph nodes.

10. ①In 20% of patients this tumour is familial forming one part of the multiple endocrine neoplasia (MEN) II complex. ②The tumour arises from the calcitonin secreting parafollicular C-cells. ③Whereas the sporadic tumour is unilateral, in familial cases it is frequently bilateral and multifocal. ④The tumour or tumours are discrete and greyish in colour. ⑤Microscopically the tumour consists of small undifferentiated cells with amyloid in the stroma. ⑥The tumour metastasises to the regional lymph nodes and later to the skeleton, liver and lungs.

11. Other than secondary changes due to hypertension, atherosclerosis and pyelonephritis, which complicate diabetes, the most important specific lesion with a high mortality, particularly in children, is diabetic glomerulosclerosis. In this condition there is deposition of eosinophilic hyaline material in the mesangium of the glomerular lobules. The deposits may be nodular or diffuse and if the latter, the appearances are not unlike those of diffuse glomerulonephritis.

12. Acute destruction of the adrenal glands was due to bacterial or viral infections, pregnancy, severe trauma and disseminated intravascular coagulation. The classic syndrome, the Waterhouse-Friderichsen, occurs following infection with purulent meningitides. Acute destruction is followed by severe hypotension, cyanosis and death. Chronic destruction of the adrenal glands was due to tuberculosis or mycotic infections, secondary malignant tumours, auto-immunity or amyloidosis usually associated with rheumatoid arthritis. Chronic destruction leads to Addison's disease.

13. Addison's is due to chronic destruction of the adrenal cortex from whatever cause. It is characterised by increasing fatigue, muscular weakness, abdominal discomfort and brown pigmentation of the buccal mucosa and the areas of skin exposed to light. This last change is due to the melanocyte stimulating action of corticotrophin which is produced in increased amounts by the pituitary. The deficiency of cortisol causes an imbalance of sodium ions and water between the intra-and extracellular compartments and thus hypotension.

14. (1) Virilism causing sexual precocity in boys and pseudohermaphroditism in girls.

(2) Feminisation leading to sexual precocity in girls and feminisation of the male.

(3) Aldosteronism.

(4) Cushing's syndrome; obesity, a "moon face", the buffalo hump, protein loss and thinning of the abdominal skin leading to the development of purple striae, osteoporosis and diabetes in many patients.

15. Cushing's syndrome is due directly to the excessive secretion of corticosteroids by an adrenal cortical adenoma, a carcinoma or adrenal hyperplasia, whereas Cushing's disease is caused by excess secretion of ACTH by a pituitary adenoma resulting in the secretion of cortisone by the stimulated adrenal.

16. Conn's syndrome is due to the excessive secretion of aldosterone by the adrenal cortex, the result of cortical hyperplasia, a cortical adenoma or, rarely, a carcinoma. This causes a number of biochemical abnormalities including a low plasma rennin, intermittently lowered serum calcium, hypokalaemia, hypernatraemia and impaired glucose tolerance. The clinical manifestations are polyuria, polydipsia and periodic muscular weakness.

17. These syndromes are characterized by hyperplastic or neoplastic proliferation of more than one endocrine gland. There are three types, all apparently inherited as autosomal dominants. MEN I (Werner's syndrome) consists of adenomata of the pituitary, pancreatic islets and parathyroid glands although the last usually shows only chief cell hyperplasia. Adenomata of the adrenal cortex and thyroid may also be present. MEN II (Sipple's syndrome) is typified by medullary carcinoma of the thyroid, pheochromocytoma and parathyroid chief cell hyperplasia. MEN III (MEN lib or Gorlin's syndrome)consists of medullary carcinoma of the thyroid, pheochromocyto-

ma, mucosal neuromata (especially of the lips), skeletal abnormalities and a marfanoid habitus.

Chapter 14   Diseases of the Nervous System

Answers and Explanations for Choose Tests
1- D   2- D   3- C   4- B

Answers and Explanations for Questions
1. See table.

	Epidemic cerebrospinal meningitis	Epidemic encephalitis B
season	winter and spring	summer and autum
organism	meningococcin,pneumococci etc.	arbovirus
infectious pathway	meniges	parenchyma
nature	suppurative inflammation	alteration inflammtion

2. Wallerian degeneration describes the changes which occur when a nerve fibre is separated from its nerve cell. Within 12 hours fragmentation of the axon can be observed, after which the myelin and the axon form ovoid bodies surrounded by proliferating Schwann cells. The rate of degeneration is determined by: ①myelination; heavily myelinated fibres degenerate more rapidly than the unmyelinated. ② function; sensory fibres degenerate faster than motor nerves. With axonal and myelin degeneration, macrophages, fibroblasts and perineural cells form continuous columns, known as von Bungner's bands. This is the architectural scaffold within which the regenerating axon grows. At the same time that these changes are taking place distal to the point of section, central chromatolysis occurs in the perikaryon of the parent nerve cell body. This leaves the nerve cell with a thin peripheral rind of Nissl substance. Such changes are not degenerative but merely a response of the nerve cell prior to regenerative activity.

3. The commonest sites for brain haemorrhage are:①the lentiform nucleus, due to bleeding from the lenticulostriate branch of the middle cerebral artery ② the pons ③ the white matter of the cerebellum, The major predisposing factors are:①hypertension causing rupture of an atherosclerotic vessel or a microaneurysm ②a preexisting brain lesion, e.g. a primary or secondary neoplasm or a septic focus. Death usually occurs following brain haemorrhage due to extension of the haematoma in the cortex or rupture into a ventricle.

4. ①Congenital defects in the media leading to the development of "berry" aneurysms, Although structural weakness in the media is common the development of an aneurysm is rare. This type of aneurysm most frequently occurs in the middle cerebral artery either at its origin or where it branches. ②Atherosclerosis. ③Hypertension. ④Mycotic, aising in patients suffering from subacute bacterial endocarditis.

5. (1) Primary tumors

1) Neuronal tend to occur in childhood and are malignant; neuroblastoma, medullo blastoma and retinoblastoma.

2) Neuroglial are all malignant but variably so. ①Gliomata are better differentiated histologically and are slower growing. They are named after the cell of origin and include astrocytoma; oligodendroglioma; ependymorea.②Anaplastic gliomata, e.g. glioblastoma multiforme are most malignant.

3）Meningioma, commonly benign.

4）Nerve sheath and nerve root tumors, all benign.①Schwannoma（neurilemmoma, acoustic neuroma）.②traumatic neuroma.③neurofibroma may become malignant when multiple（von Recklinghausen's disease）.

5）Uncommon tumors and cysts: ①angioma, a developmental.②hemangioblastoma is malignant.③epidermoid cyst.④teratoma, malignant or benign（dermoid cyst）.⑤craniopharyngioma（supracerebellar cyst）, benign.

（2）Secondary tumours are common and may be the first indication of malignant disease in almost any other part of the body.

6. Tumors derived from the Schwann cells may arise along the course of any cranial or spinal nerve. The commonest intracranial site of origin is from the eighth crunial nerve, the tumor arising just internal to the internal acoustic meatus acoustic neuroma. Normally solid, Schwann cell tumors may undergo central liquefactive necrosis. Microscopically they consist of interlacing bands of spindle aligned in parallel columns producing 'palisading'.

7. A meningioma is a tumour developing from arachnoid cell. It commonly occurs in the region of the superior sagittal sinus but may occur in the spinal canal. Meningiomata grow slowly, producing smooth or nodular, friable, encapsulated, white-coloured tumors which erode the overlying bone. They have a variable microscopic appearance. The commonest variety, the syncytial type, is composed of poorly defined polygonal cells. Less common is the transitional type composed of nests of cells arranged concentrically in whorls which calcify to form gritty psammona bodies. Malignant varieties are rare.

Chapter 15　Infectious Diseases and Parasitosis Diseases

Answers and Explanations for Choose Tests
1- E　2- A　3- A　4- E

Answers and Explanations for Questions

1. In the male, the urethra, prostate, seminal vesicles and epididymis. In the female in whom the infection is less severe, the urethra, cervix, uterine tubes and pelvic peritoneum. In prepubertal girls vaginitis may occur due to the neutral pH of the vagina. In the mature woman, due to oestrogen secretion, the pH is normally acidic and thus anti bacterial.

2. Neutrophils first appear at the site of infection and are soon replaced by macrophages and lymphocytes. As the lesion develops the following zones from centre to periphery become recognisable and constitute a tubercle: ①a central zone of caseous necrosis in which organisms may be found.②a zone composed of macrophages which, having a supposed similarity to the cells of the stratum spinosum of the skin are called epithelioid cells, scattered among which are the multinucleate giant cells, the Langhans' cells. Tubercle bacilli are most likely to be seen in this zone. ③a zone of lymphocytes beyond which may be found granulation or fibrous tissue depending on the age of the lesion, the amount of tissue loss and the stage of healing.

3. Primary and secondary tuberculosis occur at the same sites, most frequently the lung or intestine, but whereas a primary lesion tends to heal spontaneously, a post-primary lesion, in the absence of treatment, tends to progress to produce cavitation in the affected tissues. Both, however, if progressive, spread in a similar fashion but primary lesions tend to be associated with a greater degree of enlargement of the nodes draining the site than in the case of secondary lesions. Miliary

tuberculosis, the result of bloodstream dissemination of the bacilli in a susceptible individual, is more common in primary than secondary tuberculosis.

4. From the primary site of infection, lung, intestine or rarely skin, bacilli may spread to the adjacent lymph nodes via the lymphatics and then by the blood stream to the brain, meninges, the genito-urinary tract, bones and joints. When the primary focus is the lung, sputum, when swallowed may infect the bowel or, when expectorated may affect the trachea, vocal cords or tongue.

5. Renal tuberculosis arises by haematogenous spread of Mycobacterium tuberculosis from a focus else where, which may or may not be clinically evident

6. A gumma is typically the lesion of tertiary syphilis. It is an area of coagulative necrosis which can occur in almost any organ and eventually becomes fibrosed and rubbery hard (gummi in Latin = rubber). The lesion is an area of ischaemic infarction due to hypersensitivity to the spirochaete and although the necrosis is similar, to caseation, the tissue is mummified instead of undergoing crumbling (cheesy) necrosis and thus its original architecture is still discernible. Numerous inflammatory cells, lymphocytes, plasma cells, histiocytes and occasional giant cells are seen. Fibroblasts then lay down collagen. Common sites are liver, testes, subcutaneous tissues and bone.

7. Because of the rich lymphatic supply to this part of the aorta. The lymphatics provide a pathway for the treponemes from the mediastinal lymph nodes to the vessel wall. The basic lesion is an arteritis of the vasa vasorum ramifying in the adventitia.

8. The infected rectal wall epithelium is ragged and may be ulcerated. In the later stages the rectal wall becomes fibrosed and may become calcified. Multinucleate eggs are seen in the wall.

9. A hard chancre of the penis is caused by the treponema pallidum. It is initially a hard nodule in the coronal region. Superficial or deep ulceration occurs followed by spontaneous healing within 30~60 days. In all cases marked inguinal lymphadenopathy occurs. Microscopically there is an initial collection of polymorphonuclear leucocytes which is soon replaced by lymphocytes and plasma cells, tending to be most prominent around the blood vessels.

10. (1) Congenital absence or aplasia of the lymphatics, Mitroys' disease.

(2) Neoplastic permeation.

(3) Chronic lymphangitis.

(4) Invasion of the lymphatics by Wuchereria banacrofti, the adult worm blocking the lymphatics, particularly those draining lower limbs and external genitalia.

病理讨论与测验

一、病理讨论选择题

这部分的问题都有备选答案,从中选出一个最佳答案

1. 一个 58 岁的男性住院了。因为最近间断性的上腹部疼痛,病史和物理检查显示在最近的几个月体重减轻 25 斤,上腹软,无肿块,无腹水,无黄疸,最好的诊断方法和最可能的诊断是

    A. 腹部超声检查诊断为慢性肝炎

    B. 血清胆色素检测诊断为胆石症性慢性胆囊炎

    C. 内窥镜检查为十二指肠乳头胆道口壶腹部癌症

    D. 剖腹探察术诊断为胰腺头部癌

    E. CT 诊断为胰腺体部癌

2. 肾的同种异体移植的接收者发生血性腹泻,直肠活检为局灶性坏死和出血,个别的内皮细胞大,并有明显的核包涵体。可能的病原菌是

    A. EB 病毒感染　　B. 念珠菌感染　　C. 肺囊虫　　D. 弓形虫病　　E. 贾第虫

3. 30 岁的女性最近表现为渐进性进展的声音嘶哑,因为近来的上呼吸道的感染而加剧,直接喉镜检查见声带上有小的乳头状的息肉,最可能的原因是

    A. 自身免疫　　　B. 细菌　　　C. 病毒　　　D. 真菌

4. 最常见的胃良性间叶细胞肿瘤是

    A. 息肉性腺瘤　　B. 良性间质细胞瘤　C. 血管瘤　　D. 脂肪瘤　　E. 平滑肌瘤

5. 一个 60 岁的老人,有长期的稳定性心绞痛病史,胸痛的频率和严重程度进行性增加,在一次特别严重的胸痛发作 12 小时后,被送进急诊室后发现有低血压和严重的充血性心力衰竭, 心电图显示明显的 Q 波 ST 段和 T 波变化,血清酶学检查证明有明显的肌酸激酶 MB 异构酶增加,各种治疗手段没能控制住病人的低血压和心力衰竭,心跳停止后复苏失败,进行尸检,关于病人的情况,下面哪一种是符合病人的情况?

    A. 尸检中很可能发现有心内膜下心肌梗死

    B. 尸检中不可能发现冠状动脉血栓

    C. 临床表现是限制性心包炎

    D. 在尸检中可能发现小于 2cm 直径的心肌梗死的区域

    E. 在尸检中很可能发现至少有一根冠状动脉严重狭窄

6. Barrett 上皮位于消化管道的哪个部位

    A. 食管　　　　　B. 胃　　　　　C. 小肠　　　D. 大肠　　　　E. 直肠

7. 一个 1 岁的婴儿在腹泻一周后发生左面部的肿胀,体格检查显示一个温热波动性的

肿块在耳朵的下面偏外侧, 细针穿刺诊断最有可能的结果是

A. 脓肿 B. 上皮细胞的病变

C. 肉芽肿 D. 恶性细胞

8.一个 50 岁的男性,送至急诊室前有慢性咳嗽,盗汗,入院胸部 X 线显示肺尖部侵润,痰液分析没有提示,但经支气管活检显示伴巨细胞的肉芽肿, 诊断是

A. 肉瘤样结节 B. 铍中毒 C. 结核病 D. 巨细胞癌

E. 肺炎球菌的肺炎

9. 下面哪个是急性非特异性阑尾炎的特征

A. 可发生在任何年龄,但主要发生在年长者;

B. 阑尾的蛲虫蠕虫性的感染是一个重要的易感因素;

C. 在 2/3 的病例中有粪石引起的管道堵塞;

D. 透壁性的慢性炎症是特征性的结果;

E. 出现白细胞减少。

10. 一个 12 岁的男孩主诉腿部疼痛和肿胀,患侧肢体的 X 线检查显示一个典型的 Codman 三角,最可能的诊断是什么?

A. 软骨肉瘤 B. 骨化性肌炎 C. 骨肉瘤 D. 多发骨髓瘤

E. 动脉瘤性骨囊肿

11. 一个四十岁的妇女发现她的乳房上有一个肿块后,前来就诊,医生检查发现在她的右乳房外侧有一个 3cm,质硬,不规则的肿块。同时伴有表皮的酒窝形成,活检显示这个肿块为慢性炎症,坏死脂肪组织伴皂化以及局部的钙化。这些组织学发现与下列哪项诊断一致:

A. 粉刺癌 B. 脂肪坏死 C. 导管扩张 D. 肉芽肿型乳腺炎

E. 腺病

12. 哪项是与该病有关的最可能的病史

A. 未经产 B. 雌激素治疗 C. 母乳喂养 D. 以前的创伤 E. 肺结核

13. 哪种自身免疫疾病以在皮肤,肾脏,肺出现免疫复合物为特征

A. 系统性红斑狼疮(SLE) B. 干燥综合征

C. 进展性硬皮病 D. 移植物抗宿主病

E. 雷诺综合征(钙化,雷诺肺炎,管道功能紊乱,并指(趾)畸形和毛细血管扩张)

14. 一个 50 岁的妇女因其手臂上色素性皮损就诊,患者自述,这个"胎记"出生时即存在,只是最近才出现病变,检查发现一个 0.5cm 的色素结节,一侧边缘不规则,有小范围痂皮形成,周围红斑,把痣与恶性黑素瘤鉴别诊断,下列哪一个组织学特征最有利于这两个疾病的鉴别

A. 黑素细胞巢在真皮下 1/3 B. 表皮过度角化症

C. 大量核分裂 D. 多核巨细胞

E. 环绕毛干的痣细胞

15. 一个 38 岁的男子在车祸中头部受伤,当送至急诊室时,患者处于休克状态,意识丧失,需要呼吸机,患者经抢救无效死亡,尸检神经病理中最有可能发现

A. 基底动脉瘤破裂   B. Duret 出血(脑干出血)

C. 延髓离断   D. 大脑梗死

E. 动静脉畸形

16. 一个肾移植术后患者在肾移植后三个月出现发热和腺病症状,查血显示抗 EB 病毒滴度明显升高,移植物的活检中下列哪项最可能见到

A. 小血管纤维素样坏死   B. 血管硬化   C. 间质纤维化

D. 间质大量淋巴腺细胞浸润及非典型性细胞

E. 肾小管上皮细胞空泡样改变

17. 一个 62 岁男性出现胃灼热感有数年,胃镜检查显示在胃食管交界处有一红色,天鹅绒样的指状突起,有 5 厘米伸入食管腔内,活检示肠形柱状上皮。下列哪项关于该病的描述是正确的

A. 这种病变约 10% 的患者中出现食管反流症状;

B. 鳞状细胞癌是最重要的该病的癌性并发症;

C. 形态学特征为典型的念珠菌性食管炎;

D. 肠肌丛内神经节细胞缺失;

E. 气管食管瘘为常见并发症。

18~19   一个 28 岁的男子出现单侧睾丸下降,CT 可见一个 6cm 的高密度腹部包块影。

18. 这个包块最可能的诊断是

A. 转移性前列腺癌   B. 隐睾增生

C. 畸胎瘤   D. 腺瘤样瘤

E. 精原细胞瘤

19. 下列哪一项对于这个肿瘤的治疗和预后是正确的

A. 无指征的切除术   B. 肿瘤对于放疗敏感

C. 低于 5 年的生存率

D. 此病人可根据血清中特异性前列腺抗原水平来进行进一步临床治疗

E. 在下降的睾丸中没有增加恶性肿瘤发生的危险性

20. 一个 16 月的男孩出现右侧腹部肿块,X 射线检查显示,一个已部分钙化的肿瘤占据了右侧腹部的大部分,肿瘤组织镜下显示细胞排列呈菊心团样,下列哪个诊断是最可能的

A. Wilm 肿瘤   B. 肝母细胞瘤

C. 胰母细胞瘤   D. 神经母细胞瘤

E. 胰岛细胞瘤

21. 一个病人出现恶心,呕吐和少尿,血压为 180/110mmHg。尿检显示有血尿和白细胞,未查及细菌,细菌培养为阴性,血清肌酐为 3.0mg/dl,下列哪项病理学发现能解释该病人的肾脏改变?

A. 结节性肾小球硬化   B. 细胞性新月体形成

C. 基底膜钉突   D. 刚果红组织染色呈阳性

E. 弥漫性足细胞消失

22.60 岁男性的胸膜渗出液细胞学检查中发现恶性细胞,该患者最可能发现的原发性癌是

    A. 淋巴瘤   B. 间皮瘤   C. 结肠癌   D. 肺癌   E. 胰腺癌

23. 下列哪项正确描述了病毒性肝炎的病原学因子

    A. HBV 是输血后肝炎最常见的病因

    B. HDV 感染人类时需要 HBV 的辅助

    C. HCV 是引起散发性肝炎的最常见病因

    D. HBV 的基因组是显著的双链 RNA

    E. 10%~20% 慢性甲型肝炎发生于急性病毒感染的患者中

24. 下列哪项对于卡波西肉瘤(Kaposi)的描述是正确的

    A. 经典型常见于女性患者   B. AIDS 患者常会有非皮肤表现

    C. 不同的临床形式有不同的组织学特征

    D. 在肾移植病例中,停用免疫抑制治疗对于卡波西肉瘤患者是无效的

    E. 已经明确 AIDS 病毒是引起卡波西肉瘤的原因

25. 一个小孩在发生病毒性疾病后出现肾病综合征,下列哪项是正确的

    A. 肾小球中弥漫性上皮细胞足突消失

    B. 约有 50% 的新月体形成

    C. 结节性肾小球硬化

    D. 基底膜破裂

    E. 肾小球基底膜的 IgG 线形沉积

26. 一个 60 岁的女性两年前患乳腺癌,并经外科手术切除,放疗化疗,定期随访病人,虽然病人无症状出现,但她的血红蛋白浓度为 8.7g/dl,血细胞比容是 27%,下列哪项是最可能的解释

    A. 缺铁性贫血   B. 化疗引起的骨髓损伤

    C. 急性白血病   D. 乳癌转移

    E. 题中信息不适当,无法判断

27. 判断癌症预后最重要的因素是什么

    A. 肿瘤分级   B. 肿瘤分期   C. 淋巴细胞浸润

    D. 血管侵犯   E. 核分裂指数

28. 胃癌可转移到卵巢子宫的最可能肿瘤是下列哪项

    A. Brenner 瘤   B. Wilms 瘤

    C. Klatskin 瘤   D. Krukenberg 瘤

    E. Grawitz 瘤

29. 一个 57 岁的病人在结肠癌术后 7 天,感觉左腿腓肠肌胀痛,伴气促,胸片检示无异常现象,下列病理描述最可能的是哪项?

    A. 心肌肥厚,心房扩张   B. 心肌梗死

    C. 淋巴细胞性间质性肺炎   D. 近期肺栓死

30. 一个 45 岁的女性主诉加重性头痛 6 个月,并伴有右臂无力与步态不稳,外科检查发现在左枕骨部位病变,该病变病理学检查显示为脑膜瘤,该患者的预后取决于
    A. 脑膜瘤的组织学类型   B. 脑膜瘤的核分裂指数
    C. 手术切除的完全性   D. 肿瘤的血供
    E. 病人对放疗的敏感性

31. 下列哪种原发性肝肿瘤是最常见的
    A. 肝细胞癌   B. 血管肉瘤   C. 胆管癌   D. 海绵状血管瘤
    E. 灶性结节性增生

32. 一个 35 岁的男性患者按急性支气管肺炎治疗,在抗生素治疗后似有好转,然而医生注意到在一个医学生的病案记录中提到该患者在陶瓷厂工作。下一步的处理是
    A. 询问该工厂是否老厂,工厂内是否有石棉
    B. 询问患者是否服用过类固醇激素
    C. 拍胸片,看是否有空洞形成
    D. 进行铍元素的皮试
    E. 询问该患者是否做过挖煤工人

33. 接受肾脏移植患者术后 48 小时内没有排尿,影像学显示移植肾大小正常。移植配型良好。活检示血管腔内有针形结晶,以下哪项为最可能的诊断
    A. 超急性排斥反应   B. Harvest 损伤
    C. 原有的动脉栓塞性病变   D. 急性细胞排斥反应
    E. 急性血管排斥反应

34、35   一个 35 岁经产妇在新一次妊娠的头三个月内出现子宫异常增大及血中人绒毛膜促性腺激素(HCG)水平异常增高。

34. 病人的病史和下列哪个诊断最相符
    A. 宫外孕   B. 植入性胎盘   C. 平滑肌瘤
    D. 水泡状胎块   E. 绒毛膜血管瘤

35. 以下哪种病症是该病常见的并发症
    A. 输卵管破裂   B. 平滑肌肉瘤
    C. 腹膜假性黏液瘤   D. 子宫内膜息肉
    E. 绒毛膜癌

36. 一个 37 岁女性因为乳房 X 线片发现可疑现象,而进行乳房活检,该患者近五年来每年进行乳房 X 线检查。3 年前的乳房活检示纤维腺瘤及纤维囊性变,并有活跃的上皮细胞增生。当问及她相关的家族史时,患者自诉其母亲死于恶性叶状囊性肉瘤,并且她的儿子在学校体检中被发现患有男性乳腺发育。该患者这次的乳房活检显示为原位小叶癌。以下哪个最可能是增加她乳腺癌的危险性因素。
    A. 该病人先前的纤维腺瘤   B. 病人先前的上皮细胞增生
    C. 病人儿子患有男性乳腺发育症   D. 病人的 5 次乳房 X 线照射
    E. 病人的年龄

37. 32 岁的女性直肠出血,进行钡灌肠和结肠镜检查,均显示大量息肉覆盖整个结直

肠。对其中一个息肉活检显示为管状腺病。乙状结肠内的一个 3 厘米大小的肿块活检后显示为侵润性腺癌。下列哪项正确描述了该病的特征。

A. 常染色体隐性遗传

B. 腺癌通常在发生 20 年后才能被发现

C. 这个疾病的基因位点位于 14 号染色体短臂上

D. 这个病人的病症从结肠腺瘤发展到腺癌提供了一个肿瘤发生的模式

E. 在这个疾病中,未发现肠外腺瘤

38. 一个 16 岁的男孩出现鼻塞和反复鼻出血的症状,检查发现在鼻咽处有一个质硬,表面光滑紫红色息肉,对病变处进行诊断性活组织检查导致出血不止,进行输血和紧急手术,最可能的诊断是

　　A. 疣状癌　　　　B. 淋巴上皮瘤　　　C. 血管纤维瘤　　D. 鼻息肉

39. 一个 70 岁的男性患者发生两侧腹股沟疝无其他症状,在进行疝修复的手术中切除了增大的淋巴结,病理学检查显示为一个转移性腺癌。该肿瘤的原发性可通过下列哪项来确定

　　A. 钡灌肠　　　　　　　　　　　　B. 剖腹探查术

　　C. 特异肿瘤标记物的免疫过氧化物酶定位

　　D. 骨盆 CT 检查　　　　　　　　　E. 淋巴结电镜检查

40. 下列哪种病人最有可能会患有听神经瘤

　　A. 一个患有Ⅲ型多发性内分泌腺瘤综合征的 16 岁男孩

　　B. 一个 49 岁妇女,在其腋前线的皮肤出现色素斑

　　C. 一个患有头皮恶性黑素瘤的 28 岁男子

　　D. 一个 46 岁因患有垂体腺瘤进行放疗的妇女

　　E. 一个患有室间隔缺损的 3 个月大的婴儿

41~43　70 岁男性,有 50 年吸烟史伴咳嗽、呼吸困难和发绀,胸经增加,呼吸运动在下降,末端呼气性喘息。体检发现胸部 X 线检查未见肿块。

41. 吸烟引起的肺部疾病发生机制是

　　A. 减少 α_1 抗胰蛋白酶基因的转录

　　B. 肺基底膜形成透明膜　　　　C. 肺泡间隔的破坏

　　D. 产生黏液　　　　　　　　　E. 引起脱屑样间质性肺炎

42. 另外的体征还发现肝肿大致周围性水肿,提示肺心病,下列最有关的因素是

　　A. 肺静脉阻塞性疾病　　　　　B. 肺动脉高压

　　C. 弥漫性肺泡损害　　　　　　D. 支气管肺泡发育不良

　　E. 肺栓塞

43. 胸部听诊的呼气性喘息是由于除下列因素引起除外:

　　A. 肺泡间隔破坏　　　　　　　B. 肺组织弹性丧失

　　C. 慢性支气管炎　　　　　　　D. 炭末沉着症

　　E. 杯状细胞增生

44、45　60 岁女性食管出血,体检发现掌侧红斑,脐静脉曲张(海蛇头)和大量腹水,实

验室检查凝血因子异常,低蛋白血症,10 年前患者曾经输血,血清学检查表现为 HCV+ HBsAg(-),抗 HBsAg(-),抗 HAVIgG(+),抗 HAVIgM(-)

44. 下列哪些表现不是真的

  A. 输血相关的 HAV 感染后遗症最可能解释该病人的目前的临床表现

  B. 低蛋白血症的凝血异常发生于肝硬化患者中

  C. 该患者的门脉高压的临床症状

  D. 肝移植对该患者治疗有用

45. 下列各项机制均与患者腹水形成有关,除了

  A. 窦性血管阻塞与肝硬化有关

  B. 肝后血管阻塞与肝癌有关

  C. 肝前血管阻塞与门静脉血栓形成有关

  D. 窦后血管阻塞与肝硬化有关

  E. 低白蛋白血症

46. 下列各项内分泌功能紊乱都会引起高血压,除了

  A. Cushing 综合征   B. 嗜铬细胞瘤

  C. 肾上腺髓质增生   D. Addism 病

  E. Coon 综合征

47. 肺的同种异体移植物的急性排斥反应包括下列各项病理学特点,除了

  A. 呼吸道细支气管纤维组织形成致管腔闭合

  B. 血管周围淋巴细胞浸润

  C. 间质及肺泡淋巴细胞和中性粒细胞炎症

  D. 淋巴细胞性支气管炎

  E. 出血性坏死和透明膜形成

48. 下列各项均为动脉粥样硬化的特点,除了

  A. 动脉壁脂纹   B. 胆固醇结晶

  C. 出血   D. 动脉中层肉芽肿形成

  E. 淋巴细胞炎症

49. 急性心肌梗死的并发症包括下列各项,除了

  A. 纤维素性心包炎   B. 主动脉动脉瘤形成

  C. 附壁血栓   D. 心律失常

  E. 心源性休克

50. 获得性免疫缺陷综合征(艾滋)患者对下列各项疾病有高度易感性,除了

  A. 巨细胞病毒感染   B. 卡波西肉瘤

  C. 淋巴瘤   D. 肺炎球菌性肺炎

  E. 分枝杆菌感染

51. 55 岁的男性患者,在其阴茎包皮上有一个 1 cm 大小的肿块,诊断的疑难之处在于尖锐湿疣和鳞状细胞癌的鉴别。下列各项临床特点均支持癌的诊断,除了

  A. 病变处灶性溃疡形成   B. 包皮垢

C. 病变处触痛

D. 左侧腹股沟区域有一直径 2 cm 大小的硬质肿物

E. 胸片示多个肺部肿块

52. 下列各项均为由肉芽组织形成进行组织修复的正确叙述,除了

A. 开放性伤口被称为二期愈合

B. 损伤处肉芽肿形成

C. 人体自身可以修复大多数瘘管

D. 当炎症持续存在时,肉芽组织就已经开始形成了

E. 可能会形成瘢痕疙瘩

53. 下列各项关于动脉瘤的叙述都是正确的,除了

A. 梅毒性动脉瘤好发于胸主动脉

B. Berry 动脉瘤好发于小脑动脉

C. 动脉粥样硬化性动脉瘤好发于腹主动脉

D. 梭形动脉瘤是气球样动脉的扩张

E. 曲张的动脉瘤是动脉瘤样动静脉瘘

54. 死于长期高血压所致并发症的患者,其尸检心脏的可能表现包括下列各项,除了

A. 左室向心性肥大　　　　　　　B. 乳头肌肥大

C. 心脏扩大　　　　　　　　　　D. 心内膜纤维性增厚

E. 二尖瓣瓣膜脱垂

55. 下列各项关于糖尿病性肾小球硬化症的叙述都是正确的,除了

A. 糖尿病性肾小球硬化症和尿蛋白丢失有关

B. 糖尿病性肾小球硬化症在形态学上表现为结节性毛细血管硬化

C. 糖尿病性肾小球硬化症与血尿有关

D. 糖尿病性肾小球硬化症与其他部位的血管病变比如视网膜病变有关

E. 早期糖尿病性肾小球硬化症在形态学上表现为弥漫性肾小球基底膜增厚

56. 以肉芽肿性炎为特点的疾病包括下列各项,除了

A. 猫抓病　　　　B. 结核　　　　C. 梅毒　　　　D. 肉瘤样结节

E. 葡萄球菌性脓肿

57. 一名八岁女孩间歇性右下腹痛三个月,前两次急诊排除了急性阑尾炎的可能。这次就诊,在下腹部触及一肿块,鉴别诊断包括下列各项,除了

A. 阑尾周围脓肿　　　　　　　　B. 伯基特淋巴瘤

C. Crohn 病　　　　　　　　　　D. 卵巢生殖细胞瘤

E. 霍奇金淋巴瘤

58. 下列各项均是有关 DNA 流式细胞仪检测的肿瘤细胞核特点的描述,除了哪一项外都是正确的

A. 细胞核是二倍体的肿瘤可以是良性的也可以是恶性的

B. 肿瘤细胞核是异倍体的肿瘤是恶性的

C. 恶性肿瘤的细胞核可以成二倍体

D. 反映细胞核病变的应该是二倍体

59. 肉瘤病人的预后与下列各项有关,除了
　　A. 肿瘤的大小　　　　　　　　　　　B. 肿瘤的分期
　　C. 肿瘤的分级　　　　　　　　　　　D. 肿瘤在组织中的深度
　　E. 肿瘤在诊断以前存在的时间

60. 多种形式放射线与下列各项中的肿瘤相关,除了
　　A. 皮肤鳞癌　　　B. 卵巢癌　　　C. 甲状腺癌　　　D. 肉瘤　　　E. 黑色素瘤

61. 下列各项关于急性心肌梗死的叙述都是正确的,除了
　　A. 大多数心肌梗死是透壁性的
　　B. 心肌梗死常常累及左心室
　　C. 心内膜下心肌梗死常呈环状分布
　　D. 组织学改变首先出现在梗死后 24 小时
　　E. 梗死后 48~72 小时内最敏感的标记物是肌酸激酶的 MB 型同工酶

62. 下列各项关于狼疮性肾炎的叙述都是正确的,除了
　　A. 女性的发病率比男性高　　　　　　B. 形态学表现多种多样
　　C. 常有肾小球免疫复合物沉积　　　　D. 常有针对肾小球基底膜的自身抗体
　　E. 常发生肾脏累及的临床症状

63. 下列各项关于恶性纤维组织细胞瘤的叙述都是正确的,除了
　　A. 它是深部肿瘤　　　　　　　　　　B. 它是最常见的成人肉瘤
　　C. 典型的恶性纤维组织细胞瘤由形态非常奇异的细胞构成
　　D. 它也叫做纤维肉瘤
　　E. 它是腿部最常见的肿瘤

64. 下列各项关于放射线的叙述都是正确的,除了
　　A. 骨髓和淋巴系统是体内对放射线最敏感的组织
　　B. 睾丸生殖细胞瘤可以通过放疗治愈
　　C. 整个人体受到 1000rad 辐射剂量的照射将会杀死所有暴露部位的细胞
　　D. 受到照射后的肉瘤可能在 20 年后才会继续进展
　　E. 软骨和肌肉组织是对放射敏感性的组织

65. 下列各项关于致癌基因的叙述都是正确的,除了
　　A. 致癌因素的影响可以引起量变
　　B. 致癌因素的影响可以引起质变
　　C. 真核细胞包含病毒癌基因和细胞癌基因
　　D. 致癌基因代表病毒 DNA
　　E. 致癌基因编码生长因子受体

66. 下列各项都是小动脉硬化的特点,除了
　　A. 小动脉壁增生性增厚　　　　　　　B. 与高血压有关
　　C. 严重者可有小动脉壁坏死　　　　　D. 与糖尿病有关
　　E. 小动脉壁淀粉样纤维蛋白沉着

67. 下列各项关于单核-吞噬细胞的叙述都是正确的,除了
    A. 它们是固定的细胞,循环中仅有少量
    B. 它们为成纤维细胞、骨髓前体细胞和内皮细胞产生生长因子
    C. 它们产生内源性致热原IL-1
    D. 它们通常表达主要组织相容性复合物Ⅱ类抗原
    E. 它们在抗原呈递中非常重要

68、69 一名40岁妇女来急诊室就诊。该患者有充血性心力衰竭史2年,可闻及严重二尖瓣狭窄所致心脏杂音。其病史提示:该患者10岁时曾染重病,高热,充血性心力衰竭,关节疼痛并伴局部温度升高,严重咽喉疼痛2周后发生运动失调(舞蹈病)

68. 下列各项中关于该患者的叙述哪一项是错误的?
    A. 其咽喉疼痛很可能是由A组β-溶血性链球菌感染引起的
    B. 其二尖瓣瓣膜很可能发生纤维化及变形、融合
    C. 其左房有可能很大
    D. 这种疾病的发病率在几十年前较高
    E. 阿少夫小体是该患者童年所患疾病的典型组织学特点

3年后,该患者由于充血性心力衰竭再次到急诊室就诊。此次发病,该患者有高达40℃的峰形热,并伴有可变性心脏杂音。血培养可见α-溶血性链球菌。心内膜炎诊断确定。该患者的病程包括右侧进行性轻偏瘫。

69. 下列各项中关于该患者临床表现的叙述哪一项是错误的?
    A. 感染性心内膜炎作为慢性风湿性心脏病的并发症已被公认
    B. 在心脏瓣膜有缺损的患者中,α-溶血性链球菌感染是一种不常见的引起心内膜炎的原因
    C. 该患者右侧轻偏瘫很可能是由来自感染的二尖瓣上的栓子脱落引起的
    D. 心脏瓣膜的赘生物中含纤维蛋白,中性粒细胞和革兰阳性球菌
    E. 感染性赘生物常位于二尖瓣

70. 软组织病变在大体和镜下观察都有很重要的特点,下列各项关于这种病变的叙述都是正确的,除了
    A. 周围组织浸润不一定提示为肉瘤
    B. 在肉瘤中,通过肉眼观察可能发现包裹现象的存在
    C. 良性肿瘤的典型表现为坏死
    D. 在肉瘤中,肿瘤的大小是一个重要的预后因素
    E. 肉瘤的预后很差

71. 下列各项关于肾细胞癌的叙述都是正确的,除了
    A. 患者会出现血尿   B. 肺和脑是常见的转移部位
    C. 转移主要通过血行播散   D. 发病高峰在60岁左右
    E. 男性患者与女性患者之比为1:2

72. 一般T细胞的功能包括下列各项,除了
    A. 直接细胞溶解作用   B. 增强B细胞活性

C. 抑制 T 细胞活性　　　　　　D. 抗原呈递

E. 产生淋巴因子

每组题目是由多个备选答案和多个问题组成。对于每个问题,从备选答案中选出一个最合适、最正确的答案。每个备选答案可选一次、几次,或一次也不选。

73~77　选出与每种疾病相对应的维生素缺乏或过量

A. 维生素 A　　　B. 维生素 B_{12}　　　C. 维生素 C　　　D. 维生素 D　　　E. 烟酸

73. 脊髓亚急性联合变性

74. 佝偻病

75. 坏血病

76. 干眼病

77. 巨幼细胞贫血

78~82　对于下面所列出的肿瘤,选出最可能的原因

A. 食物中的脂肪　　B. 氯乙烯　　　C. 石棉　　　D. 吸烟

E. 环己烷氨基磺酸盐

78. 肝血管肉瘤

79. 膀胱移行细胞癌

80. 结肠癌

81. 间皮瘤

82. 肺癌

83~87　把不同的免疫功能和具有这种功能的特殊类型的细胞相配对

A. 巨噬细胞　　　B. T 淋巴细胞　　　C. B 淋巴细胞

D. 杀伤细胞　　　E. 自然杀伤细胞

83. 抗体依赖性细胞毒作用

84. 抗原呈递

85. 肿瘤细胞自发性破坏

86. 产生免疫球蛋白

87. 产生淋巴因子

88~92　对于下列各种肉瘤,选出其组织来源

A. 内皮细胞　　　B. 脂肪组织　　　C. 结缔组织　　D. 骨骼肌　　　E. 施万细胞

88. 横纹肌肉瘤

89. 神经纤维肉瘤

90. 血管肉瘤

91. 脂肪肉瘤

92. 纤维肉瘤

93~97　把各种超微结构与最可能的肿瘤相配对

A. 类癌　　　B. 横纹肌肉瘤　　　C. 黑素瘤　　　D. 腺癌

E. 鳞形上皮细胞癌(SCC)

93. 伸长的颗粒

94. 致密核心的神经内分泌软粒

95. 微绒毛

96. 张力细丝

97. Z 带

98~102 对于下列各种临床或病理学特点,选出最与之相关的白血病类型

 A. 慢性髓细胞性白血病(CML) B. 急性髓细胞性白血病(AML)

 C. 急性早幼粒细胞性白血病 D. 红白血病

 E. 慢性淋巴细胞性白血病(CLL)

98. 出血素质

99. 费城染色体

100. 淋巴细胞增多

101. 牙龈增生

102. 成熟 B 细胞来源

103~107 把下列各项对皮肤损害的描述与相应的皮损名称配对

 A. 斑疹 B. 丘疹 C. 结节 D. 风团 E. 水疱

103. 局限性的,与周围皮肤平齐但颜色不同的损害

104. 可触及的,质硬的,圆形或类圆形损害,深达真皮或皮下组织

105. 局限、质硬、隆起的皮肤损害

106. 小圆形皮肤隆起内含浆液

107. 真皮上层局部水肿引起的短暂的皮肤局限性隆起

108~112 下面列出的各种肿瘤,选出与之相关的病因学原因

 A. 外部辐射 B. 紫外线 C. 人乳头状瘤病毒(HPV)

 D. EB 病毒(EBV) E. 雌激素

108. 甲状腺乳头状癌

109. 宫颈鳞癌

110. 伯基特淋巴瘤

111. 乳腺癌

112. 恶性黑色素瘤

Pathological Discussion and Tests

Directions : **Each of the numbered items or incomplete statements in this section is followed by answers or by completions of the statement. Select the one lettered answer or completion that is best in each case.**

1. A 58-year-old man is hospitalized for evaluation of recent intermittent upper abdominal pain. History and physical examination reveal a 25-lb weight loss over recent months and upper abdominal tenderness without evidence of a mass, ascites, or jaundice. The best diagnostic approach and most likely preliminary diagnosis would be

   A. abdominal ultrasonography for the diagnosis of chronic hepatitis

   B. serum bilirubin measurement for the diagnosis of chronic cholecystitis with cholelithiasis

   C. endoscopy for the diagnosis of carcinoma of the ampulla of Vater

   D. laparotomy for the diagnosis of carcinoma of the head of the pancreas

   E. computed tomography (CT) for the diagnosis of carcinoma of the body of the pancreas

2. A renal allograft recipient develops bloody diarrhea. A colonic biopsy shows focal necrosis and hemorrhage. Individual endothelial cells are large with prominent nuclear inclusions. The expected copathogen is

   A. Epstein-Barr virus (EBV)   B. Candida

   C. Pneumocystis   D. toxoplasmosis

   E. Giardia

3. A 30-year-old woman presents with a gradual onset of hoarseness exacerbated by a recent upper respiratory tract infection. Direct laryngoscopy reveals small papillary excrescences of the true vocal cords. Of the following, the most likely etiology is

   A. autoimmune   B. bacterial   C. viral   D. fungal

4. What is the most common benign mesenchymal tumor of the stomach?

   A. Polypoid adenoma   B. benign stromal tumor

   C. Glomus tumor   D. Lipoma   E. Leiomyoma

5. A 60-year-old man with a long history of stable angina complains of a progressive increase in the frequency and severity of his chest pain. About 12 hours after one particularly severe episode of chest pain, he is brought to the emergency room where he is found to be hypotensive and in severe congestive heart failure. An electrocardiogram (ECG) demonstrates significant Q waves as well as ST-segment and T-wave changes. Serum cardiac enzymes demonstrate a markedly elevated MB isoenzyme of creatine kinase (CK). Appropriate medical intervention fails to control the patient's hypotension and cardiac failure. Cardiac arrest ensues, and attempts at resuscitation fail. An autopsy is performed.Which one of the following statements about this patient's condition is true?

    A. A subendocardial myocardial infarct is likely to be found at autopsy

    B. A coronary artery thrombus is unlikely to be found at autopsy

    C. The clinical presentation is classic for constrictive pericarditis

    D. An area of myocardial infarction less than 2cm in diameter is likely to be found at autopsy

    E. Severe narrowing of at least one coronary artery is an expected finding at autopsy

6. Barrett's epithelium is found in what part of the gastrointestinal tract?

    A. Esophagus   B. Stomach

    C. Small intestine   D. Large intestine

    E. Rectum

7. A 1-year-old child develops swelling of the left side of the face following a 1-week episode of diarrhea. Examination of the infant reveals a warm fluctuant mass just lateral and inferior to the ear. What would most likely be revealed by fine-needle aspiration ?

    A. Pus   B. Cells with epithelial lesions

    C. Granulomas   D. Malignant cells

8. A 50-year-old male ,before presenting to the emergency room with a chronic cough and night sweats, he is admitted and a chest X-ray shows apical infiltrates. Sputum analysis is unrevealing, but a transbronchial biopsy reveals granulomas with giant cells. The diagnosis is

    A. sarcoidosis   B. berylliosis

    C. tuberculosis   D. giant cell carcinoma

    E. pneumococcal pneumonia

9. Which feature characterizes acute nonspecific appendicitis?

    A. It primarily affects the elderly but can occur at any age

    B. Enterobius vermicularis infestation of the appendix is an important predisposing condition

    C. Luminal obstruction by fecaliths is found in two-thirds of cases

    D. Transmural Chronic inflammation is a characteristic consequence

    E. Leukopenia is present

10. A 12-year-old boy complains of leg pain and swelling, and an X-ray of the affected limb shows the classic sign of Codman's triangle. What is the most likely diagnosis?

    A. Chondrosarcoma   B. Osteomyelitis

    C. Osteosarcoma   D. Multiple myeloma

    E. Aneurysmal bone cyst

Questions 11～12

A 40-year-old woman comes to her physician after noticing a lump in her breast. Physical examination reveals a 3-cm, firm, irregular mass in the lateral aspect of the right breast with dimpling of the overlying skin. A subsequent biopsy of this mass reveals chronic inflammation, necrotic adipose tissue with saponification, and areas of calcification.

    11. These histologic findings are consistent with the diagnosis of

        A. comedocarcinoma   B. fat necrosis

        C. duct ectasia   D. granulomatous mastitis

        E. adenosis

12. What is the most likely history associated with this lesion?

    A. Nulliparity   B. Estrogen therapy

    C. Breast-feeding   D Previous trauma

    E. Pulmonary tuberculosis

13. Which autoimmune disease is characterized by immune complex deposition in the skin, kidney, and lung?

    A. Systemic lupus erythematosus (SLE)

    B. Sjögren's syndrome

    C. Progressive scleroderma

    D. Graft versus host (GVH) disease

    E. CREST (i.e., calcinosis, Raynaud's phenomenon, esophageal dysfunction, syndactyly, and telangiectasia) syndrome

14. A 50-year-old woman presents with a pigmented skin lesion of her arm. She states that she has had this "mole" all of her life, but it has been bothering her lately. Examination reveals a 0.5cm pigmented nodule with an irregular border on one edge, a small area of crusting, and surrounding erythema. The differential diagnosis is nevus versus malignant melanoma. Which histologic feature is the most useful in distinguishing between these two entities?

    A. Nests of melanocytes in the lower one-third of the dermis

    B. Epidermal hyperkeratosis

    C. Numerous mitoses

    D. Multinucleate giant cells

    E. Hair shafts surrounded by nevus cells

15. A 38-year-old man is injured in a head-on automobile collision. When he is brought to the emergency room, he is in shock, unconscious, and requires mechanical respiratory assistance. Despite efforts to save the patient, he dies. Neuro-pathologic examination on autopsy is most likely to disclose

    A. ruptured basilar artery aneurysm   B. Duret's hemorrhages

    C. severed medulla oblongata   D. cerebral infarct

    E. arteriovenous (AV) malformation

16. A renal allograft recipient presents with fever and adenopathy 3 months after engraftment. Serum studies show markedly elevated anti-Epstein-Barr virus (EBV) titers. A biopsy of the allograft is most likely to show

    A. fibrinoid necrosis of the small vessels

    B. vascular sclerosis   C. interstitial fibrosis

    D. a dense lymphoplasmacytic interstitial infiltrate with cytologic atypia

    E. isometric vacuolar change in the tubular epithelial cells

17. A 62-year-old man presents with a several year history of heartburn. Upper endoscopy reveals red, velvety, fingerlike projections beginning in the region of the gastroesophageal junction and extending 5cm into the esophagus. A biopsy reveals intestinal-type columnar epithelium. Which statement about this patient's disorder is true?

    A. This disorder complicates reflux esophagitis in about 10% of patients

    B. Squamous cell carcinoma (SCC) is the most important neoplastic complication of this disorder

C. The morphologic features are typical of Candida esophagitis

D. Ganglion cells within the myenteric plexus are absent

E. Tracheoesophageal fistula (TEF) is a common complication

Questions 18~19　A 28-year-old man presents with a Single descended testis and a 6-cm solid abdominal mass seen by computed tomography (CT).

18. The most likely diagnosis of the mass is

A. metastatic prostate cancer　　　B. hyperplastic cryptorchid testis

C. teratoma　　　D. adenomatoid tumor

E. seminoma

19. Which one of the following statements is true regarding the treatment and prognosis of this tumor?

A. Resection is not indicated　　　B. The tumor is radiation sensitive

C. There is a poor 5-year survival rate

D. The patient can be followed clinically by measurement of serum levels of prostate-specific antigen

E. There is no increased risk of malignancy in the descended testi

20. A 16-month-old boy presents with a right-sided abdominal mass, which X-ray reveals to be a partially calcified tumor occupying most of the right abdomen. Microscopic examination of tumor tissue shows cells in rosette patterns. What is the most likely diagnosis?

A. Wilms' tumor　　　B. Hepatoblastoma

C. Pancreatoblastoma　　　D. Neuroblastoma

E. Pancreatic islet cell tumor

21. A patient complains of nausea, vomiting, and decreased urinary output. Blood pressure is 180/110mmHg. Urinalysis shows hematuria and white blood cells (WBCs), but no bacteria. Cultures are negative. Serum creatinine is 3.0 mg/dl. Which pathologic finding can be expected from this patient's kidney?

A. Nodular glomerulosclerosis　　　B. Cellular crescent formation

C. Basement membrane "spikes"　　　D. Positive tissue staining for Congo Red

E. Diffuse podocyte effacement

22. Cytologic examination of a pleural effusion in a 60-year-old man reveals the presence of malignant cells. The most likely primary cancer to be found in this man is

A. lymphoma　　　B. mesothelioma

C. carcinoma of the colon　　　D. carcinoma of the lung

E. carcinoma of the pancreas

23. Which statement accurately describes the etiologic agents of viral hepatitis?

A. Hepatitis B virus (HBV) is the most common cause of post-transfusion hepatitis

B. Hepatitis D virus (HDV; delta agent) requires help from HBV in order to infect humans

C. Hepatitis C virus (HCV) is the most common cause of sporadic cases of hepatitis

D. The genome of HBV is predominantly double-stranded RNA

E. Chronic hepatitis A develops in 10%~20% of patients acutely infected with the virus

24. Which statement about Kaposi's sarcoma is true?

A. The classic form is common in women

B. Noncutaneous manifestations are common in patients with acquired immune deficiency syndrome (AIDS)

C. The histology of the different clinical forms varies

D. Stopping immunosuppressive therapy has no effect on Kaposi's sarcoma in renal transplant cases

E. The AIDS virus has been shown to cause Kaposi's sarcoma

25. A child presents with nephrotic syndrome after a viral illness. Which pathology can be expected.

A. Diffuse effacement of the visceral epithelial podocytes

B. About 50% crescent formation

C. Nodular glomerulosclerosis

D. Basement membrane spikes

E. Linear deposition of IgG on the glomerular basement membrane (GBM)

26. A 60-year-old woman with a history of breast carcinoma that had been treated with surgical excision, radiation, and chemotherapy 2 years ago is undergoing routine follow-up. Although she is asymptomatic, her hemoglobin concentration is 8.7 g/dl and hematocrit is 27%. The most likely explanation is

A. iron deficiency anemia   B. chemotherapy-induced marrow injury

C. acute leukemia   D. metastatic breast cancer

E. inadequate data are given for a conclusion

27. The most important prognostic factor for human cancer is

A. tumor grade   B. tumor stage

C. lymphocytic infiltration   D. vascular invasion

E. mitotic index

28. A gastric carcinoma that metastasizes to the ovary is most likely to be referred to as a

A. Brenner tumor   B. Wilms' tumor

C. Klatskin's tumor   D. Krukenberg's tumor

E. Grawitz's tumor

29. A 57-yeah-old man develops swelling and tenderness in his left calf 7 days after undergoing colectomy for colon cancer. He develops acute shortness of breath. A chest X-ray is normal. Which one of the following pathologic descriptions is most likely?

A. Myocardial hypertrophy and chamber dilatation

B. Myocardial infarction

C. Lymphocytic interstitial pneumonitis

D. Recent pulmonary embolus

30. A 45-year-old woman complains that for 6 months she has experienced increasingly severe headaches associated with right arm weakness and an unsteady gait. Evaluation and subsequent surgery disclose a lesion in the left occipital area, which pathologic examination shows to be a meningioma. The maior prognostic determinant in this case is

A. the histologic subtype of the meningioma

B. the mitotic index of the tumor

C. the completeness of surgical removal

       D. tumor vascularity

       E. the patient's amenability to radiation therapy

31. Which one of the following primary hepatic tumors is the most common?

       A. Hepatocellular carcinoma   B. Angiosarcoma

       C. Cholangiocarcinoma   D. Cavernous hemangioma

       E. Focal nodular hyperplasia

32. A 35-year-old man has been treated for acute bronchopneumonia and appears to be getting better on antibiotics. However, the physician notices a medical student's note in the chart stating that the patient works in a ceramic factory, The next step is to

       A. ask if the factory is old and has asbestos in it

       B. ask if the patient has been taking steroid hormones

       C. reorder a chest X-ray to look for cavitation

       D. perform a skin test for beryllium

       E. ask the patient if he has ever been a coal miner

33. A renal allograft recipient fails to produce urine in the first 48 hours after engraftment. Imaging studies reveal that the allograft is normal size. The graft is well matched.A biopsy is performed and shows needle-shaped crystals within vascular lumens. What is the most likely diagnosis?

       A. Hyperacute rejection   B. "Harvest injury"

       C. Preexisting atheroembolic disease   D. Acute cellular rejection

       E. Acute vascular rejection

Questions 34~35

A 35-year-old multiparous woman in the first trimester of a new pregnancy experiences an abnormally rapid increase in uterine size and has an abnormally high serum human chorionic gonadotropin (hCG) level.

34. This clinical history is most compatible with which of the following disorders?

       A. Ectopic pregnancy   B. Placenta accreta

       C. Leiomyomas   D. Hydatidiform mole

       E. Chorioangioma

35. Which of the following disorders is a well-known complication of this disease process?

       A. Rupture of the fallopian tube   B. Leiomyosarcoma

       C. Pseudomyxoma peritonei   D. Endometrial polyps

       E. Choriocarcinoma

36. A 37-year-old woman comes to a surgeon for a breast biopsy because of a suspicious mammogram. She has had mammograms annually for 5 years. A breast biopsy 3 years ago showed a fibroadenoma and fibrocystic changes, with florid epithelial hyperplasia. When questioned about her relevant family history, she stated that her mother had died of a malignant cystosarcoma phylloides tumor, and that her son had gynecomastia, which was discovered during a physical examination for school sports. Her current breast biopsy reveals lobular carcinoma in situ. Which factor most in-creases her risk of breast cancer?

       A. Her previous fibroadenoma   B. Her previous epithelial hyperplasia

       C. Her son's gynecomastia   D. Her five mammogram exposures

E. Her age

37. A 32-year-old woman presents with rectal bleeding, workup includes a barium enema followed by colonoscopy, both procedures demonstrate numerous polyps carpeting the entire colorectum. Biopsy of one of these reveals a tubular adenoma. A 3cm mass located in the sigmoid colon is also biopsied, revealing invasive adenocarcinoma. Which statement correctly characterizes this patient's disorder?

A. It is inherited as an autosomal recessive trait

B. Adenocarcinoma is usually detected by the second decade

C. The genetic locus for this disease has been mapped to the short arm of chromosome 14(14p)

D. This patient's disorder serves as a model for the adenoma to carcinoma sequence of colorectal carcinoma

E. Extracolonic adenomas are not found in this disorder

38. A 16-year-old boy presents with symptoms of nasal obstruction and recurrent epistaxis. Examination reveals a firm, smooth, red-purple polyp in the nasopharynx. An attempted biopsy of the lesion results in uncontrolled bleeding requiring transfusion and emergency surgery, The most likely diagnosis is

A. verrucous carcinoma   B. lymphoepithelioma

C. angiofibroma   D. nasal polyp

39. A 70-year-old asymptomatic man is found to have bilateral inguinal hernias. At operation for hernia repair, an enlarged lymph node is removed. Pathologic evaluation discloses a metastatic adenocarcinoma. The primary site of such a tumor can best be determined by

A. barium enema   B. exploratory laparotomy

C. immunoperoxidase (IP) localization of specific tumor markers

D. computed tomography (CT) of the pelvis

E. electron microscopic (EM) examination of the node

40. Acoustic neuroma is most likely to be found in which of the following patients?

A. A 16-year-old boy with type III multiple endocrine neoplasia (MEN)

B. A 49-year-old woman with pigmented macules of the axillary skin

C. A 28-year-old man with malignant melanoma of the scalp

D. A 46-year-old woman who received radiation for pituitary adenoma

E. A 3-month-old boy with ventricular septal defect

Questions 41~43　A 70-year-old man with a 50-year history of cigarette smoking presents with a productive cough, dyspnea, and cyanosis. An increased chest diameter, decreased respiratory excursion, and endexpiratory wheezes are found during physical examination. No masses are seen on chest radiograph.

41. Cigarette smoke contributes to the pathogenesis of this pulmonary disorder by

A. reducing α_1-antitrypsin gene transcription

B. causing pulmonary basement membrane hyalinization

C. inducing destruction of interalveolar septa

D. reducing mucus production

E. causing desquamative interstitial pneumonitis

42. Additional physical findings of hepatomegaly and peripheral edema suggest cor pulmo-

nale. An expected related finding would be

A. pulmonary veno-occlusive disease   B. pulmonary arterial hypertension

C. diffuse alveolar damage   D. bronchopulmonary dysplasia

E. pulmonary embolism

43. The expiratory wheezes heard on the chest auscultation may be contributed to by all of the following EXCEPT

A. interalveolar septal destruction   B. loss of lung tissue elasticity

C. chronic bronchiolitis   D. anthracosis

E. goblet cell hyperplasia

Questions 44 ~ 45   A 60-year-old woman presents with bleeding esophageal varices. Physical examination reveals palmar erythema, caput medusae, and massive ascites. Laboratory data reveals clotting abnormalities and hypoalbuminemia. The patient had a blood transfusion 10 years ago. Serologic studies reveal the following: anti-hepatitis C virus (anti-HCV), positive; anti-hepatitis B surface. antigen (anti-HBsAg) negative; HBsAg, negative; anti-hepatitis A virus (anti-HAV) immunoglobulin G (IgG), positive; anti-HAV IgM, negative.

44. Which one of the following statements is NOT true?

A. Sequelae from blood transfusion-related hepatitis A virus (HAV) infection is most likely responsible for this patient's clinical presentation

B. Hypoalbuminemia and clotting abnormalities are common findings in patients with cirrhosis

C. This patient has clinical evidence of portal hypertension

D. Liver transplantation is a treatment option for this patient

45. All of the following mechanisms would be likely to he causally related to the patient's ascites EXCEPT

A. sinusoidal vascular blockade related to underlying cirrhosis

B. posthepatic vascular blockade related to hepatocellular carcinoma

C. prehepatic vascular blockade related to portal venous thrombosis

D. postsinusoidal vascular blockade related to underlying cirrhosis

E. hypoalbuminemia

46. Hypertension is found in all of the following endocrine disorders EXCEPT

A. Cushing's syndrome   B. pheochromocytoma

C. adrenal medullary hyperplasia   D. Addison's disease

E. Conn's syndrome

47. Acute rejection in lung allografts includes all of the following pathologic features EXCEPT

A. fibrosing obliteration of respiratory bronchioles

B. perivascubr lymphocytic infiltrate

C. interstitial and alveolar lymphocytic and neutrophilic inflammation

D. lymphocytic bronchitis

E. hemorrhagic necrosis and hyaline membrane formation

48. All of the following features are characteristic of atherosclerosis EXCEPT

A. fatty streaks   B. cholesterol clefts

C. hemorrhage   D. medial granulomas

E. lymphocytic inflammation

49. Complications of acute myocardial infarction include all of the following EXCEPT
    A. fibrinous pericarditis   B. aortic aneurysms
    C. mural thrombi   D. cardiac arrhythmia
    E. cardiogenic shock

50. Acquired immune deficiency syndrome (AIDS) patients have an increased susceptibility
    to all of the following diseases EXCEPT
    A. cytomegalovirus (CMV) infection   B. Kaposi's sarcoma
    C. lymphoma   D. pneumococcal pneumonia
    E. mycobacterial infection

51. A 55-year-old man presents with a 1cm exophytic mass on the prepuce of his penis. The
    differential diagnosis is condyloma acuminatum versus squamous cell carcinoma. Each of
    the following clinical features favors the diagnosis of carcinoma EXCEPT
    A. focal ulceration of the lesion
    B. the presence of smegma
    C. elicitation of pain with palpation of the lesion
    D. a firm 2cm mass in the left inguinal region
    E. multiple lung masses on a chest radiograph

52. True statements concerning tissue repair by granulation tissue formation include all of the
    following EXCEPT
    A. a wound left open is called secondary healing
    B. granulomas can develop at the site
    C. the body can repair most fistula tracts
    D. granulation tissue formation begins white inflammation is ongoing
    E. a keloid may form

53. All of the following statements about aneurysms are true EXCEPT
    A. syphihtic aneurysms usually occur in the thoracic aorta
    B. berry aneurysms are common in small cerebral arteries
    C. atherosclerotic aneurysms often occur in the abdominal aorta
    D. fusiform aneurysms are balloon-shaped arterial dilatations
    E. cirsoid aneurysms are aneurysmic arteriovenous fistulas

54. Possible autopsy findings in the heart of a patient who died from complications of long-
    standing hypertension include all of the following EXCEPT
    A. concentric left ventricular hypertrophy
    B. papillary muscle hypertrophy
    C. cardiomegaly   D. endocardial fibrous thickening
    E. floppy mitral valve

55. All of the following statements about diabetic glomerulosclerosis are true EXCEPT
    A. diabetic glomerulosclerosis is consistently associated with urinary protein loss
    B. diabetic glomerulosclerosis is morphologically characterized by nodular intercapillary
       sclerosis
    C. diabetic glomerulosclerosis is associated with hematuria
    D. diabetic glomerulosclerosis is usually associated with vasculopathy at other sites such

as the retina

E. early diabetic glomerulosclerosis is morphologically characterized by diffuse glomerular basement membrane (GBM) thickening

56. Disorders characterized by granulomatous inflammation include all of the following EXCEPT

   A. cat-scratch disease   B. tuberculosis
   C. syphilis   D. sarcoidosis
   E. staphylococcal abscess

57. An 8-year-old girl has a 3-month history of intermittent right lower quadrant pain. Two previous visits to the emergency room have ruled out acute appendicitis. At this visit, a mass is palpated in the lower abdomen. The differential diagnosis includes all of the following conditions EXCEPT

   A. periappendiceal abscess   B. Burkitt's lymphoma
   C. Crohn's disease (CD)   D. ovarian germ cell tumor
   E. Hodgkin's lymphoma

58. All of the following statements concerning the nuclear characteristic of tumors, as determined by DNA flow cytometry, are true EXCEPT

   A. a diploid lesion can be benign or malignant
   B. an aneuploid tumor is a malignant tumor
   C. a malignant tumor can be diploid
   D. reactive lesions should be diploid

59. The prognosis for a patient with sarcoma is related to all of the following EXCEPT

   A. size   B. stage   C. grade   D. depth in the tissues
   E. tumor duration before diagnosis

60. Radiation, in one form or another, is linked to all of the following cancers EXCEPT

   A. squamous cancers of skin   B. ovarian cancer
   C. thyroid cancer   D. sarcoma
   E. melanoma

61. All of the following statements regarding acute myocardial infarction are true EXCEPT

   A. most myocardial infarctions are transmural
   B. myocardial infarctions usually involve the left ventricle
   C. subendocardial infarctions usually are circumferential
   D. histologic evidence is seen first at about 24 hours postinfarction
   E. the most sensitive marker within 48 to 72 hours postinfarction is an elevation of the MB isoenzyme of creatine kinase (CK)

62. All of the following statements about lupus nephritis are true EXCEPT

   A. it occurs more frequently in women than in men
   B. variable morphology is the rule
   C. glomerular immune complex deposition is common
   D. autoantibodies to glomerular basement membrane (GBM) are common
   E. clinical evidence for renal involvement often develops

63. All of the following statements about malignant fibrous histiocytoma (MFH) are true EXCEPT

A. it is a deep tumor　　　　　　　　B. it is the most common adult sarcoma

C. it typically is made up of very bizarre cells

D. it is also called fibrosarcoma

E. it is the most common tumor of the thigh

64. All of the following statements concerning radiation are true EXCEPT

A. the marrow and lymphoid system are the most radiosensitive tissues of the body

B. a testicular germ cell tumor may be cured by radiotherapy

C. a dose of 1000 rad of total body radiation would kill all members of an exposed population

D. postradiation sarcomas may develop after a 20-year interval

E. cartilage and muscle tissue are relatively radiosensitive

65. All of the following statements about oncogenes are thought to be true EXCEPT

A. quantitative change can be brought about by carcinogenic influence

B. qualitative change can be brought about by carcinogenic influence

C. eukaryotic cells contain v-oncs and c-ones

D. oncogenes represent viral DNA

E. oncogenes appear to code for growth factor receptors

66. All of the following are characteristic of arteriolosclerosis EXCEPT

A. proliferative thickening of the arteriole wall

B. association with clinical hypertension

C. necrosis of the arteriole wall in severe cases

D. association with diabetes

E. deposition of amyloid fibrils in the arteriole wall

67. All of the following statements regarding mononuclear phagocytes are true EXCEPT

A. they generally are fixed cells with little proponsity for circulation

B. they produce growth factors for fibroblasts, myeloid precursors, and endothelial cells

C. they produce interleukin-1 (IL-l), which acts as an endogenous pyrogen

D. they normally express major histocompatibility complex (MHC) class II antigens

E. they are important in antigen presentation

Questions 68~69. A 40-year-old woman comes to the emergency room. She has a 2-year history of congestive heart failure. A murmur characteristic of severe mitral stenosis is heard. Her medical history reveals that at 10 years of age, she developed a severe illness characterized by fever; congestive heart failure; painful, warm joints; and a movement disorder (chorea) 2 weeks after the onset of a severe sore throat.

68. Which one of the following statements about this patient's condition is FALSE?

A. Her sore throat most likely was caused by infection with group A β-hemolytic streptococci

B. Her mitral valve is likely to be quite fibrotic and deformed, with fused commissures

C. Her left atrium is likely to be quite large

D. The incidence of this patient's disorder has increased dramatically before the last several decades

E. The Aschoff body is the classic histologic feature of her childhood illness.

Three years later, the patient returns to the emergency room in congestive heart failure. At this time, she is found to have a spiking fever to 40℃ and a changing cardiac murmur. Blood cultures grow α-hemolytic (viridans) streptococci. A diagnosis of endocarditis is made. The patient's clinical course includes the development of a right hemiparesis.

69. Which one of the following statements regarding the patient's clinical course is FALSE?

   A. Infective endocarditis is a well recognized complication of chronic rheumatic heart disease

   B. Infection with α-hemolytic (viridans) streptococci is an uncommon cause of endocarditis in patients with damaged heart valves

   C. The patient's right hemiparesis most likely resulted from embeli arising from an infected mitral valve

   D. The valvular vegetations contain fibrin, neutrophils, and gram-positive cocci

   E. The mitral valve is a likely site for the infected vegetations

70. Soft tissue lesions have important features that can be seen grossly or microscopically. All of the following statements about these lesions are true EXCEPT

   A. infiltration of surrounding structures does not necessarily imply sarcoma

   B. encapsulation may be seen in a sarcoma on gross examination

   C. a benign tumor typically shows necrosis

   D. size is an important prognostic feature in a sarcoma

   E. Sarcomas have a very poor prognosis

71. All of the following statements about renal cell carcinoma are true EXCEPT

   A. patients may present with hematuria

   B. lungs and brain are common sites for metastasis

   C. metastatic spread is principally via the blood stream

   D. peak incidence is in the sixth decade of life

   E. the ratio of men to women with renal cell carcinoma is 1 ·2

72. Usual T-cell functions include all of the following EXCEPT

   A. direct cytolysis   B. promotion of B-cell activities

   C. suppression of T-cell activities   D. antigen presentation

   E. lymphokine production

Questions 73~77. Match each disorder with the associated vitamin lack or excess.

   A. Vitamin A   B. Vitamin B_{12} C. Vitamin C   D. Vitamin D   E. Niacin

73. Subacute combined degeneration of the spinal cord

74. Rickets

75. Scurvy

76. Xerophthalmia

77. Megaloblastic anemia

Questions 78~82. For each tumor listed below, select the purported causative agent.

   A. Dietary fat   B. Vinyl chloride   C. Asbestos   D. Cigarette smoking

   E. Cyclamates

78. Angiosarcoma of the liver

79. Transitional cell carcinoma of the bladder

80. Carcinoma of the colon

81. Mesothelioma

82. Carcinoma of the lung

Questions 83 ~ 87. Match each immune cell function to the specific type of cell that performs it.

    A. Macrophage   B. T lympocyte

    C. B lymphocyte   D. Killer（K）cell

    E. Natural killer（NK）cell

83. Antibody-dependent cytotoxicity

84. Antigen presentation

85. Spontaneous destruction of tumor cells

86. Production of immunoglobulins

87. Production of lymphokines

Questions 88 ~ 92. For each type of sarcoma that follows, select the tissue that it recapitulates.

    A. Endothelium   B. Adipose tissue   C. Connective tissue

    D. Skeletal muscle   E. Schwann cell

88. Rhabdomyosarcoma

89. Neurofibrosarcoma

90. Angiosarcoma

91. Liposarcoma

92. Fibrosarcoma

Questions 93 ~ 97. Match each ultrastructural finding with the tumor type that is most likely to demonstrate it.

    A. Carcinoid tumor   B. Rhabdomyosarcoma

    C. Melanoma   D. Adenocarcinoma

    E. Squamous cell cancer（SCC）

93. Elongated granules

94. Dense core neurosecretory granules

95. Microvilli

96. Tonofilaments

97. Z-bands

Questions 98 ~ 102. For each clinical or pathologic characteristic, select the most closely associated type of leukemia.

    A. Chronic myelogenous leukemia（CML）

    B. Acute myelogenous leukemia（AML）

    C. Acute promyelocytic leukemia

    D. Erythroleukemia

    E. Chronic lymphocytic leukemia（CLL）

98. Bleeding diathesis

99. Philadelphia chromosome

100. Absolute lymphocytosis

101. Thickened gums

102. Mature B-cell origin

Questions 103 ~ 107. Match each description of a skin lesion with the name of the lesion.

A. Macule   B. Papule   C. Nodule   D. Wheal   E. Vesicle

103. A circumscribed, flat area of skin distinguished by color from the surrounding skin

104. A palpable, solid, round or ellipsoid lesion situated deep in the skin or in the subcutaneous tissue

105. A well-circumscribed solid elevation of the skin

106. A small, circumscribed elevation of the skin containing serum or other fluid

107. A short-lived, circumscribed area of elevated skin produced by focal edema of the upper dermis

Questions 108 ~ 112. For each tumor listed below, select the etiologically, related agent.

A. External irradiation   B. Ultraviolet light

C. Human papilloma virus (HPV)   D. Epstein-Barr virus (EBV)

E. Estrogen

108. Papillary carcinoma of the thyroid

109. Squamous cell carcinoma (SCC) of   the cervix

110. Burkitt's lymphoma

111. Breast carcinoma

112. Malignant melanoma

答案与解释

一、选择题答案

1. 答案 E　这个病人有腹痛和体重减轻史,这些提示胰腺癌的存在。CT 是可以获得最多诊断信息,而对病人伤害最小的技术,CT 能准确的发现小块的病变,慢性胆囊炎不会出现新近才发作的症状以及明显的消瘦。壶腹部癌及胰头癌最可能引起临床上显著的黄疸,而病人并没有出现黄疸。

2. 答案 B　结肠活检示巨细胞病毒性结肠炎出血、坏死与巨细胞性病变有关伴核与胞浆包涵体,这些是巨细胞病毒性结肠炎的特征。霉菌的反复感染,尤其是念珠菌,在CMV感染的免疫病人中很常见。

3. 答案 C　关于这个病变的描述与良性乳头状瘤病或其他肿瘤的过程都相符。因为肿瘤未出现在选项中,那么最合适的回答就是一个病毒病因学方面的原因,反映了乳头状瘤与人乳头瘤病毒感染之间的联系。细菌与霉菌感染很少形成散在的乳头状小结,而且这些病变与自身免疫无关。

4. 答案 B　胃肠间质细胞肿瘤是一种最常见的良性胃间叶性瘤。这些肿瘤的大小从 1cm 到 20cm 不等;大于 3cm 的肿瘤常引起疼痛或出血。大于 6cm 时需要排除恶性肿瘤的可能(这种肿瘤通常是在壁内的);有一些肿瘤通过一个细的蒂连接到固有肌层上,这样伸入到网膜中。镜下:肿瘤细胞由梭形细胞和上皮样间叶细胞组成。对这些肿瘤的组织发生现象现在还有争议,但是大多数人倾向于认为有平滑肌的分化的证据。腺瘤是上皮性的,不是间叶性的;血管球瘤,脂肪瘤以及平滑肌瘤很少发生于胃。

5. 答案 E　病人的临床表现为典型的大面积透壁性心肌梗死(累及 40% 以上的左心室心肌),引起心源性休克,透壁性的心肌梗死与冠状动脉血栓形成相关,而后者可能是由粥样斑块的破裂所引起。

6. 答案 A　在 Barrete 上皮组织(也称为 Barrete 食管)食管末端的柱状上皮取代了正常的鳞状上皮,是化生的结果,慢性消化性溃疡可能发生于 Barrete 食管。虽然柱状黏膜相似于胃黏膜和肠黏膜,但它是非常容易发生不典型增生肠的类型。3%~ 10% 的 Barrete 食管患者会发生或后来发展为食管腺癌。

7. 答案 A　细针抽吸活检显示脓液。体检扪及病灶处温暖的、波动性包快,提示腮腺的化脓性病变。脱水的小孩是急性化脓性腮腺炎的典型病史。病毒性腮腺炎,如流行性腮腺炎中所见的通常是双侧性的,当单侧发病时,不是化脓性的。肉芽肿性腮腺炎与脓液形成无关,发生在婴儿腮腺的原发性恶性性肿瘤是罕见的,而且不会出现典型的化脓性病变。

8. 答案 C　肺浸润在所有的疾病中均可见,但仅有肉瘤样结节铍毒症,以及结核病可引起肉芽肿形成。出现肺尖部的浸润在结核病中是常见的。

9. 答案 C 急性非特异性阑尾炎主要发生在年轻人,通常由于粪石阻塞引起腔壁局部缺血而引发。虽然在3%阑尾中发现了蛲虫,但蛲虫极少引起阑尾炎。在组织学上,急性阑尾炎是以黏膜溃疡形成和不同程度的腔壁坏死以及中性粒细胞弥漫性浸润为特征。慢性阑尾炎的概念尚有争议,白细胞增多通常发生。

10. 答案 C 当骨肉瘤穿透骨皮质,它使骨膜掀起。掀起的骨膜通常与其下面的正常骨皮质形成一个"锐角",这一现象称为 Codman 三角。Codman 三角作为一种明显的 X 线表现对骨源性肉瘤的诊断有参考价值。

11、12. 11- B. 12- D 乳房的脂肪坏死能形成一个相似于癌的肿块,伴有表皮的皱缩。这种病变集中在脂肪组织,不伴有导管扩张。此处没有发生在乳腺粉刺癌中的恶性上皮增生。

虽然在脂肪坏死的慢性机化过程中出现巨噬细胞,但肉芽肿性炎并不是脂肪坏死的主要病因,腺病指的是小叶增生而不是脂肪坏死的重要特征。

乳房的脂肪坏死通常继发于损伤后,损伤的脂肪细胞死亡,类脂降解为皂化。组织学上表现为细胞质同源嗜酸性的鬼影细胞。在脂肪坏死的慢性阶段,继发坏死组织的钙化和机化,并出现巨噬细胞和单核细胞的积聚。未产妇、雌激素治疗、母乳喂养以及肺结核与脂肪坏死没有直接联系。

13. 答案 A 系统性红斑狼疮是一种典型的,与免疫复合物多器官沉积相关的疾病,这种现象会影响多克隆 B 细胞的活性。干燥综合征,硬皮病,移植物抗宿主反应以及雷诺综合征(例如,钙质沉着病,雷诺现象,食管功能障碍,并趾畸形,毛细血管扩张),这些疾病与免疫复合物沉淀没有特定的联系。

14. 答案 C 一个成年人病变黑素细胞病变中,出现大量核分裂,是恶性的标志。多核巨细胞,真皮深层的黑素细胞巢以及表皮的改变,可见于良性或恶性黑素细胞的病变中围绕毛干的痣细胞也是良性先天性痣的特征。

15. 答案 B 像这个病人一样严重的头部外伤会导致大脑与颅骨之间的损伤。脑水肿接踵发生,伴有中脑和桥脑的移位。小脑幕切迹疝之后发生。后者会导致脑干动静脉的拉伸和撕裂,引起脑干实质的出血(Duret 出血),虽然动脉瘤破裂和动静畸形会引起于 Duret 出血相似的症状,但这些诊断并不适用这个病例。延髓离断和大脑梗死都不是符合这个病人。

16. 答案 D 移植物接受者有发生各种机会感染的危险。EBV 病毒感染伴移植后淋巴增生性病变(PTLD)就是一个并发症。在 PTLD 中,免疫抑制的宿主会有原发的或再发的感染。EBV 病毒给 B 细胞施加了增殖的压力。在缺乏 T 细胞调控时,B 细胞可能扩增并产生克隆性增生(如淋巴瘤)。

17. 答案 A 远端食管的红色天鹅绒样改变是 Barrett 食管的标志。其中远端食管的改变在组织学上以柱状黏膜为特征(尤其是肠型或"特异"的类型)。大约10%该病患者会发生反流性食管炎,柱状黏膜进行性异型增生可以导致腺癌的发生,发生概率为3%到10%。每年须行活组织检查监测病情。如果出现高级别异型增生或黏膜内癌,那么就要考虑行食管切除术。念珠菌性食管炎以酵母和假菌丝出现为特征,它们经常侵及食管鳞状上皮黏膜。神经节细胞以正常数目出现在 Barrett 食管中,在食管弛缓不能时,神经节细胞减少或缺失。

气管食管瘘(TEF)不是 Barrett 食管并发症,虽然它可由 Barrett 腺癌引起。

18~19. 18- E 19- B 阴囊中单个睾丸出现的临床表现与单睾丸者(先天性一侧睾丸缺失)或隐睾症(睾丸未下降)相关。在这个部位一个腹部包块的存在很可能是发生于一个隐睾的生殖细胞瘤,因为睾丸一般只会萎缩不会发生肥大。最常见的生殖细胞瘤是精原细胞瘤,存在实性肿块的 X 线证据有力支持了精原细胞瘤的诊断,因为畸胎瘤通常有囊性成分。前列腺癌在年轻人中很罕见,腺瘤样瘤通常是发生于附睾的小肿瘤。

精原细胞瘤选用的治疗是切除原发病变,再辅以放疗。精原细胞瘤对放疗高度敏感。精原细胞瘤的预后较好,有 90%~98% 的 5 年生存率。前列腺特异性抗原是前列腺癌的标记,对精原细胞瘤的诊断无效。在发生一侧睾丸精原细胞瘤的病人中有 2% 可能引起另一侧睾丸的精原细胞瘤。

20. 答案 D 最有可能的诊断是神经母细胞瘤,由于病人的年龄尚小,可以直接排除胰岛细胞瘤的可能性。神经母细胞瘤是幼儿和儿童最常见的颅外实体性恶性肿瘤,常发生钙化。Wilms 肿瘤,肝母细胞瘤和胰母细胞瘤并没有这样的特征,从病理上,菊心团样结构以及神经纤维细胞形成是神经母细胞瘤的特定表现。

21. 答案 B 该病人出现恶心,呕吐,少尿,血尿,高血压和血肌酐浓度升高,这些症状可能是由肾炎引起的。肾炎的基本病理学特征是肾小球大量增殖及活动性炎症。细胞性新月体是由于毛细管攀破裂,血浆蛋白质溢出到肾小囊腔而引起的肾小囊壁层细胞增生。而其他选项只是肾病综合征的形态学特征,例如:结状性肾小球硬化(糖尿病),基底膜钉突(膜性肾小球肾病),嗜刚果红染色组织(淀粉状蛋白),弥漫性足细胞消失(微小病变性肾病)。

22. 答案 D 大量的研究表明,当胸腔渗出液内出现腺癌细胞而不知是什么恶性肿瘤细胞时,统计学显示,该部位的肿瘤细胞女性是乳腺癌,男性是肺癌最多见。

23. 答案 B HBV 辅助 HDV 在肝细胞内装配成完整的病毒颗粒,完整的 HDV 病毒颗粒是由 HBSAg 的外壳和 HDV 的 RNA 核心组成。HBV 是散发性肝炎和暴发性肝炎最常见的原因。HCV 是输血后肝炎最常见的病因。HBV 的基因组主要是双链 DNA 而非 RNA。在慢性乙型肝炎中,HBV 基因组可能是以游离或整合状态存在,也可能两种状态同时存在,急性甲型肝炎不会发展成为慢性肝病。

24. 答案 B 卡波西肉瘤曾经不常见,但现在发病率在增加,因为该病与 AIDS 有关,但 AIDS 病毒并不会引起恶性肿瘤,无同源性的病毒 DNA 被发现。在 AIDS 患者中,卡波西肉瘤常是黏膜和淋巴结上的小肿瘤,这些肿瘤可能没有典型的皮肤病变。虽然卡波西肉瘤以不同的临床特征,但他们有共同的组织学特征,经典型卡波西肉瘤见于老年的东欧犹太教徒,90% 的患者为男性。卡波西肉瘤很少发生在接受免疫抑制治疗的肾移植患者身上;停止了免疫抑制治疗就会使肿瘤发生退化。

25. 答案 A 对于儿童肾病综合征最常见的原因为微小病变。在这种情况下,肾变病有时会在免疫接种或感染后发生,病理上仅仅发现有弥漫性足细胞足突消失,因此命名为微小病变肾病。

26. 答案 E 缺铁性贫血,化疗诱导的骨髓(造血功能)损伤,急性白血病以及转移性乳腺癌对这个 60 岁妇女的低血色素值都是可以解释的。没有详细的外周血涂片的形态学检查和进一步的实验室诊断数据,诊断不能最终确定。老年人可能因为饮食不佳而出现营养缺乏,另一个可能性是不明原因的胃肠道失血(如癌症)。化疗会抑制和损伤骨髓(造血功能)导致贫血,在这一些情况下,骨髓(造血功能)的损伤可能是长期的,化疗后也可发生急性白血病。最后骨髓转移瘤可产生一种骨髓代替型贫血。

27. 答案 B 在大多数人类的癌症中,肿瘤的分期是判断预后最重要的因素。分期涉及肿瘤大小播散的广度和深度(比如:局限的,局部的或远处的)。肿瘤分级(比如分化),核分裂计数以及于肿瘤分期相关的侵袭程度,因此高分级(比如:低分化)肿瘤和高度侵袭性肿瘤往往是高度分期的肿瘤。

28. 答案 D 大多数卵巢转移灶来源于胃腺癌,由印戒细胞组成,因此符合 Krukenberg 瘤的定义。Krubenberg 瘤通常是双侧的。这些肿瘤最常见的原发灶是胃,少数情况下,可能从结肠、乳房、阑尾或其他部位播散而来。Brenner 肿瘤是卵巢的原发性上皮肿瘤,组织学上与泌尿道上皮类似。肾细胞癌有时被称为 Grawitz 肿瘤。Klatskin 肿瘤(肝门胆管肿瘤)是一种胆管癌,它发生左右肝管的连接处。Wilms 肿瘤,也被称为肾母细胞瘤,是一种常发生于儿童的原发性肾肿瘤。

29. 答案 D 深部静脉血栓是在外科手术中和手术后卧床时的一种并发症,处于小静脉深处的血栓物质可以脱落移行到肺部形成肺栓塞,引起缺氧和呼吸困难。

30.答案 C 脑膜瘤由于位置比较特殊,所以在外科手术中常不能完全将其切除,故可能导致复发,由于这样的原因,手术时病灶是否被完全切除是这个肿瘤预后最重要因素。如果肿瘤没有被完全切除,那么检查所得出的组织参数(例如,组织学亚型,核分裂指数,肿瘤血供)就都没有价值。进行放疗暗示着不能进行手术治疗,预后较差。

31. 答案 D 海绵状血管瘤是一种最常见的原发性肝肿瘤。这些病变经常会在尸检和剖腹手术时被偶然发现,或是在检查其他一些不相关的疾病时被 X 线检查到。海绵状血管瘤好发于所有年龄段的人。其症状最常见于一些患有腹痛的妇女。海绵状血管瘤极少发生破裂,但一旦发生破裂,它通常发生在巨大海绵窦状血管瘤中。

32. 答案 D 易感性个体,吸入带有铍的灰尘可引起急性支气管肺炎。这些病人可表现为皮肤超敏反应,是慢性铍中毒的典型特征。石棉沉积症不表现为支气管肺炎,而表现为间质病变。类固醇激素很少引起肺病疾病,除非长期使用导致免疫抑制和间质性肺炎。但是,如果发生以上情况,病人不能通过常规的抗生素治疗而治愈,因为抗生素是用于合并细菌感染的患者。空洞形成是肺结核的典型表现,在 X 线片上可见小的或大的结节性肉芽肿。虽然煤矿工人可以发生支气管肺炎,但这例关键的因素是他现在在陶瓷厂工作,已知在那里能接触铍元素。

33. 答案 C 15%的供体肾在采集前就有前期损伤的改变。动脉性栓子在病理学上被定义为微血管内的针样空隙。动脉栓塞与供体严重的动脉粥样硬化斑块和导管插入术或血管手术有关。但是,移植肾的"原发性无功能"可继发于各种原因。采集过程中的缺血性损伤(即采集损伤)最常见。针对供体组织产生的抗体常在移植前交叉配对试验中被忽略,而导致急性排斥,但这种情况不常见。

34~35. 答案 34- D, 35- E 葡萄胎是来自病理性卵子的异常绒毛,能在子宫增殖和变大,人绒毛膜促性腺激素的分泌水平比正常妊娠要高。异位妊娠的人绒毛膜促性腺激素水平是正常的,但子宫不增大。胎盘粘连是植入性胎盘的特征,但子宫不增大,人绒毛膜促性腺激素也不过高分泌。妊娠期合并子宫平滑肌瘤时子宫异常增大,但无人绒毛膜促性腺激素 hCG 的水平的升高。绒毛膜血管瘤是胎盘的良性血管源性肿瘤,子宫不异常增大,人绒毛膜促性腺激素的分泌也无异常。

绒毛膜癌可继发于正常妊娠或流产,但最常继发于以前有或现在合并葡萄胎的妊娠。绒毛膜癌能穿透子宫到达周围组织或远处转移。输卵管破裂与异位妊娠有关,能导致出血而危及生命;而不继发于宫内葡萄胎性妊娠。腹膜假黏液瘤是卵巢、间皮和消化道黏液上皮瘤的并发症。子宫内膜息肉常与雌激素刺激,由良性子宫内膜腺体和间质组成。

36. 答案 B　活跃上皮的增生和患乳癌危险性增加相关;纤维腺瘤(除非有上皮增生)则不与乳腺癌相关。乳腺癌的家族病史是一个危险因素,但男性乳腺发育的病史则不是。37 岁的病人处于低危险的年龄组。接收少量的射线,即使经过多次乳房 X 线摄片也不会增加危险性。

37. 答案 D　患者患有家族性多发性腺瘤息肉病(FAP),它以无数个(超过 100 个)结肠直肠腺瘤为特征。腺瘤在小肠(特别是十二指肠)和胃很少见。FAP 很好的证明了结肠直肠腺瘤发展为腺癌的过程。FAP 的遗传基因定位于 5 号染色体的长臂(5q)。腺瘤通常发生于 20~30 岁,十年后出现临床症状。在临床症状出现之前,约 2/3 的病人发展为结肠直肠癌。癌很少发生在 30 岁前。如果在 20 岁之前没有实施预防性的结肠切除术,那么实际上所有的病人最终都会发生腺癌。腺癌也可以在结肠外发生。

38. 答案 C　四种病变中,只有血管纤维瘤含有血管成分,导致活检并发症。血管纤维瘤的特征性颜色和组成可与普通鼻息肉区别。疣状癌,正如其名,并不表现为光滑的病灶。

39. 答案 C　如问题中描述那样,在老年人,转移性肿瘤最可能的原发部位是前列腺。前列腺酸性磷酸酶(一种肿瘤标记的酶)或前列腺特异抗原的免疫化学定位,是损伤最小、比较经济的检测这种肿瘤的技术。其他选择——钡灌肠,剖腹术,X 线电子计算机断层摄影(CT)和电子显微镜(EM)检查并无特异性,更昂贵,且检查起来令病人感觉不适。

40. 答案 B　听神经瘤发生于中老人,女性比男性多见。神经纤维瘤病的特征是皮肤上多发性咖啡色斑点性病变。听神经纤维瘤最可能发生于腋前线有色素斑的 49 岁女性。Ⅲ型多发性内分泌腺瘤病患者可有结肠神经节瘤病,但没有明显增加听神经纤维瘤发生的机会。患黑素瘤(一种与神经病变无关的肿瘤)的病人,患中枢神经系统肿瘤的倾向没有增加。其他系统无论是暴露于射线还是先天异常,都与听神经纤维瘤发生率增加无关。

41~43. 答案 41-C, 42-B, 43-D　病史和临床表现与慢性阻塞性肺疾病(COPD)的诊断一致,该病的特征是肺气肿和慢性支气管炎两种病同时发生。吸烟对该病是一个慢性刺激因子,它能诱发炎症并能降低蛋白水解酶活性,导致肺实质的损伤。吸烟不会影响 α_1-抗胰蛋白酶基因活性。在 COPD 中,肺基底膜通常增厚,而脱屑性间质性肺炎不是本病的特征。继发性肺动脉高压可发生于 COPD,当严重的 COPD 时,会导致右心衰(肺源性心脏病)。肺静脉闭塞性疾病与肺血栓栓塞也可以导致肺源性心脏病的发生,但与 COPD 无特定的联系。弥漫性肺泡损伤涉及于肺透明膜病以及 Ⅱ 型肺细胞增生可见于急性呼吸窘迫综合征中。支气管肺发育不良是新生儿呼吸窘迫综合征的后遗症。

可在 COPD 患者身上听到的呼气喘鸣是由气管狭窄引起的,这是由于气管塌陷来证实。慢性细支气管炎是通过水肿和纤维化引起气管的狭窄;杯状细胞异常增生黏液分泌增加引起气道狭窄。在呼气相,胸腔内正压造成的气管塌陷,是由于肺气肿肺弹性缺失所致。炭末沉着症是碳色素在肺巨噬细胞中的积聚,它不会引起气管狭窄。

44~45. 答案 44- A, 45- C　这个病人最可能发生与丙肝病毒(HCV)感染相关的肝硬化,丙肝病毒可能是该病人在以前输血过程中被感染。这个病人的甲肝病毒(HAV)血清证明了有先前的 HAV 感染,这在成年人中常见,但是 HAV 不引起慢性肝病。对于这些患有晚期肝病的患者来说,肝移植是一个可供选择的治疗方法,即使再发性 HCV 感染常见。门静脉高压是肝硬化上的一种常见临床结果。

在大部分病例中,门静脉高压引发的腹水与窦状血管,窦后性或肝后的血管阻塞有关。这些血管阻断导致肝淋巴回流的增加,使淋巴液从肝表面流入腹腔。低白蛋白血症和继发性醛固酮增多症促进腹水形成。与丙肝病毒(HCV)相关的肝硬化增加了发展为肝细胞肝癌的危险性,这肿瘤可能广泛侵入到肝静脉导致肝后血管阻塞。

46. 答案 D　患有 Addism 综合征的病人常出现血压过低,这是由于肾上腺皮质的破坏使肾上腺皮质激素(醛固酮)缺乏所致。Cushing 综合征会引起高血压,它是由垂体后叶素,肾上腺病变或过量摄取糖皮质激素所引起。Conn 综合征,通常由肾上腺皮质腺瘤产生,与过量的醛固酮产生相关,它的结果是引起高血压。由于儿茶酚胺的过量释放,嗜铬细胞瘤以及肾上腺髓质增生引起高血压。

47. 答案 A　闭塞性细支气管炎(OB)指的是假膜性支气管与呼吸性细支气管的一种进行性纤维化病变。这种慢性改变可在排斥现象中看到,但也见于感染、缺血或移植物抗宿主反应中。肺的急性细胞排斥的特征取决于排斥病变的严重性。在早期排斥反应中,淋巴细胞性炎症局限于血管周隙内,随着严重性增加,炎症就会渗出到间质和肺泡腔中,并可见到更多的中性粒细胞浸润。严重的排斥反应可能出现出血,坏死并伴有透明膜的形成。

48. 答案 D　中层肉芽肿不是动脉粥样硬化的特征。脂肪纹和粥样斑块(内膜的斑点)是动脉粥样硬化的典型病变。当粥样斑块形成溃疡,钙化,血栓形成,斑块内出血或轻度淋巴细胞性炎症,他们被称为"复合性斑块"。脂纹期发生于儿童,引发一个关于动脉粥样硬化可能始发于很小年龄的思考。

49. 答案 B　主动脉瘤不是急性心肌梗死的并发症,但常是动脉粥样硬化、不同的感染性因素、结缔组织异常或先天性缺陷的结果。心肌梗死的并发症很多而且各不相同,一些发生在梗死后 1 小时以内,而另一些则发生在急性期后数月或更长时间。其中一些并发症(例如,室性心律失常、心源性休克、心脏破裂)非常严重并且是心肌梗死病人常见的死亡原因。

50. 答案 D　获得性免疫缺陷综合征(AIDS)的特点是进行性细胞介导的免疫缺陷。大多数严重影响的是辅助性 T 细胞——该类细胞辅助 B 细胞及其他 T 细胞对抗原作出适当的反应。辅助性 T 细胞的缺失使宿主易患各种感染(特别是原虫、真菌、分枝杆菌以及病毒的感染)和恶性肿瘤。对细菌感染的抵抗多数是由体液免疫介导。因此,肺炎球菌性肺炎的发病率在艾滋病患者中并没有增高。

51. 答案 B　虽然有假说认为包皮垢的长期刺激易致阴茎鳞状细胞癌的发生,但体检中发现包皮垢并不能区分尖锐湿疣和癌。溃疡和疼痛是癌的表现。腹股沟和肺部肿块提示癌的局部和远处转移。

52. 答案 C　组织常通过肉芽组织形成对自身进行修复,该过程最终导致纤维化(瘢痕组织)代替损伤所致的缺损。肉芽组织在炎症发生后不久就开始形成并且在 100 小时内生长成熟,除非病人患有恶性肿瘤或者存在营养不良、老年、糖尿病及感染因素。肉芽组织不是肉芽肿,虽然缝合外科手术伤口的缝线会致异物肉芽肿的形成(在此过程中,发生 Ⅰ 期愈合)。有时,一个开放性的伤口不能通过外科手术缝合,因此,属于 Ⅱ 期愈合,形成的瘢痕大而不规则。如果一个患者具有敏感体质,瘢痕组织增生过度,形成瘢痕疙瘩。炎症可以导致瘘管形成(例如,两种结构的异常连接,常与体表与空腔脏器相通,像肠皮肤瘘(肛瘘)或直肠阴道瘘)。由于炎症或者感染的持续刺激,机体往往很难修复这些结构,这就需要外科手术来解决。

53. 答案 D　Berry 动脉瘤是小的囊状(气球样)动脉瘤,大多数是先天性的,并且存在于较细的大脑动脉中。梭形动脉瘤是动脉的梭形膨胀。继发于动脉粥样硬化的动脉瘤是最常见的类型,它常常位于腹主动脉肾动脉分支起始点以下。由于 Ⅲ 期梅毒的发病率下降,梅毒性动脉瘤在今天已不常见。这些动脉瘤几乎都是发生在胸主动脉的上行和横向部分。曲张的动脉瘤是由动静脉瘘的扩张形成。

54. 答案 E　在二尖瓣脱垂中可见二尖瓣下垂,但它并不是高血压性心脏病的表现。长期高血压可以导致严重的终末器官效应,特别是心和肾。心脏主要的形态学改变包括心脏肥大,左室向心性肥厚以及乳头肌肥厚。心内膜纤维性增厚偶有发生。

55. 答案 C　血尿不是糖尿病性肾小球硬化症的主要特点,糖尿病性肾小球硬化症是糖尿病肾病的一种形式。糖尿病性肾小球硬化症以早期弥漫性肾小球基底膜增厚为特点。其晚期,毛细管间的肾小球系膜基质扩展(弥漫性糖尿病性肾小球硬化症),最终转变为结节(结节型糖尿病肾小球硬化)。这种扩展累及肾小球毛细血管腔。糖尿病性肾小球硬化症在临床上表现为微白蛋白尿,蛋白尿,最终发展为肾衰竭。糖尿病性肾小球硬化症总是伴有其他部位的小血管病变,比如糖尿病视网膜病变。

56. 答案 E　细菌性疾病常引起脓肿的产生,它是中性粒细胞的聚集。而肉芽肿不会产生这种现象。几种不同的传染原可以引起具有不同形态学特点的肉芽肿性炎。肉芽肿为直径 1~2 mm 的小结节由巨噬细胞(组织细胞)构成,该细胞可转化成类上皮样细胞,单核细胞浸润包围这些上皮样组织细胞,在此典型肉芽肿中有大量的淋巴细胞。虽然结核是感染性肉芽肿性疾病的经典例子,许多其他感染性疾病亦以肉芽肿形成为特点,包括猫抓病、梅毒、某种真菌感染(例如,组织胞浆菌病,球孢子菌病)以及性病性淋巴肉芽肿。结节病,一种未明原因的疾病,是肉芽肿性炎的另一个例子,与其他三种疾病相比,在结节病中没有干酪性不形成坏死性肉芽肿。

57. 答案 E　霍奇金淋巴瘤几乎不累及胃肠道或生殖器官。然而,伯基特淋巴瘤常累及胃肠道,特别是在儿童中。题中所述病人,要考虑阑尾周围脓肿复发的可能。Crohn 病(CD)可以产生炎性纤维素性物质。最后,卵巢生殖细胞肿瘤好发于年轻女孩,在这例患者的诊断中要考虑其可能性。

58. 答案 B　异倍体的细胞核并不等同于恶性肿瘤,虽然大多数异倍体的细胞是肿瘤性的,但是也有例外。流式细胞仪可以用来测定肿瘤细胞核的具体情况,在某些情况下,也可以提供有意义的预后信息。这种做法有其局限性,但是,重要的是他们可以知道细胞 DNA

的相关信息。一个二倍体的结果并不意味着病变一定是良性的,二倍体的病变可以是良性的或者恶性反应性的或者肿瘤性的。但一个反应性的或良性病变细胞几乎都是二倍的。

59. 答案 E 肉瘤的分级是建立在肿瘤分化程度基础上的预后标准。低度恶性的(高分化)肿瘤与高度恶性的(高有丝分裂)肿瘤相比发展较慢。分期同样也是一个预后指标,它与肉瘤的分级相关(Ⅰ,Ⅱ,Ⅲ期)并且与局部骨骼或血管累及和转移有关(Ⅳ期)。如果其他因素是等同的,那么一个肉瘤越大,其预后越差。肉瘤浸润的深度是另外一个重要的影响因素,位于皮下的表浅性肿瘤与位于肌肉内的深在性肿瘤相比预后要好很多。肿瘤持续存在的时间是肿瘤确诊以前可以被看到或感觉到的时间,它与预后无关。

60. 答案 B 通常皮肤癌[鳞状细胞癌(SCC)]和黑素瘤与长期暴露于阳光的紫外线有关。放疗性肿瘤可以在不同的部位发生,包括甲状腺、软组织或骨骼,发生于软组织和骨的肿瘤称肉瘤。然而,内部器官,如卵巢、肝脏及肾脏是最不易受到自然或治疗性射线影响的。

61. 答案 D 虽然在急性心肌梗死后第一小时内就可以发现超微结构(电镜下的)改变,但组织学表现在梗死后 5~12 小时(不是 24 小时)后出现。这些变化以凝固性坏死为特点,包括细胞质玻璃样变和嗜酸性,横纹缺失,核固缩以及核碎裂。毛细血管内中性粒细胞边集,24 小时左右进入组织。急性心肌梗死的另外一个标志是梗死后 48~72 小时内血清肌酸激酶(CK)MB 型同工酶的水平。大多数心肌梗死是透壁性的(例如,它常累及心室壁的全层)并且常累及左心室。心内膜下(非透壁性的)心肌梗死常累及心室壁厚度的1/3到1/2呈环状。

62. 答案 D 狼疮性肾炎用于描述在系统性红斑狼疮(SLE)中所发生的一组肾小球肾炎。在狼疮性肾炎中可以发现大量针对不同抗原的自身抗体。但是,针对肾小球基底膜的抗体显著不同。大约 50% 到 80% 的患者具有不同程度的肾脏改变的临床表现。对肾脏疾病的认识往往是在系统性疾病发生后的 2 年以内。狼疮性肾炎的标志是广泛的肾小球免疫复合物沉积。广泛多样的组织病理学损伤形式与疾病的严重程度相关。狼疮性肾炎常见于女性患者。

63. 答案 D 恶性纤维组织细胞瘤(恶纤组 MFH)是很常见的成人肿瘤,该肿瘤几乎总是发生在深部和多形性(具有奇异的细胞)。这种肿瘤好发于大腿。事实上,恶性纤维组织细胞瘤是成人腿部最常见的肿瘤。虽然该肿瘤是由纤维母细胞和肌纤维母细胞组成,但由于其含有组织细胞样细胞所以不能称纤维肉瘤。纤维肉瘤在儿童中较为常见,是非多形性(均一的)肿瘤。

64. 答案 E 软骨和肌肉组织是相对抗放射性的。体细胞受电离辐射的影响,与它们的更新率成正比,与它们分化的程度成反比。因此,很少进行分裂的分化成熟软骨和肌肉组织的细胞与具有很高更新率的骨髓和淋巴系统细胞相比,相对受到辐射的影响较小。其他关于放射线的叙述都是正确的。

65. 答案 C 致癌基因是反转录病毒(病毒癌基因 v-oncs)和真核生物细胞(细胞癌基因 c-oncs)中特殊的 DNA 核苷酸序列。病毒被认为是在整合入宿主细胞的过程中从同源染色体 c-oncs 中获得 v-oncs。致癌基因在细胞生长中发挥一定的作用,因为许多 v-oncs 编码作为生长因子受体的酶。由于 c-oncs 在真核生物的进化过程中是保守的,它们在细胞增殖、细胞分化或两者中可能具有很重要的生物学作用。在动物中,病毒癌基因可以诱发恶性肿瘤。虽然在人类,还没有明确地发现某种致癌基因能产生癌症,但是某种 c-oncs 被发现与特定的人类肿瘤,特别是那些与染色体异常也相关的肿瘤有关(例如伯基特淋巴瘤)。

66. 答案 E   在动脉硬化中,没有发现淀粉状纤维蛋白。动脉硬化是小动脉和微动脉内膜增生及管壁硬化的过程。动脉硬化的类型分两种——玻璃样动脉硬化和增生性动脉硬化——二者都和高血压有关。玻璃样动脉硬化在糖尿病中也很常见。在玻璃样动脉硬化中,所发现的物质是血浆蛋白在微动脉壁中的沉积。在增生性动脉硬化中,动脉壁向心性逐层增厚并且常伴有纤维蛋白沉积和坏死。

67. 答案 A   单核巨噬细胞系统(也叫做网状内皮系统)的细胞在体内广泛分布,并且根据其所在部位而具有不同的名称。这些细胞具有明显的向损伤部位迁移的倾向,它们受到趋化因子的刺激而迁移。单核巨噬细胞系统的细胞具有许多功能。它们是重要的吞噬细胞,它们处理外源性抗原并把它提呈给 T 细胞,它们表达 Ⅱ 类主要组织相容性复合物抗原(MHC),它们产生调节炎症过程的许多物质[例如白介素-1(IL-1),促进成纤维细胞、骨髓前体细胞以及内皮细胞生长的生长因子、干扰素-α(IFN-α)]。

68~69. 答案 68-D,69-B   该患者童年曾患有急性风湿热,导致了成年后的慢性风湿性心脏病。风湿性心脏病的发病率在过去的几十年里已经显著下降。风湿热是系统性的、非化脓性的,由 A 组 β-溶血性链球菌引起的未治疗的咽部感染性炎性的并发症。在慢性风湿性心脏病患者中,瓣叶增厚变形(纤维化的结果)、瓣膜粘连为其典型表现。由于严重的二尖瓣狭窄或关闭不全导致左房扩张。在风湿病中,阿少夫小体是典型的组织学表现。

链球菌,特别是 α-溶血性链球菌,感染占了累及心瓣膜的感染性心内膜炎的 65%,通常瓣膜已有病变存在。虽然在感染性心内膜炎的部分病例中,风湿性心脏病曾经被认为是引起潜在的瓣膜损害的最常见的原因。但现在二尖瓣脱垂也是最常见的瓣膜异常。由于该例患者存在二尖瓣狭窄,其二尖瓣瓣膜易受到心内膜炎的影响。来自瓣膜赘生物的脓毒性栓子可能会引起脑、心、肾、脾的败血性梗死。赘生物通常含有纤维蛋白,炎性细胞和感染的微生物。

70. 答案 E   浸润虽然是肉瘤的典型表现,但不一定仅表现在恶性肿瘤,浸润同时也是局部侵袭性纤维瘤病的典型表现。在大体和镜下,良性肿瘤常可以看到包膜。但是,在肉眼检查中肉瘤也可以看到包膜(例如,假包膜),通过镜检可以发现其侵袭性。病变处的坏死常提示为恶性,良性软组织肿瘤很少发生坏死。肿瘤的大小不能区分其良恶性,但是一旦肉瘤的诊断明确,其大小对预后非常重要。肿瘤较小(< 5 cm)的患者其预后比肿瘤大的患者好。患有多种肉瘤的患者其 5 年生存率可以很高,因此,肉瘤并不一定预后很差。

71. 答案 E   肾细胞癌在男性的发病是女性的两倍。它表现为血尿,疼痛和腰部包块。肾细胞癌是最常见的转移性肿瘤之一,它主要通过血道转移。肺和脑是常见的转移部位。肾细胞癌常发生于 60 岁左右的男性。

72. 答案 D   T 细胞具有很多重要的免疫功能。但是,只有外源性抗原被巨噬细胞接受、处理然后提呈给 T 细胞,T 细胞才能对抗原进行识别。一组 T 细胞——辅助性 T 细胞,可以增强 T 细胞和 B 细胞的活性;另一组细胞亚群——抑制性 T 细胞——抑制 T 细胞及 B 细胞反应。T 细胞通过直接与靶细胞接触而溶解靶细胞。同时,T 细胞通过产生淋巴因子,比如白介素-2(IL-2)来参加免疫应答。

73~77. 答案 73-B,74-D,75-C,76-A,77-B　亚急性脊髓联合变性与维生素 B_{12} 缺乏有关。维生素 B_{12} 和叶酸的缺乏会导致巨幼细胞性肿瘤。巨幼变可以发生在骨髓中所有的细胞系,但以红系为主。但是,在亚急性脊髓联合变性中,只有维生素 B_{12} 缺乏。

佝偻病属于儿童骨骼疾病,它是缺乏维生素 D 引起的。佝偻病以儿童生长期类骨质过度增生,骨骼发育畸形为特点。在成人表现为骨软化症。

坏血病是维生素 C(抗坏血酸)缺乏引起的疾病。结缔组织结构和功能的异常引起点状皮下出血和牙龈出血。

眼球干燥症与维生素 A 缺乏有关,它表现为结膜极度干燥,偶致结膜溃疡。

78~82.答案 78-B,79-D,80-A,81-C,82-D　一种少见的肝脏肿瘤(血管肉瘤)和过度接触氯乙烯之间的相关性已经得到确认。这又由肿瘤不常见的组织学表现的流行病学证明。

政府研究显示了在用大量环己烷氨基磺酸盐喂养的动物与胆囊癌的发生有关,但在人类,这种联系还不清楚。与人类膀胱癌发生有关的因素包括暴露于苯胺染料中的致癌物质以及吸烟。

世界各地区的流行病学调查揭示了饮食和结肠肿瘤的关系。其中一个饮食因素是脂肪。在饮食中脂肪含量丰富的国家结肠癌的发病率较高。

很多种癌症,特别是肺癌,与暴露于石棉暴露有关。然而,在暴露于石棉的个体中,间皮瘤的发生是不成比例的。人群中间皮瘤的低发病率支持它与石棉的成因性联系。

吸烟和肺癌(通常为鳞状细胞癌和小细胞癌)的关系已经明确并且很有意义,因为吸烟人群很庞大。

83~87. 答案 83-D,84-A,85-E,86-C,87-B　免疫系统的细胞具有精细的、高度特异性的防御机制。当这些细胞遇到抗原时,就会发生协调有序的免疫应答,可以是体液性的,也可以是细胞介导的,或二者均发生。免疫应答中最初涉及的细胞是淋巴细胞,它主要分为两大类:T 淋巴细胞(T 细胞)和 B 淋巴细胞(B 细胞)。第三类淋巴细胞叫做裸细胞,分为自然杀伤(NK)细胞,杀伤(K)细胞和淋巴细胞激活的杀伤细胞(LAK)。巨噬细胞除了在急性炎症反应中的作用,同样在免疫应答中也发挥重要的作用。

抗体依赖性靶细胞的溶解是 K 细胞的主要功能。在抗体依赖性细胞毒反应中,抗体(通常为免疫球蛋白 G)与 K 细胞 Fc 受体以及靶细胞的抗体结合位点相结合。

在由细胞介导的对某种微生物(例如,结核分枝杆菌)的免疫应答中,活化的巨噬细胞是首先与抗原接触的细胞。它摄取有机物,对抗原进行处理,使其成为 T 细胞可以识别的形式。然后巨噬细胞与其表面的主要组织相容性复合物(MHC)分子一起把抗原提呈给 T 细胞,这种活动叫做抗原呈递。

与 K 细胞相反,NK 细胞对靶细胞的杀伤作用不需要抗体信号。NK 细胞可以在体外杀伤几种肿瘤细胞系,并且不需要事先致敏。NK 细胞通过受体与靶细胞相连,该过程不需要二价钙离子。

B 细胞在抗原、T 细胞以及其他细胞的刺激下分化成为浆细胞。浆细胞产生五种类型的免疫球蛋白。每个浆细胞只产生一种免疫球蛋白。

在免疫反应中,特别是细胞介导的免疫反应和抗体应答,致敏 T 细胞产生并释放大量可溶性物质(称为淋巴因子)。淋巴因子通过许多途径发挥调节及加强免疫应答的功能。白介素-2(IL-2)和干扰素是淋巴因子的两个代表。

88~92.答案 88- D,89- E,90- A,91- B,92- C　大多数肉瘤的组织学类型概括了一种特殊类型的间叶组织,并且肿瘤的命名也源自这些组织。因此,横纹肌肉瘤源自横纹肌(骨骼肌);神经纤维肉瘤源自神经细胞(施万细胞);血管肉瘤源自血管(血管内皮);脂肪肉瘤源自脂肪细胞(脂肪组织);以及纤维肉瘤源自纤维细胞(结缔组织)。虽然一些权威人士认为大多数肉瘤源自全能间叶干细胞。但表型的精确性(例如,平滑肌肉瘤在患者的病程中保持其可识别性)无法用该理论来解释。因此,肉瘤的细胞来源或组织来源尚未清楚并且是一个需要探讨的问题。

93~97. 答案 93- C,94- A,95- D,96- E,97- B　超微结构的分析通过提供有关肿瘤性质及细胞起源的信息而有助于肿瘤的诊断,电子显微镜(EM)可以显示细胞水平的各种变化,包括发生在细胞核,连接复合体,表面微绒毛,颗粒以及指状突起形成过程的一系列变化。

电子显微镜有助于黑色素瘤的诊断,它可以显示伸长颗粒(前黑色素小体)的特点。如果黑色素瘤是未分化的(例如,色素不明显),诊断就比较困难。

类癌是低度恶性的神经内分泌肿瘤,就像黑色素瘤一样,在超微结构上它也含有颗粒。在类癌中,这种颗粒电子显微镜下呈高密度核心颗粒。

腺癌具有微绒毛,在间皮瘤中发现的绒毛很长。在鳞状细胞癌(SCCs)中发现的具有诊断意义的超微结构是大量的张力丝,它可能是束状分布的细胞角蛋白丝。

骨骼肌源性肿瘤横纹肌肉瘤在电镜下可见 Z 带。

98~102.答案 98- C,99- A,100- E,101- B,102- E　急性早幼粒细胞白血病的特征是,出现大量原始细胞质颗粒正如出现在正常早幼粒细胞中的一样。由于这种颗粒释放具有促凝血酶原激酶活性的促凝血因子,75%的患者具有明显的出血素质或者在治疗中出现这种情况。

慢性髓细胞性白血病(CML)是骨髓源性的肿瘤,它主要包括各成熟期的粒细胞。白细胞计数(WBCs)常常超过 $5×10^{10}$/L。90%的患者骨髓中出现费城染色体。

慢性淋巴细胞性白血病(CLL)是成熟小淋巴细胞的病变并且具有较低的增殖率。98%的病例是 B 细胞源性的。这种白血病常影响年长者,伴有脾肿大以及与肿瘤有关的症状。大多数患者淋巴细胞显著增多(超过 $2×10^{10}$/L)。

急性髓细胞性白血病(AML)主要影响成人,并且在发病前几天或几个星期有乏力、出血,高热等前驱症状。体检可见皮肤瘀点,胸骨压痛,牙龈增生,淋巴结肿大,脾肿大和肝脏肿大。不经治疗,这种类型的白血病患者常于 1 到 3 个月内死亡。

红白血病是急性髓细胞性白血病的特殊亚型,在这种白血病中,骨髓示红细胞的前体细胞极度增生,同时还有髓母细胞增殖。

103~107. 答案 103- A,104- C,105- B,106- E,107- D　斑疹、丘疹、结节、风团和水疱都是不同皮肤病损名称。例如,位于胫骨前表皮的有触痛的红色结节,是结节性红斑的典型表现,结节性红斑是一种皮肤和皮下组织的炎性疾病。传染性软疣是痘病毒感染引起的疾病,它以皮肤上形成肉色的表面光滑的丘疹为特点。花斑癣中的斑疹颜色从白到褐色不等——由圆形酵母感染引起。风团和水疱以不同的皮肤疹为特点,这种皮肤疹是口服或胃肠外给药引起的。

108~112.答案 108- A,109- C,110- D,111- E,112- B 颈部的外部照射(常为低剂量)可能引起甲状腺乳头状癌,尽管这种照射剂量足以破坏甲状腺而不致产生致瘤效应。很多研究报道,当儿童期就暴露于放射线时,甲状腺癌和放射线的关系是非常明显的。

肿瘤形成的病原学强烈提示病毒与之有关。流行病学、血清学及生物化学方面的证据表明子宫颈癌与人乳头状瘤病毒(HPV)密切相关。另外一个病毒相关性肿瘤是伯基特淋巴瘤和 EB 病毒(EBV),虽然二者具有相关性的证据不如宫颈癌与乳头状瘤病毒相关性的证据充分,但仍然很有意义。

乳腺导管癌是女性常见的肿瘤,很多确诊的病人中曾经使用过雌激素。

黑色素瘤可能与紫外线有关,因为流行病学调查表明该肿瘤在阳光照射强烈的地区很常见,在澳大利亚该肿瘤几乎就是一种流行病。

Answers and Explanations

1. The answer is E　This patient's history of abdominal pain and weight loss is suggestive of pancreatic cancer. The least invasive technique that is likely to yield the most diagnostic information is computed tomography (CT), which can detect small mass lesions with great accuracy. The diagnosis of chronic cholecystitis is unlikely in view of the relatively recent onset of symptoms and the marked weight loss. Carcinoma of the ampulla of Vater and the head of the pancreas would most likely produce clinical evidence of jaundice, which is not present in this patient.

2. The answer is B　The pathologic description of the colonic biopsy is that of cytomegalovirus (CMV) colitis. Hemorrhagic necrosis related to cytomegalic change, with nuclear and cytoplasmic inclusions, is characteristic of CMV colitis. Superinfection with fungus, in particular, Candida, is common in CMV infection in immunocompromised patients.

3. The answer is C　The lesions described are consistent with either benign papillomatosis or another neoplastic process. Since neoplasia is not a choice, the best answer is a viral etiology, reflecting the association between papillomatosis and human papillomavirus (HPV) infection. Bacterial and fungal infections do not usually form discrete papillary nodules, and such lesions are not associated with an autoimmune process.

4. The answer is B　Gastin stromal tumor(GST) is the most common benign meseochymal tumor of the stomach. These tumors vary in size from 1 to 20 cm; those larger than 3 cm often cause pain or bleeding. Tumors larger than 6 cm need to be extensively evaluated to rule out the possibility of malignancy. The tumors usually are intramural; some are attached to the muscularis propria by a thin pedicle and, thus, project into the omentum. Microscopically, they consist of spindle and epithelioid mesenchymal cells. The histogenesis of these tumors currently is controversial but most appear to demonstrate some primitive evidence of smooth muscle differentiation. Adenomas are of epithelial, not mesenchymal origin; glomus tumors, lipomas, and leiomyoma are distinctly uncommon in the stomach.

5. The answer is E　The patient's clinical presentation is typical for a massive transmural myocardial infarct (involving more than 40% of the left ventricular myocardium) that resulted in cardiogenic shock. Transmural infarcts are typically associated with coronary artery thrombosis, which may result from rupture of an atheromatous plaque.

6. The answer is A　In Barrett's epithelium (also called Barrett's esophagus), columnar epithelium replaces the normal squamous epithelium of the distal esophagus as a result of metaplastic change. Chronic peptic ulcers may develop in the setting of Barrett's epithelium. Although the columnar mucosa may resemble either gastric or intestinal mucosa, it is the intestinal, or "specialized" type that most frequently develops dysplastic changes. From 3% to 10% of patients with Barrett's epithelium have or subsequently develop esophageal adenocarcinoma .

7. The answer is A　Fine-needle aspiration would likely reveat pus. The physical findings of a warm fluctuant mass in this location are suggestive of a suppurative lesion of the parotid gland.

The history of a young child with an illness predisposing to dehydration is a typical setting for acute suppurative parotitis. Viral parotitis, such as that seen in mumps, is usually bilateral, and when it is unilateral, it is not suppurative. Granulomatous parotitis also is not associated with pus formation. A primary malignancy of the parotid gland in an infant is extremely rare and would not typically present as a suppurative process.

8. The answer is C   Lung infiltrates are found in all the disorders, but only sarcoidosis, berylliosis, and tuberculosis cause granulomas. Apical pulmonary infiltrates are common in tuberculosis.

9. The answer is C   Acute nonspecific appendicitis primarily affects young adults and most commonly is caused by mural iscbemia induced by impacted fecaliths. Although enterobius vermicularis (pinworm) may be found in 3% of appendixes, it only rarely causes appendicitis. Histologically, acute appendicitis is characterized by mucosal ulceration and a variable degree of mural necrosis and neutrophihc diffuse infiltration. The concept of chronic appendicitis is controversial. Leukocytosis often is present.

10. The answer is C   When an osteogenic sarcoma (osteosarcoma) penetrates the bone cortex, it elevates the periosteum. This periosteal elevation usually produces an acute angle with the underlying remaining cotical bone, which is known as Codman's triangle. As a significant radiographic sign, Carman's triangle aids in the diagnosis of osteogenic sarcoma.

11、12. The answers are: 11- B, 12- D   Fat necrosis in the breast can form a mass that simulates carcinoma clinically, with retraction of the overlying skin. The lesion is centered in the adipose tissue and does not include ductal dilatation, which occurs in duct ectasia. There is no malignant epithelial proliferation, which occurs in comedocarcinoma.

Although macrophages are present in the chronic organizing phase of fat necrosis, granulomatous inflammation is not the primary etiology of fat necrosis. Adenosis refers to the proliferation of lobules and is not a primary feature of fat necrosis.

Fat necrosis of the breast is usually secondary to previous trauma. The injured lipocytes die, and the lipids undergo a degradative process known as saponification. The histologic correlate of this is cell ghosts with a homogeneous eosinophilic appearance to the cytoplasm. Secondary calcification and organization of necrotic tissue, with accumulation of macrophages and mononuclear cells, occur in the chronic phase of the process. Nulliparity, estrogen therapy, breast-feeding, and pulmonary tuberculosis are not directly associated with fat necrosis.

13. The answer is A   Systemic lupus erythematosis (SLE) is the prototype disease associated with immune complex deposition in multiple organs. This occurrence reflects polyclonal B-cell activation. Sjögren's syndrome, scleroderma, graft versus host (GVH) disease, and CREST (i.e., calcinosis, Raynaud's phenomenon, esophageal dysfunction, syndactyly, and telangiectasia) syndrome are not particularly associated with immune complex deposition.

14. The answer is C   Numerous mitoses in a melanocytic lesion of an adult are almost always an indication of malignancy. The presence of multinucleated giant cells, nests of melanocytes deep in the dermis, and epidermal changes can be seen in both benign and malignant melanocytic lesions. The presence of nevus cells surrounding pilar units in an otherwise benign lesion is characteristic of a congenital nevus.

15. The answer is B   Severe head trauma, as would be expected in this patient, leads to bruising of the brain against the skull. Cerebral edema ensues, with consequent caudal displace-

ment of the midbrain and pons; transtentorial herniation then takes place. The latter results in stretching and tearing of brain stem arteries and veins, producing parenchymal hemorrhages (Duret's hemorrhages). Although a ruptured aneurysm and an arteriovenous (AV) malformation could result in findings similar to Duret's lesion, these diagnoses would not apply in this instance. Neither a severed medulla oblongata nor a cerebral infarct would be expected findings.

16. The answer is D   Transplant recipients are at risk for a variety of opportunistic infections. Epstein-Barr virus (EBV) infection with posttransplant lymphoproliferative disorder (PTLD) is one such complication. In PTLD, the immunosuppressed host suffers from primary or reactivated infection. EBV exerts a proliferative pressure on the B cells. In the absence of regulatory T-cell control, B cells may expand and develop clonal populations (i.e., lymphoma).

17. The answer is A   The presence of a red, velvety, distal esophagus that is characterized histologically by a columnar mucosa (particularly the intestinal or "specialized" type) is the hallmark of Barrett's esophagus. This disorder complicates reflux esophagitis in about 10% of patients. Progressive dysplasia of the columnar mucosa may result in the development of adenocarcinoma, which complicates 3% to 10% of cases. Surveillance biopsies are generally performed annually. If high-grade dysplasia or intramucosal carcinoma is found, esophagectomy may be considered for suitable surgical candidates. Candida esophagitis is characterized by the presence of yeasts and pseudohyphae, which often invade the esophageal squamous mucosa. Ganglion cells are present in normal numbers in Barrett's esophagus; they are decreased or absent in achalasia. Tracheoesophageal fistula (TEF) is not a complication of Barrett's esophagus, although a fistula could potentially complicate a Barrett's adenocarcinoma.

18、19. The answers are: 18- E,19- B   The clinical finding of a single lestis in the scrotum is consistent with either monorchid (congenital absence of one testis) or cryptorchidism (undescended testis). The additional finding of an abdominal mass in this setting is highly suggestive of a germ cell tumor arising in a cryptorchid testis, since such gonads are normally atrophic and do not undergo hypertrophy. The most common germ cell tumor is seminoma, and the radiographic evidence of a solid mass is most consistent with such a diagnosis since teratomas usually have a cystic component. Prostate cancer is rare in young men, and adenomatoid tumors usually are small tumors of the epidermis.

The treatment of choice for seminoma is resection of the primary lesion followed by radiation therapy. The tumor is exquisitely sensitive to radiation. There is good prognosis for seminoma patients, with a 90%~98% 5-year survival rate. Prostate-specific antigen is a marker of prostate cancer and is not useful in the management of seminoma. Patients with seminoma in one testis have a 2 % risk of having a second seminoma in the other testis.

20. The answer is D   The most likely diagnosis is neuroblastoma. Because of the young age of the patient, pancreatic is let cell tumor can be virtually eliminated as a diagnosis. Neuroblastoma, which is the most common extracranial malignant solid tumor of infancy and childhood, frequently is characterized by calcification; Wilms' tumor, hepatoblastoma, and pancreatoblastoma do not reveal this feature.Pathologically, the presence of rosettes plus neurofibril formation is pathognomonic for neuroblastoma.

21. The answer is B   A patient who presents with nausea and vomiting, oliguria, hematuria, hypertension, and elevated serum creatinine probably suffers from nephritis. Basic pathologic features of nephritis are glomerular proliferation and active inflammation. Cellular crescents are ext-

racapillary glomerular proliferation in response to capillary loop rupture and spillage of plasma proteins into Bowman's space. The other choices are morphologic features associated with nephrotic syndrome [i. e., nodular glomerulosclerosis (diabetes), basement membrane spikes (membranous glomerulopathy), tissue congophilia (amyloid), diffuse podocyte effacement (minimal change disease)].

22. The answer is D   Numerous studies have shown that most pleural effusions contain adenocarcinoma cells when the effusions are caused by malignant disease in patients without known cancer. Statistically, the usual primary sites for such tumors are the breast in women and the lung in men.

23. The answer is B   The hepatitis D virus (HDV; delta agent) requires the hepatitis B virus (HBV) to act as a helper within the hepatocyte in order to be able to assemble complete viral particles. The complete HDV particle consists of an outer coat of hepatitis B surface.antigen (HBsAg) with the RNA. core of HDV. HBV is the most common cause of sporadic and fulminant hepatitis. Hepatitis C virus (HCV) is the most common cause of posttransfusion hepatitis. The genome of HBV is predominantly double-stranded DNA, not RNA. In chronic hepatitis B, the HBV genome may be in the episomal state, the integrated state, or both. Patients with acute hepatitis A do not develop chronic liver disease.

24. The answer is B   Kaposi's sarcoma, once uncommon, is increasing in incidence because it is one of the problems associated with acquired immune deficiency syndrome (AIDS). However, the AIDS virus does not cause the malignancy; no homology to the viral DNA has been found. In AIDS patients, Kaposi's sarcoma often causes small tumors of the mucous membranes or lymph nodes; these may occur without the more typical cutaneous lesions. Although Kaposi's sarcoma occurs in different clinical forms, the histology is always the same. The classic form of Kaposi's sarcoma is seen in elderly Eastern European Jews; over 90% of patients are men. Rarely, Kaposi's sarcoma develops in renal transplant patients receiving immunosuppressive therapy; stopping this therapy results in regression of the tumor.

25. The answer is A   The most common cause of nephrotic syndrome in children is minimal change disease. In this condition,nephrosis sometimes follows an immunization or infection. The only pathologic finding is diffuse foot process effacement, thus, the name " minimal change" disease.

26. The answer is E   Iron deficiency anemia, chemotherapy-induced marrow injury, acute leukemia, and metastatic breast cancer are all possible explanations for the low blood values of the 60-year-old woman described. Without detailed peripheral smear morphology and further laboratory data, the diagnosis cannot be determined definitively. Elderly people may have nutritional deficiencies from a poor or inadequate diet; another possibility is gastrointestinal blood loss from an undefined condition (e.g., a cancer). Chemotherapy can depress and injure marrow, producing anemia; and, in some cases, the marrow injury may be prolonged. Cases of postchemotherapy acute leukemia also occur. Finally, metastatic tumors of the bone marrow can produce a marrow-replacement type of neoplasia.

27. The answer is B   In most human cancers, the stage of the disease is the most important prognostic factor. Stage refers to the extent, or degree of spread, of the disease in the patient (Le., localized, regional, or distant). Tumor grade (i.e., differentiation), mitotic count, and extent of invasion correlate with the stage of the tumor, in that highergrade (i.e., less differentiated) tumors

and highly invasive tumors tend to be higher-stage lesions.

28. The answer is D   The maiority of ovarian metastases from gastric adenocarcinoma are composed of signet-ring cells and, thus, conform to the definition of Krukenberg's tumor. Krukenberg's tumors usuafiy are bilateral. By far the most common source for these tumors is the stomach; less commonly, they may disseminate from the colon, breast, appendix, or some other site. A Brenner tumor is a primary epithelial tumor of the ovary, which histologically resembles epithelium found in the urinary tract. A renal cell cancer sometimes is called a Grawitz's tumor. A Klatskin tumor is a bile duct cancer that arises at the junction of the left and right hepatic ducts. Wilms' tumor, also known as nephroblastoma, is a primitive renal tumor generally found in pediatric patients.

29. The answer is D   Deep venous thrombosis is a complication of surgery and bedrest. Thrombus material in the deep veins may dislodge and travel to the lungs as pulmonary emboli, causing hypoxia and shortness of breath.

30. The answer is C   Because of their location, meningiomas are not always completely re-moved surgically and, therefore, may recur. For this reason, the completeness of removal at initial surgery is the most important prognostic feature in the case described. None of the histologic pa-rameters (i.e., histologic subtype, mitotic index, tumor vascularity) are significant if surgery is not complete. The need for radiation therapy implies in-adequacy of surgery and, thus, a poorer prognosis.

31. The answer is D   The cavernous hemangioma is the most common primary hepatic tumor. These lesions usually are incidental findings at autopsy or lapamtomy, or they are detected radiographically in the workup for some other unrelated disorder. Cavemous hemangiomas occur at all ages. When symptomatic, they most commonly are found in women who complain of ab-dominal pain. Rupture is distinctly uncommon; but when it occurs, it usually is in a giant cavern-ous hemangioma.

32. The answer is D   In susceptible individuals, exposure to beryllium dust may cause an acute bronchopneumonia. These individuals may show a hypersensitive skin reaction, which is very characteristic of chronic berylliosis. Asbestosis does not present as broncho-pneumonia but, rather, as interstitial disease.Steroid hormones rarely cause pulmonary prob-lems unless long-term use has resulted in immunosuppression and pneumocystis pneumonia. However, if that situation had occurred, the patient would not be recovering on ordinary anti-biotics, which were used in this case to cover bacterial infection. Cavitation is typical of tu-berculosis, which causes small or large nodular granulomas on X-ray. Although coal miners may develop bronchopneumonia, the key factor in this case is the current work in a ceramic factory, where exposure to beryllium is known.

33. The answer is C   About 15 % of donor kidneys show changes related to preexisting damage prior to harvest. Atheroemboli are pathologically recognized as needlelike spaces within the microvasculature. Atheroembolism is associated with severe atheromatous plaque in the donor vasculature and invasive procedures such as catheterization or vascular surgery. "Primary non-function" in a renal allograft may be secondary to a variety of causes. Ischemic damage during harvest (i.e., "harvest injury") is most common. Preformed antibody directed against donor tissue can occasionally be missed during pretransplant crossmatch testing and cause hyperacute re-jection, but this situation is uncommon.

34、35. The answers are: 34- D,35- E   Hydatidiform moles are the abnormal villi from a pathologic ovum that can proliferate and enlarge to expand the uterus, and secrete human chorionic gonadotropin (hCG) in levels higher than those associated with a normal pregnancy. The levels of hCG in an ectopic pregnancy are normal, and the uterus is not abnormally enlarged. Placenta accreta is characterized by an abnormally invasive placenta, but it does not abnormally enlarge the uterus or secrete excess hCG. Leiomyomas may enlarge during pregnancy, leading to an unexpectedly large uterus, but do not elevate the hCG level. Chorioangioma is a benign vascular tumor of the placenta that does not appreciably increase its size or alter hCG secretion.

Choriocarcinoma can follow a normal pregnancy or an abortion but is most commonly associated with previous or concomitant molar pregnancies. Choriocarinoma can invade through the uterus into the surrounding structures or can metastasize to distant sites. Tubal rupture is associated with ectopic pregnancies and can cause life-threatening hemorrhage; it is not associated with intrauterine molar pregnancies. Pseudomyxoma peritonei is a complication of mutinous epithelial tumors of the ovary, megothelium, and gastrointestinal tract. Endometrial polyps are usually found in the clinical setting of unopposed estrogen stimulation and are composed of benign endometrial glands and stroma.

36. The answer is B   Florid epithelial hyperplasia is associated with an increased risk of breast cancer; fibroadenomas (unless they contain epithelial hyperplasia) are not. A family history of breast cancer is a risk factor, but a history of gynecomastia is not. The patient's age of 37 years places her in a low-risk age-group. The low dose of radiation received, even after multiple mammographies, does not increase risk.

37. The answer is D   This patient's disorder is familial adenomatous polyposis (FAP), which is characterized by innumerable (more than 100) colorectal adenomas. Less frequently, adenomas are found in the small bowel (partic-ularly the duodenum) and stomach. FAP gives strong support to the adenoma-carcinoma sequence of colorectal neoplasia. FAP is inherited as an autosomal dominant trait with genetic linkage to the long arm of chromosome 5 (5q). Adenomas usually occur in the second and third decades, with symptoms appearing one decade later. By the time the symptoms have occurred, roughly two-thirds of patients have developed colorectal carcinoma.Carcinoma only rarely occurs prior to the third decade, if colectomy is not performed prophylactically (usually by age 20), then virtually all patients eventually will develop adenocarcinoma. Adenocarcinoma may also occur at extracolonic sites.

38. The answer is C   Of the four lesions, only angiofibroma would contain the vascular component that has led to the unfortunate complications of the biopsy. The characteristic color and consistency of the angiofibroma serve as a warning to distinguish it from the more common nasal polyp. A verrucous carcinoma, as its name implies, would not present as a smooth lesion.

39. The answer is C   The most likely primary site for a metastatic lesion in an elderly man, as described in the question, is the prostate gland. Immunochemical localization of prostatic acid phosphatase (an enzyme that acts as a tumor marker) or prostate-specific antigen is the least invasive and least expensive technique for determining the site of such a tumor. The other choices-barium enema, laparotomy, computed tomography (CT), and electron microscopic (EM) examination-are less specific, more expensive, and more uncomfortable for the patient.

40. The answer is B   Acoustic neuromas occur in middle-aged to elderly people, they affect women more often than men, and they are found commonly in patients with evidence of Von

Recklinghausen's disease (neurofibromatosis). Neurofibromatosis is characterized by the presence of multiple coffee-colored (cafe au lait) spots on the skin, Thus, acoustic neuroma is most likely in the 49-year-old woman who presents with pigmented mac-ules of the axillary skin. The patient with type III multiple endocrine neoplasia (MEN) may have colonic ganghoneuromatosis, but he has no apparent increased chance of developing acoustic neuroma. The patient with melanoma (a tumor that is unrelated to neural lesions) would not have an increased propensity for a central nervous system (CNS) tumor. Neither radiation nor congenital abnormalities of other systems are associated with an increased frequency of acoustic neuroma.

41、43. The answers are: 41 - C, 42 - B, 43 - D   The history and clinical findings are consistent with a diagnosis of chronic obstructive pulmonary disease (COPD), with features of both emphysema and chronic bronchiolitis. Cigarette smoking is a chronic irritant that induces inflammation and also reduces antiproteolytic activity, leading to destruction of pulmonary parenchyma, Cigarette smoke does not affect α_1-antitrypsin gene activity. The pulmonary basement membrane is usually increased in COPD, and desquamative interstitial pneumonitis is not a feature of the disease.

Secondary pulmonary hypertension can occur in COPD, and when it is severe, it can lead to right-sided heart failure (cor pulmonale). Pulmonary veno-occlusive disease and pulmonary thromboembolism can also cause cor pulmonale but are not specifically associated with COPD. Diffuse alveolar damage refers specifically to the hyaline membranes and type II pneumonocyte hyperplasia seen in acute respiratory distress syndromes, bronchopulmonary dysplasia refers to the chronic sequelae of neonatal respiratory distress syndrome.

Expiratory wheezes heard in COPD patients are produced by narrowing of the airways, which is pronounced by airway collapse. Chronic bronchiolitis causes narrowing of the airways by edema and fibrosis; goblet cell hyperplasia contributes to airway narrowing by mucus secretion. The collapse of the airways by positive intrathoracic pressure during expiration is caused by the loss of lung elasticity found in emphysema due to the destruction of interalveolar septa. Anthracosis refers to the accumulation of carbon pigment within pulmonary macrophages and does not contribute to narrowing of the airways.

44、45. The answers are: 44- A, 45- C   This patient most likely has cirrhosis related to infection by the hepatitis C virus (HCV), which she probably contracted through her prior blood transfusion. The patient's hepatitis A virus (HAV) serologies demonstrate prior infection, which is common in the adult population, but HAV does not cause chronic liver disease.Liver transplantation is a treatment option for some patients with end-stage liver disease, although recurrent HCV infection is common. Portal hypertension is a common clinical consequence of cirrhosis.

In most cases, ascites results from portal hypertension related to siousoidal, postsinusoidal, or posthepatic vascular blockade. These forms of vascular blockade lead to increased hepatic lymph flow and weeping of lymph from the liver surface into the peritoneal cavity. Hypoalbuminemia and secondary hyperaldosteronism may contribute to ascites formation. Patients with hepatitis C virus (HCV)-related cirrhosis are at increased risk for development of hepatocellular carcinoma; this tumor may extensively invade the hepatic vein, leading to posthepatic blockade.

46. The answer is D   Patients with Addison's disease often are hypotensive because of destruction of the adrenal cortex and, thus, mineralocorticoid (aldosterone) deficiency. Cushing's syndrome, which is caused by pituitary or adrenal lesions or by excessive glucocorticoid intake,

results in hypertension. Conn's syndrome, which usually is produced by an adrenocortical adenoma, is associated with excessive production of aldosterone; the result is hypertension. Pheochromocytoma and adrenal medullary hyperplasia characteristically produce hypertension by excessive release of catecholamines.

47. The answer is A   Obliterative bronchiolitis (OB) refers to a progressive fibrosing lesion of the membranous and respiratory bronchioles. This chronic change may be seen in rejection, but it can also be seen in infection, ischemia, or graff-versus-host (GVH) disease.The features of acute cellular rejection in the lung depend on the severity of the rejection process. In early rejection, lymphocytic inflammation is confined to the perivascular space. With increasing severity, the inflammation spills into the interstitium and alveolar spaces, and more neutrophils are seen. Severe rejection may have hemorrhage and necrosis accompanied by hyaline membrane formation.

48. The answer is D   Medial granulomas are not characteristic of atherosclerosis. Fatty streaks and atheromas (intimal plaques) are the classic lesions of artherosclerosis. When atheromas develop ulceration, calcification, thrombosis, intraplaque hemorrhage, or mild lymphocytic inflammation, they are referred to as "complicated plaques." Fatty streaks have been found in children, leading to the speculation that atherosclerosis may begin at a very early age.

49. The answer is B   Aortic aneurysms are not a complication of acute myocardial infarction but usually are the results of atherosclerosis, various infectious agents, connective tissue abnormalities, or congenital defects. The complications of myocardial infarction are numerous and varied; some may occur within the first hour after the onset of infarction, whereas others may be delayed for months or longer after the acute event. A few (e.g., ventricular arrhythmia, cardiogenic shock, myocardial rupture) are extremely serious and represent common causes of death in patients with myocardial infarction.

50. The answer is D   Acquired immune deficiency syndrome (AIDS) is characterized by a progressive deficiency in cell mediated immunity. Most severely affected are the helper T cells-cells responsible for "helping" B cells and other T cells to respond appropriately to antigen. Depletion of the helper T-cell population leaves the host susceptible to a variety of infections (especially protozoal, fungal, mycobacterial, and viral) and to secondary malignancies. Resistance to bacterial infections most often is mediated through humoral mechanisms. Therefore, the incidence of pneumococcal pneumonia is not increased in AIDS patients.

51. The answer is B   Although chconic irritation by smegma is a postulated predisposing factor to squamous cell carcinoma, its presence during physical examination is not useful in distinguishing clinically between the lesions of condyloma and carcinoma. Ulceration and pain are attributes of carcinoma. The presence of inguinal and lung masses are suggestive of local and distant metastases of carcinoma.

52. The answer is C   Tissues often repair themselves by granulation tissue formation, a process that eventually leads to fibrosis (scar tissue) replacing the defect left by the injury. Granulation tissue begins to form shortly after the onset of inflammation and is well established within 100 hours unless the patient has a malignancy or is malnourished, very old, diabetic, or infected. Granulation tissue does not imply granulomas, although foreign-body granulomas can form in the presence of sutures used to close a surgical wound (in which primary healing is occurring).

Sometimes an open wound cannot be closed surgically and, so, undergoes secondary healing, with creation of a large irregular scar. if a person is susceptible, the scar can be excessive, leading to a keloid. Inflammation can lead to fistula formation (i.e., abnormal connection of two structures, often with connection to a lumen, as in an enterocutaneous or a rectovaginal fistula). The body usually cannot heal these structures, which are exposed to continuous insult from inflammation or infection, and surgery is needed to correct the problem.

53. The answer is D   Berry aneurysms are small saccular (balloon-shaped) aneurysms that most often are congenital and present in the smaller cerebral arteries. Fusiform aneurysms are spindle-shaped dilatations of an artery. Aneurysms secondary to atherosclerosis are the most common type and usually are located in the abdominal aorta below the origin of the renal arteries. Syphilitic aneurysms are relatively infrequent today because of the decrease in the incidence of tertiary syphilis. These aneurysms nearly always are confined to the ascending and transverse portions of the thoracic aorta. Cirsoid aneurysms are dilatations of arteriovenous fistulas.

54. The answer is E   A floppy mitral valve is seen in mitral valve prolapse, but is not a component of hypertensive cardiac disease.Long-standing hypertension leads to serious end-organ effects, particularly involving the heart and kidneys. The major morphologic changes seen in the heart include cardiomegaly, concentric hypertrophy of the left ventricle, and hypertrophied papillary muscles. Endocardial fibrous thickening may occasionally be present.

55. The answer is C   Hematuria is not a prominent feature of diabetic glomerulosclerosis, a form of diabetic nephropathy. Diabetic glomerulosclerosis is characterized in its early stage by diffuse glomerolar basement membrane (GBM) thickening, in later stages of diabetic glomerulosclerosis, intercapillary mesangial matrix expansion (diffuse diabetic glomerulosclerosis) eventually becomes nodular (nodular diabetic glomerulosclerosis). This expansion compromises the glomerular capillary lumens. Diahetic glomerulosclerosis is clinically associated with a sequence of microalbuminuria, proteinuria, and eventual renal failure. Diabetic glomerulosclerosis is always found in association with small vessel changes in other sites, such as occur in diabetic retinopathy.

56. The answer is E   A bacterial disease typically causes an abscess, which is a collection of netarophils; a granuloma does not. Several infectious agents cause the distinctive morphologic pattern of inflammation known as granulomatous inflammation. The granulomas consist of nodules that are 1 to 2mm in diameter and are composed of macrophages (histiocytes) that have been modified to be epithelioid in nature. These epithelioid histiocytes are surrounded by a mononuclear cell infiltrate, which typically is composed mainly of lymphocytes. Although tuberculosis is the classic example of an infectious granulomatous disease, a variety of other infectious disorders are characterized by granuloma formation, including cat-scratch disease, syphilis, certain fungal infections (e.g., histoplasmosis, coccidioidomycosis), and lymphogranuloma venereum. Sarcoidosis, a disease of unknown cause, is another example of a granulomatous inflammatory disorder; in contrast to the other three disorders, noncaseating or nonnecrotizing granulomas are formed in sarcoidosis.

57. The answer is E   Hodgkin's lymphoma almost never involves the gastrointestinal tract or the reproductive (pelvic) organs. However, Burkitt's Lymphoma commonly involves the gastrointestinal tract, especially in children. In the patient described, the possibility of a smoldering periappendiceal abscess must be considered. Crohn's disease (CD) can produce inflammatory fibrous masses. Finally, ovarian germ cell tumors may occur in young girls and must be considered

in the diagnosis of this patient.

58. The answer is B   An aneuploid result does not equate with malignancy. Although most aneuploid lesions are neoplastic,there are exceptions. Flow cytometry can be used to evaluate the nuclear details of a tumor and, in some cases, can provide significant prognostic information. The procedure does have limitations, however, and they are particularly important to know given the relative newness of DNA flow cytometry. A diploid result does not mean that a lesion of benign; diploid lesions may be benign or malignant reactive or neoplastic. A reactive and benign lesion, however, almost always is diploid.

59. The answer is E   The grade of a sarcoma is a prognostic index based on the tumor's degree of differentiation; low-grade (more-differentiated) tumors tend to have a more indolent course than high-grade (highly mitotic) tumors. Stage also is a prognostic indicator, which is related to the grade of the sarcoma (stages I, Il, and Ⅲ) and to local involvement of bone or vessels and metastatic disease (stage Ⅳ). If other factors are equal, the larger a sarcoma, the less favorable the prognosis. Depth is another important factor; superficial tumors in the subcutaneous area carry a far more favorable prognosis than is associated with deep intramuscular tumors. Tumor duration indicates how long a neoplasm could be seen or felt as a lump before diagnosis but has nothing to do with prognosis.

60. The answer is B   Regular skin cancers [squamous cell carcinoma (SCC)] and melanoma ane associated with prolonged exposure to the ultraviolet radiation of the sun. Postradiation therapy tumors may develop in a variety of sites, including the thyroid, soft tissues or bone; the latter tumors are called sarcomas. However, internal organs, such as the ovary, liver, and kidney, are the least likely to be affected by natural or therapeutic radiation.

61. The answer is D   Although ultrastructural (electron microscopic) changes can be seen during the first hour after an acute myocardial infarction, the first histologic evidence is seen at about 5 to 12 hours postinfarction (not 24 hours). These changes are characterized by coagulative necrosis, including cytoplasmic hyaline change and eosinophilia, loss of cross-striations, nuclear pyknosis, and karyorrhexis. Neutrophils marginate within capillaries, then exit into the parenchyma at about 24 hours. Another sign of acute myocardial infarction is a serum elevation of the MB isoenzyme of creatine kinase (CK) during the first 48 to 72 hours postinfarction. Most myocardial infarctions are transmural (i.e., they involve virtually,the full thickness of the ventricular wall) and involve the left ventricle. Subendocardial (nontransmural) intarctions usualy involve one third to half the thickness of the ventricular wall and are circumferential.

62. The answer is D   Lupus nephritis is a term used to describe a range of glomerular nephritides that can occur in systemic lupus erythematosus (SLE). Autoantibodies to a wide variety of antigens can be found in lupus nephritis; however, antibody to glomerular basement membrane (GBM) is distinctly unusual. About 50% to 80% of patients develop some degree of clinical evidence of renal change. The recognition of renal disease usually occurs within 2 years of the onset of systemic illness. The hallmark of lupus nephritis is the extensive glomerular immune complex deposition. A wide variety of histopathologic damage patterns correlate with the severity of the disease.Lupus nephritis is most common in women.

63. The answer is D   Malignant fibrous histiocytoma (MFH) is a very common adult tumor, which almost always is deep and pleomorphic (with bizarre cells). The thigh is a typical site for this tumor; in fact, MFH is the most common tumor of the thigh in adults; Although the

tumor is composed of fibroblasts and myofibroblasts, it is not referred to as a fibrosarcoma because it also has histiocyte-like cells. Fibrosarcoma is seen more often in children and is a nonpleomorphic (uniform) tumor.

64. The answer is E   Cartilage and muscle tissue are relatively radioresistant. Body cells are affected by ionizing radiation in direct proportion to their rate of turnover and in inverse proportion to their degree of specialization. Thus, the cells of mature cartilege and muscle, which rarely divide, would be relatively less affected by irradiation than the cells of the bone marrow and lymphoid system, which have a high turnover rate. The other statements about radiation are correct.

65. The answer is C   Oncogenes are specific DNA nucleotide sequences found in retroviruses (v-oncs) and in eukaryote cells (c-oncs). The viruses are thought to have acquired v-oncs from homologous c-oncs during integration host cells. Oncogenes are thought to play a role in cell growth, since many v-oncs code for enzymes that seem to serve as growth factor receptors. Because c-oncs have been conserved in eukaryotes throughout evolution, they are presumed to have an important biologic role, perhaps in cell growth, cell differentiation, or both. Viral oncogenes are known to induce malignancies in animals. Although no oncogene is definitely known to produce cancer in humans, certain c-oncs are found in association with specific human malignancies, particularly in those also associated with chromosomal abnormalities (e.g., Burkitt's lymphoma).

66. The answer is E   In arteriolosclerosis, no amyloid fibrils are found. Arteriolosclerosis refers to a process of intimal proliferation and sclerosis found in the walls of small arteries and arterioles. Two types of arteriolosclerosis have been described-hyaline arteriolosclerosis and hyperplastic arteriolosclerosis-both of which show a relationship with hypertension. Hyaline arteriolosclerosis also is common in diabetes. In the hyaline type of arteriolosclerosis, the material found is an insudate of plasma constituents into the arteriole wall. In hyperplastic arteriolosclerosis, concentric, laminated thickening of the arteriole wall often is accompanied by fibrin deposits and necrosis.

67. The answer is A   Cells of the mononuclear phagocyte system (also known as the reticuloendothelial system) are widely distributed throughout the body and are named differently depending on location. These cells have a marked propensity for migration toward a site of injury, being stimulated to migrate by chemotatic factors. Cells of the mononuclear phagocyte system perform a variety of functions. They are important phagocytic cells; they process and present foreign antigens to T cells, they express class II major histocompatibility complex (MHC) antigens; and they produce a variety of substances that regulate the inflammatory process [e.g., interleukin-1(IL-1); growth factors for fibroblasts, myeloid precursors, and endothelial cells; alpha-interferon (IFN-α)].

68、69. The answer are: 68 - D, 69 - B   The patient's childhood condition was acute rheumatic fever, leading to chronic rheumatic heart disease in adult life. The incidence of rheumatic heart disease has decreased dramatically over the past several decades. Rheumatic fever is a systemic, nonsupprative inflammatory complication of untreated pharyngeal infection with group A β-hemolytic streptococci . A typical finding in patient with chronic rheumatic heart disease is that of thickened and deformed valve leaflets (as a result of fibrosis) and of fused commissures. Left atrial dilatation, as a result of severe mitral stenosis or insufficiency, may result. The Aschoff body is a classic histologic finding in rheumatic disease.

Streptococci, particularly the hemolytic (viridans) variety, account for 65% of cases of infective endocarditis occurring on native heart valves.Typically, the valves have been damaged by prior valve disease. Although rheumatic heart disease was previously the most common cause of the underlying valvular damage found in some cases of infective endocarditis, mitral valve prolapse currently is the most common predisposing valvular abnormally. Because this patient had mitral stenosis, her mitral valve is likely to be affected by the endocarditis. Septic emboli, which originate from the valvular vegetation, may lead to septic infarct in the brain, heart, kidneys, or spleen. The vegetations generally consist of fibrin, inflammatory cells, and the offending organism.

70. The answer is E   Infiltration, although typically seen in sarcomas, is not sufficient evidence for a diagnosis of malignancy; infiltration also is very typical of the locally aggressive fibromatosis. Benign tumors are encapsulated as a rule, both grossly and microscopically. However, the appearance of encapsulation can be seen in a sarcoma on gross examination (i.e., pseudocapsule), and invasion can be seen under microscopic examination. Necrosis in a lesion practically always signifies malignancy, and it is rarely present in a benign soft tissue tumor, Size cannot distinguish between a benign or malignant tumor, but it is very important prognostically once a sarcoma diagnosis is made. Patients with smaller tumors (< 5 cm) do better than patients with larger tumors. Patients with many sarcoma types have good 5-year survival rates and, thus. sarcomas do not necessarily have a very poor prognosis.

71. The answer is E   Renal cell carcinoma affects men twice as often as it affects women. The carcinoma presents with hematuria, pain, and flank mass. Renal cell carcinoma is one of the most frequently metastasizing tumors, with a major route of metastasis via the bloodstream. Lungs and brain are two of the favorite landing sites. Renal cell carcinoma most frequently affects men near the sixth decade.

72. The answer is D   T cells perform many important immunologic functions; however, T cells have the ability to recognize foreign antigens only alter the antigens have been taken up, processed, and "presented" to them by macrophages. One set of T cells-helper T cells-promotes the activities of both T cells and B cells; another subset-suppressor T cells-suppresses T-and B-cell respnnses. T cells lyse target cells by direct contact. T cells also participate in the immune response through the production of lymphokines, such as interleukin-2 (IL-2).

73 ~ 77. The answers are: 73- B, 74- D,75- C, 76- A , 77- B   Subacute combined degeneration of the spinal cord is associated with deficiency of vitamin B_{12}. Both vitamin B_{12} deficiency and folic acid deficiency can result in megaloblastic neoplasia. The megaloblastic changes are seen in all cell lines of the bone marrow, but they are especially prominent in the red cell series, However, subacute combined degeneration of the spinal cord is seen only in vitamin B_{12} deficiency.

Rickets is the bone disease seen in children with a deficiency of vitamin D. Rickets is characterized by overgrowth of osteoid and the development of bone deformities as the child is growing. The similar bone condition in adults is osteomalacia.

Scurvy is a disease of vitamin C (ascorbic acid) deficiency. The resultant functional and structural abnormalities of connective tissue cause petechial hemorrhages and bleeding gums.

Xerophthalmia, which is associated with vitamin A deficiency, is a condition of extreme conjunctival dryness, leading occasionally to ulceration of the conjunctiva.

78 ~ 82. The answers are: 78- B,79- D, 80- A, 81- C, 82- D   An association between a very rare liver tumor （angiosarcoma） and occupational exposure to vinyl chloride has been established. The epidemiology is indicated by the unusual histology of the tumor.

Although furor raged over governmental studies showing the development of bladder cancer in animals fed large amounts of cyclamates, this association in man is far from clear. Factors that have been linked to urinary bladder cancers in humans include exposure to carcinogens contained in aniline dyes and cigarette smoke.

Epidemiologic studies from many areas of the world have indicated an association between diet and colonic neoplasia. One dietary agent implicated is fat; the incidence of colon cancer is high in countries in which the diet is rich in fat.

Asbestos exposure has been implicated in a variety of cancers, especially cancer of the lung. Mesothelioma, however, develops in a disproportionate number of individuals who bare been exposed to asbestos. The rarity of mesothelioma in the general population supports a theory of "causative" association with asbestos.

The link between cigarette smoking and lung cancer （usually squamous and small cell types） is well established and is of major significance because the number of cigarette smokers is large.

83 ~ 87. The answers are: 83- D, 84- A, 85- E, 86- C, 87- B   The cells of the immune system represent an elaborate and highly specialized defense mechanism. When an antigen is encountered by these cells, a well-coordinated immune response follows, which may be humoral, cell-mediated, or both. The primary cells involved in the immune response are lymphocytes, of which there are two major types:T lymphocytes （T-cells） and B lymphocytes （B cells）. A third group of lymphocytes,termed null cells, divide into natural killer （NK） cells, killer （K） cells, and lymphocyte activated killer （LAK） cells. Macrophages—in addition to their functions in the acute inflammatory response-also play an important role in the immune response.

Lysis of target cells that are antibody-dependent is the main function of K cells, in antibody-dependent cytotoxic reactions, the antibody （usually immunoglobulin G） binds to the Fe receptor on the K cell and to the antibody combining site on the target cell.

In the cell-mediated immune response to certain microorganisms （e.g., Mycobacterium tuberculosis）, activated macrophages are the first cells to come in contact with the antigen. The macrophage ingests the organism and "processes" the antigen into a form recognizable to T cells. It then presents the antigen to T cells in conjunction with major histocompatibility complex （MHC） molecules on the macrophage surface.This activity is called antigen presentation.

NK cells, in contrast to K cells, kill target cells without an antibody signal. NK cells are capable of killing several tumor cell lines in vitro, and they do so without prior sensitization. NK cells attach to target cells via a receptor, in a process that does not require divalent calcium.

B cells—with stimulation by antigen, T cells, and other cells—differentiate into plasma cells. Plasma cells are responsible for the production of the five types of immunoglobulins; each plasma cell produces only one type of immunoglobulin.

Sensitized T cells produce and release a variety of soluble substances （called lymphokines） during immune reactions, particularly cell-mediated immune reactions and antibody responses. Lymphokines function in many ways is to regulate and intensify the immune response. Interleukin-2 （IL-2） and interferon are examples of lymphokines.

88~92. The answers are: 88- D, 89- E, 90- A, 91- B, 92- C   The histologic pattern of most sarcomas recapitulates a particular type of mesenchymal tissue, and the tumors originally were named for such tissues. Thus, rhabdomyosarcoma is a sarcoma that recapitulates striated (skeletal) muscle; neurofibrosarcoma, nerve (Schwann) cells; angiosarcoma, blood vessels (endothelium); liposarcoma, fat cells (adipose tissue); and fibrosarcoma, fibrocytes (connective tissue). Although some authorities believe that most sarcomas arise from a totipotential mesenchymal stem cell, phenotypic fidelity (i.e., leiomyosarcoma remaining recognizable as such throughout a patient's course) would not be explained by that theory. Suffice it to say that the cell of origin or histiogenesis of sarcomas is unclear and a subject of debate.

93~97. The answers are: 93- C, 94- A, 95- D, 96- E, 97- B   Ultrastructural analysis can help in the diagnosis of neoplastic diseases by disclosing information about the nature of a neoplasm and the cells of its origin. Electron microscopy (EM) can reveal a variety of changes at the cellular level, including changes in nuclei, junctional complexes, surface villi, granules, and interdigitating processes.

The diagnosis of melanomas can be aided by EM, which reveals characteristic elongated granules (premelanosomes). If the melanoma is undifferentiated (i.e., has inconspicuous pigment), diagnosis can be difficult.

Carcinoid tumors are low-grade neuroendocrine carcinomas that, like melanomas, have ultrastructura granules. In carcinoids, the granules are present in a dense core that can be recognized by EM.

Adenocarcinomas display microvilli, whereas the villi seen in mesotheliomas are quite long. The diagnostic ultrastructural finding in squamous cell cancers (SCCs) is the presence of abundant tonofilaments, which probably represent sheaves of cytokeratin filaments.

The skeletal muscle tumor rhabdomyosarcoma recapitulates the normal cell by exhibiting Z-bands on EM.

98~102. The answers are: 98- C, 99- A, 100- E, 101- B, 102- E   Acute promyelocytic leukemia is characterized by prominent primary cytoplasmic granules, as seen in normal promyelocytes. Due to granule release of a procoagulant factor with thromboplastin activity, 75 % of patients either present with a significant bleeding diathesis or develop this condition during therapy.

Chronic myelogenous leukemia (CML) is a marrow-derived neoplasm composed principally of granulocytic cells in various stages of maturation. White blood cell counts (WBCs) usually are greater than $50,000/\mu l$. The Philadelphia chromosome is present in the bone marrow in 90% of patients.

Chronic lymphocytic leukemia (CLL) is a lesion of the mature small lymphocyte and has a low proliferative rate.Fully 98% of cases are of B-cell origin. This common form of leukemia affects the elderly, who present with splenomegaly and symptoms related to neoplasia. Most patients present with a marked lymphocytosis (above $20,000/\mu l$).

Acute myelogenous leukemia (AML) primarily affects adults and is preceded by a few days to weeks of weakness, bleeding, and fever. Physical examination shows petechiae, sternal tenderness, thickened gums, adenopathy, splenomegaly, and hepatomegaly. Untreated, this form of leukemia causes death in 1 to 3 months.

Erythroleukemia is a special subtype of AML in which the marrow shows vastly increased numbers of erythroid precursors in addition to the myeloblastic proliferation.

103～107. The answers are: 103- A, 104- C, 105- B, 106- E, 107- D   Macule, papule, nodule, wheal, and vesicle are all terms that describe the lesions that are produced by various diseases of the skin. For example, tender red nodules, which are found in the pretibial skin surfaces are the classic findings in erythema nndosum, an inflammatory disease of the skin and subcutaneous tissue. Molluscum contagiosum is a poxvirus infection characterized by flesh-colored, smooth papules of the skin. Macules varying from white to brown are seen in tinea versicolor—a yeast infection caused by Pityrosporum orbiculare. Wheals and vesicles characterize the various eruptions that may follow oral or parenteral administration of a drug.

108～112. The answersare: 108- A, 109- C, 110- D, 111- E, 112- B   External irradiation to the neck (usually low dose) has been implicated in papillary thyroid cancer, although doses of radiation high enough to destroy the thyroid gland do not have this neoplastic effect. Most series have reported that the association of thyroid cancer and radiation is strongest when the radiation exposure occurred in childhood.

There are strong indications for a viral etiology of neoplasia. Epidemiologic, serologic, and biochemical evidence closely link cervical cancer and human papillomavirus (HPV). Another neoplastic-viral association is Butkitt's Lymphoma and Epstein-Barr virus (EBV); although the evidence for the association is less strong than that for cervical cancer and papillomavirus, it is nonetheless intriguing.

Ductal carcinoma of the breast is a very often tumor in women. When a series of these tumors was diagnosed, epidemiologic evidence showed that the some patients of breast cancers had been used to estrogen.

Melanoma may be related to ultraviolet light, since epidemiologic studies indicate that the tumor is more common in areas of strong sunlight; it is almost epidemic in Australia.

参 考 文 献

陈莉,孔庆兖,冯振卿.2003.病理学考试指导.第 2 版.上海:第二军医大学出版社

陈莉.2006.病理学.修订版.北京:科学出版社

高雄医学大学病理学科.高医病理学科教学光碟.2005.http://pathology.class.kmu.edu.tw

李玉林.2004.病理学.第 6 版.北京:人民卫生出版社

杨光华.2001. 病理学.第 5 版.北京:人民卫生出版社

Cotran RS, Kumar V, Collins T. 1999. Robbins Pathology Basis of Disease. 6th ed. Philadelphia:WB Saunder Company

Cowen PN, Smiddy FG.1996.Pocket Examiner in Pathology.2nd ed. New York:Churchill Livingstone Inc

Kuwar V, Cortran RS ,Robbins SL .1997. Basic Pathology. 6th ed. Philadelphia : WB Saunders Company

Robbins SL ,Cotran RS , Kumar V .1991. Pocket Companion to Robbins Pathologic Basis of Disease. Philadelphia: WB Saunders Company

Rosai J. 2004. Rosai and Ackerman's Surgical Pathology.9th ed.Volume 1~2.London:Mosby

Vinay KF, Ramzi SC, Stanley LR.2003.Basic Pathology.7th ed.Philadelphia:WB Saunder Company

Virginia AL , Maria JM , Johu SJ ,et al.1994.Pathology. 3th ed.London:Harwal Publishing A Waverly Company